Implant Dentistry

Implant Dentistry

Editor: Preston Bailey

AMERICAN
MEDICAL PUBLISHERS
www.americanmedicalpublishers.com

AMERICAN
MEDICAL PUBLISHERS
www.americanmedicalpublishers.com

Cataloging-in-publication Data

Implant dentistry / edited by Preston Bailey.
p. cm.
Includes bibliographical references and index.
ISBN 979-8-88740-206-2
1. Dental implants. 2. Dental implants--Complications.
3. Mouth--Surgery. 4. Implants, Artificial. 5. Dentures.
6. Dentistry. I. Bailey, Preston.

RK667.I45 I47 2023
617.693--dc23

American Medical Publishers,
41 Flatbush Avenue,
1st Floor, New York,
NY 11217, USA

ISBN 979-8-88740-206-2 (Hardback)

Contents

Preface

I am honored to present to you this unique book which encompasses the most up-to-date data in the field. I was extremely pleased to get this opportunity of editing the work of experts from across the globe. I have also written papers in this field and researched the various aspects revolving around the progress of the discipline. I have tried to unify my knowledge along with that of stalwarts from every corner of the world, to produce a text which not only benefits the readers but also facilitates the growth of the field.

A dental implant is a prosthesis that connects to the bone of jaw or skull to support a dental prosthesis, like crown, bridge, denture, and facial prosthesis. The biological process called osseointegration, in which materials like titanium or zirconia develop an intimate contact with bone, is the foundation of modern dental implants. The health of the person receiving treatment, medicines that impact osseointegration, and the health of the tissues in the mouth play a crucial role in the success or failure of implants. The fundamental use of dental implants is to support dental prosthetics. The risks and problems associated with implant dentistry are divided into three categories. These include complications that arise during the surgery process, complications occurring within six months of the surgery and long-term effects like peri-implantitis and mechanical failures. After the implant procedure, implants must be cleaned with a periodontal scaler for removing any plaque. Different evaluations, techniques and advanced studies on implant dentistry have been included in this book. It will help the readers in keeping pace with the rapid changes in this field.

Finally, I would like to thank all the contributing authors for their valuable time and contributions. This book would not have been possible without their efforts. I would also like to thank my friends and family for their constant support.

Editor

1

Virtual Planning for Dental Implant Placement Using Guided Surgery

Vinicius Nery Viegas, Celso Gustavo Schwalm Lacroix,
Rogério Miranda Pagnoncelli and Marília Gerhardt de Oliveira
Pontifícia Universidade Católica do Rio Grande do Sul
Brazil

1. Introduction

Technical and scientific advances in diagnostic and therapeutic methods in the biomedical field have substantially increased the predictability and longevity of the outcomes of restorative surgical procedures. In contemporary oral implantology, bioprototyping techniques based on computer-aided design and computer-aided manufacturing (CAD/CAM) technology have proven to be valuable aids in diagnosis, treatment planning, and surgical intervention. Among other aspects, use of these technologies improves preoperative planning, makes it easier for patients to understand proposed procedures, increases the predictability of treatment, and may reduce surgical morbidity.

The preliminary stages that precede dental implant surgery are as important as the actual operative intervention itself, or even more so. Inadequate placement of implants may injure important anatomical structures or lead to aesthetic or functional compromise of the prosthetic stage of oral rehabilitation.

Implant planning and placement can be based solely on computed tomography data and surgical guides fashioned after diagnostic models. However, direct three-dimensional visualization of the surgical site and real-model simulation of the intended surgical procedure can play a significant role in obtaining outcomes that are more consistent with the original treatment plan. Biomedical prototypes, or biomodels, provide faithful reproductions of the patient's bone condition, thus enabling this type of assessment.

Likewise, the surgery itself can be made safer and less invasive with use of individualized surgical guides for implant placement. The development of software programs for implant placement planning and the integration of these software packages with rapid prototyping methods have made fabrication of such guides possible.

The process of obtaining and reformatting computed tomography (CT) data, planning implant placement over a virtual model, fabricating a surgical guide with prototyping methods, and using this guide or template during dental implant surgery with specifically designed systems may be referred to as guided implant surgery.

2. Principles of guided surgery

Guided implant surgery is based on the combination of virtual surgical planning and prototyping techniques. Rapid prototyping can be defined as a set of technology-based

processes that enable fabrication of three-dimensional, concrete objects from a computer-aided design (CAD) project. The objective of rapid prototyping is to create a real model with the same geometric features of the virtual model, which can then undergo real-world manipulation for a variety of purposes (James et al., 1998; Peltola et al., 2008).
The greatest challenges in the surgical and prosthetic stages of dental implant surgery are due to diagnostic failure and poor case planning (Lal et al., 2006).
The American Academy of Oral and Maxillofacial Radiology (AAOMR) recommends that any evaluation of the available bony architecture for diagnosis and planning of extensive implant-based oral rehabilitation include CT imaging (Almog et al., 2006).
In this context, Jacobs et al. (1999) assessed the reliability of two-dimensional CT images for implant placement planning. The Jacobs study was performed on 100 partially or fully edentulous patients who underwent CT scanning and subsequent implant placement. Available bone height was measured below the maxillary sinus and nasal fossa and above the mandibular canal, and a 1.5 mm safety margin was respected. Planning took into account implant number, location, and size, available bone height, and possible anatomic complications, such as bony dehiscences and fenestrations, maxillary sinus perforation, absence of primary stability, and poor implant positioning in light of the required biomechanical and cosmetic outcome. The authors found that, in some cases, placement of implants according to plan was impossible, mostly due to intraoperative findings that had been missed or underestimated on CT images. Agreement between planned and intraoperative implant number and sites was satisfactory. Of the 416 planned implants, 395 were successfully placed. However, the authors found weak agreement between the size of the planned implant and that of the implant actually placed (44%). Implants were shorter or longer than planned in 110 and 74 of the 395 successful cases respectively.
According to the authors, CT images can be used for preoperative planning of the number of implants, as well as for choice of implant sites. However, CT scans are not sufficiently reliable for precise determination of implant size or for prevention of intraoperative anatomic complications, and can thus reduce the predictability of the implant placement procedure (Jacobs et al., 1999).
Thus, in light of the need for implementation of available treatment planning resources in implantology, virtual planning and rapid prototyping techniques have come to provide an excellent choice in the search for satisfactory outcomes with lower intra- and postoperative complication rates (Choi et al., 2002; Almog et al., 2006).
Biomedical prototypes and virtual evaluation provide the ability to visualize and manipulate the surgical sites, measure the patient's bony structures, and simulate the surgical intervention itself. These preoperative procedures increase predictability of the chosen technique, improve applicability of the surgical plan, and can shorten operative time (Choi et al., 2002; Sarment et al., 2003a; Sarment et al., 2003b; Meurer et al., 2008).
Erickson et al. (1999) surveyed the opinions of oral and maxillofacial surgeons about the use of stereolithographic models for diagnosis, treatment planning, preoperative surgical simulation, and construction of alloplastic implants for anatomical reconstruction. Seventy-six models were constructed in the study period. Prototypes were used by 69% of respondents as a diagnostic aid during the planning phase, and played a role in treatment planning in 92% of cases. Seventy-three percent of respondents used the models to instruct patients as to the planned procedure. Preoperative surgical simulation was employed in 38% of cases. Seventy-seven percent of surgeons reported reductions in operative time when

prototypes were used, 38% reported improvement in surgical access, and 46% noted that more complex procedures were made safer and more predictable by preoperative study of prototype models. Despite the wide applicability of biomodels (in 96% of treatment phases) only 15% of surgeons that responded to the survey believed that rapid prototyping had played an essential role in proper treatment. Nevertheless, the authors stressed the validity of prototypes as a tool for obtaining more predictable and lasting results.

In a similar study, Erben et al. (2002) interviewed 38 oral and maxillofacial surgeons to determine the main indications for biomodels and the key benefits provided by their use in preoperative planning. Models were used in planning placement of osseointegrated implants and other procedures. Surgeons noted that use of biomedical prototypes improved the quality of diagnosis, enabled preoperative simulation of planned interventions, made it easier for patients to understand the procedure and provided intraoperative guidance.

Wulf et al. (2003) published a study conducted between September 1999 and April 2002 in order to assess the relevance of biomedical prototypes in the preoperative, intraoperative, and postoperative stages of maxillofacial surgery. Fifty-four surgeons described their experiences on a total of 466 cases. This study corroborated the advantages of biomodel use described in the aforementioned investigations.

In dental implantology, bioprototyping techniques are not limited to model construction and analysis. With the advent of sophisticated data acquisition methods and image manipulation and virtual planning software, fabrication of rapid-prototyped surgical guides and templates have made it possible to achieve more reliable agreement between the planned and final position of dental implants. This improved predictability of implant and prosthesis positions is based on the concepts of guided surgery (Garg, 2006; Rosenfeld et al., 2006).

3. Guided surgery in dental implantology

Fabrication of a surgical guide that faithfully reproduces planned implant positions can play an essential role in the success of implant-based oral rehabilitation (Ganz, 2003).

Surgical templates fashioned using conventional methods have some drawbacks that can make successful aesthetic and functional outcomes more difficult to achieve. The diagnostic models on which these guides are based provide a rigid, non-functional representation of the soft tissues that cover the alveolar ridge, which prevents visualization of the underlying bone anatomy of the region of interest and consequently makes it impossible to decide on a definitive orientation for implants (Lal et al., 2006).

Guided surgery can be used in rehabilitation of fully or partially edentulous patients, or even for single teeth. Likewise, guides can be mucosa-supported (tissue-borne), tooth-supported (tooth-borne), or bone-supported (bone-borne).

In guided surgery for rehabilitation of fully edentulous arches, certain steps must be followed prior to implant position planning:

a. placement of diagnostic models on a semi-adjustable articulator;
b. diagnostic wax-up;
c. duplicate of wax-up for fabrication of acrylic-resin CT guide;
d. placement of at least six 1.5 to 2 mm-diameter holes on the vestibular region of the guide and filling with radiopaque material;

e. interocclusal registration with addition or condensation silicone for guidance during CT scanning;
f. occlusal CT view of guide and interocclusal record;
g. isolated scan of guide (for flapless procedures) (Parel & Triplett, 2004; Balshi et al., 2006; Marchack, 2007; Sanna et al., 2007; Van Assche et al., 2007).

CT slices acquired in the DICOM file format must be converted with the aid of a specific software package prior to manipulation and reformatting into 3D images. During this process, the isolated radiographic guide scan is superimposed onto its occlusal view, using the radiopaque points as landmarks (Parel & Triplett, 2004; Balshi et al., 2006; Marchack, 2007; Sanna et al., 2007; Van Assche et al., 2007). The threshold for the case is also defined during this stage (Souza et al., 2003).

Files obtained during this step can then be opened in implant position planning software. These applications provide axial, panoramic, and three-dimensional reconstructions of CT slices (Marchack, 2007; Sanna et al., 2007; Van Assche et al., 2007). They also enable manipulation of the panoramic reconstruction curve on the axial plane, providing orthogonal slices for assessment of alveolar ridge thickness in the vestibulolingual or vestibulopalatal direction (Parel & Triplett, 2004; Sanna et al., 2007; Van Assche et al., 2007).

Virtual planning gives implantologists the ability to choose the precise location, orientation, and dimensions of implants, abutments and other fixtures. Implant emergence and the relationship of the implant to the future prosthesis can also be visualized and adjusted as convenient. In short, virtual planning can overcome the limitations of conventional surgical guides (Lal et al., 2006).

Several virtual planning and guided surgery systems are available on the market. Each has its own particularities that should be taken into account by the implantologist, according to therapeutic indication, cost-benefit ratio, and learning curve for clinical use.

The final stage of planning consists of defining the sites for placement of two or more anchor pins for the surgical guide, which are inserted through the vestibular aspect of the guide, between the implants (Balshi et al., 2006; Marchack, 2007; Sanna et al., 2007).

After planning is complete, files are sent to a medical prototyping facility, where they will be converted into an appropriate format for prototype fabrication (Parel & Triplett, 2004; Marchack, 2007; Sanna et al., 2007; Van Assche et al., 2007).

With implant positions established, a surgical guide is designed on the basis of the virtual model and sent to the prototyping station, where it is then fabricated (Lal et al., 2006).

Three types of surgical guides or templates can be manufactured with rapid prototyping methods to improve the predictability of osseointegrated implant-based oral rehabilitation. Bone-supported (or bone-borne) guides are placed after the mucoperiosteal flap has been raised. Their advantages include positional stability during implant placement and the possibility of direct visualization of anatomical structures. The need for broader surgical exploration, however, may be regarded as a drawback of this type of guide, which is usually reserved for partially or fully edentulous arches (Tardieu et al., 2003; Garg, 2006; Lal et al., 2006).

In mucosa-supported (or tissue-borne) surgical guides, templates, anchor pins are placed transmucosally. The drilling sequence for implant placement begins with a tissue punch or extractor, with the guide in place (Parel & Triplett, 2004; Marchack, 2007; Sanna et al., 2007). These guides are indicated in fully edentulous patients. Use of the double-scan technique, in which two independent scans of the radiographic guide—individually and in occlusion—are obtained, is mandatory in these cases. The key advantage of this method is the possibility of performing allows minimally invasive flapless procedures, which make for an easier intraoperative and postoperative period (Garg, 2006).

Tooth-supported (or tooth-borne) surgical guides, as the name implies, are supported by the patient's remaining teeth. They are indicated in rehabilitation of single teeth or partially partially edentulous regions, and provide good outcomes when used for minimally invasive flapless surgery (Garg, 2006).

Once the prototyped guide is ready, implant placement may proceed as recommended for each system (Figures 1 and 2).

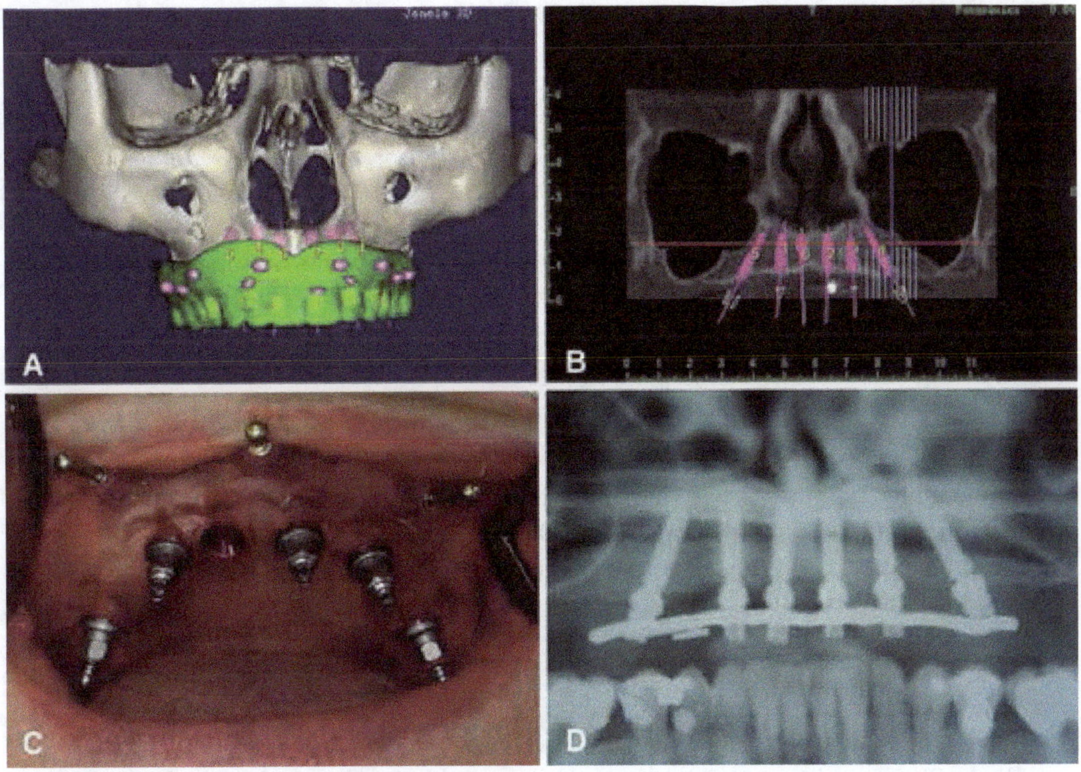

Fig. 1. Guided surgery for complete upper arch rehabilitation. a) Three-dimensional view of preoperative planning. Note radiopaque markers used to superimpose scans of the guide (isolated and in occlusion). Dentaslice® software package (Bioparts®, Brazil). b) Preoperative implant positioning. c) Five implants in place. Note insertion of anchor pins into stereolithographic guide. Neoguide® system (Neodent®, Brazil). d) Postoperative panoramic radiograph. Note similarity to virtual planning.

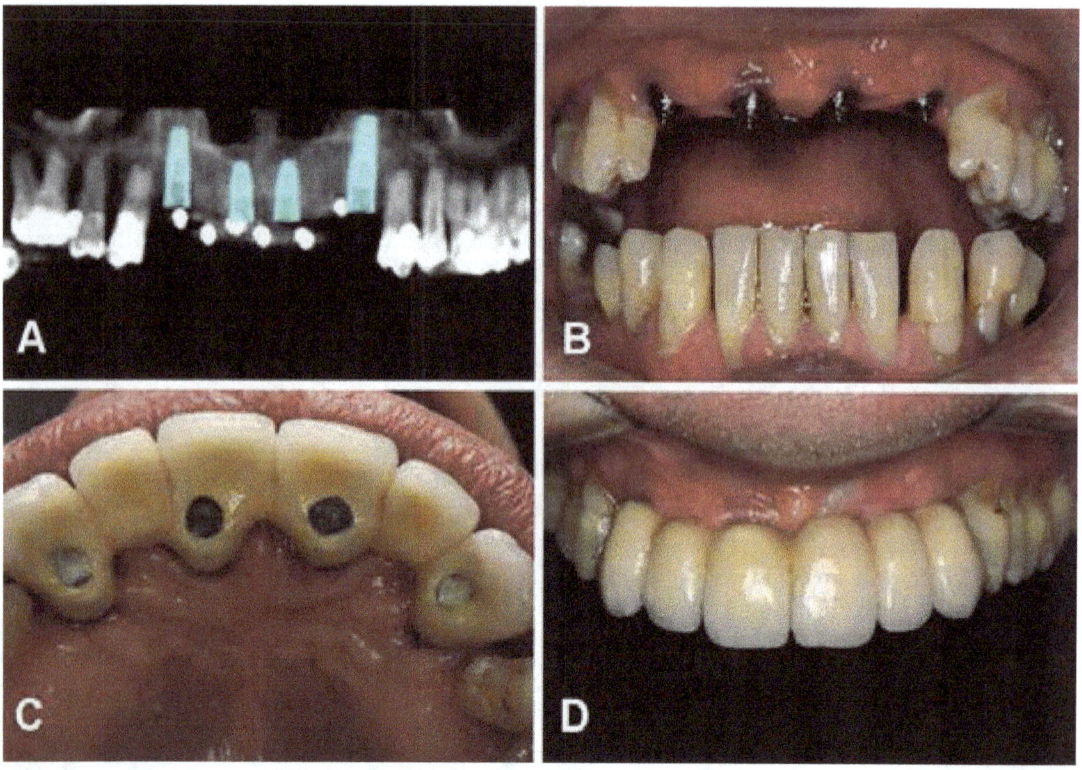

Fig. 2. Guided surgery for partial anterior-superior rehabilitation. a) Preoperative planning. Nobelguide® software system (Nobel Biocare®, Sweden) b) Implant position, immediately after surgery. c) Palatal emergence of implants, in accordance with virtual planning. d) Final result: porcelain-fused-to-metal restoration.

4. Final remarks

Implant planning has always been a major challenge of dental practice. CT is often unable to provide precise definitions of implant size and will not always be useful in preventing anatomical complications during surgery. Loubele et al (2007) found that bony dimensions were underestimated on the basis of measurements taken from several CT scans. Likewise, Suomalainen et al. (2008) reported errors in measurement of bone dimensions on CT images. These setbacks are even more critical when planning implants for patients with little available bone tissue.

The advent of virtual planning and rapid prototyping techniques has led to a shift in this paradigm. Biomedical prototypes have made it possible for the implantologist to visualize and directly manipulate areas of interest, thus narrowing the gap between pre- and intraoperative findings (Choi et al., 2002; Sarment et al., 2003a; Meurer et al., 2008). Virtual planning permits three-dimensional analysis of implant position. Its clinical application—guided surgery—optimizes intra- and postoperative outcomes, as it can reduce surgical morbidity and improve the predictability of the proposed treatment plan.

Studies on guided surgery have gained prominence in the dentistry literature since the early 2000s. Gateno et al. (2003) studied the fit precision of stereolithographic surgical splints and that of conventional acrylic resin splints. Their results indicated that stereolithographic splints had a high degree of accuracy of seating, thus enabling transfer of virtual treatment plans directly to the patient during surgery.

Van Assche et al. (2007) evaluated the precision of transfer of computer-based planning for implant placement in four partially edentulous human jaws with soft tissues present. All stages of guided surgery were performed on the anatomical specimens, from molding and diagnostic wax-up to placement of implants (a total of 12).

Postoperative cone-beam CT scans were obtained and superimposed onto preoperative scans in a virtual environment. Placed implants had a mean angular deviation of 2 degrees (range, 0.7 - 4 degrees) from the planned position, whereas mean linear deviation was 1 mm (0.3 – 2.3 mm) at the hex and 2 mm (0.7 – 2.4 mm) at the apical implant tip.

The authors conclude that cone-beam CT images can be used in computer-based implant planning for guided implant surgery with rapid-prototyped guides (Van Assche et al., 2007).

Viegas et al. (2010) conducted an experiment on 11 dry human mandibles to assess transfer of virtual implant position planning to surgery. Implant positions were standardized and simulated in an appropriate software package, using preoperative cone-beam CT scans as a basis. Models and surgical guides for each mandible were fabricated using stereolithography methods. Simulated surgeries, including implant placement and removal, were first performed on each prototype. Implants were then placed into the mandible replicas. Analysis of results was based on standardized postoperative CT scanning of prototypes and replicas for visualization of the implant beds. Superposition of pre- and post-operative three-dimensional models enabled assessment of the linear distance and angle between the long axes of planned and placed implants. Linear measurements made directly on models were used to assess the validity of prototype-simulated procedures as a tool for treatment planning in oral implantology. The variations in distance between the coronal, central, and apical regions of the 22 implants evaluated in this study were, on average, <0.41 mm. Mean deviation in angle was 1.45 ± 0.89 degrees for implants placed on the right and 0.70 ± 0.30 degrees for implants placed on the left. Comparison of samples by means of Student's *t* test, using a reference value of zero, showed statistically significant differences for all measurements ($p < 0.05$). The correlation between implant bed positions in each mandible was fair to very good, depending on the distance analyzed and on the method used for interpretation of measurements. This study found that real-life deviation from planned dental implant positions determined by means of virtual planning and simulated surgery on a biomedical prototype were within a range that indicates the reliability of guided surgery as a method of dental implant placement.

In a clinical study, Nickenig and Eitner (2007) evaluated transfer of virtual implant plans to the operative field by means of the guided surgery technique. A total of 102 patients took part in the study (250 implants). Implants were placed into the posterior area of the mandible in 55.4% of cases. Eighteen cases (7.2%) involved rehabilitation of fully edentulous arches.

Computer-based virtual planning based on cone-beam CT scans was used in all cases. Flapless surgery was used for placement of 147 implants (58.8%) and all patients had uneventful intraoperative courses. In 98.4% of patients, there were no issues with surgical guide fit or instrumentation. Reduced interocclusal distance limited applicability of the technique in four patients.

Initial plans were changed in eight cases, when raising the mucoperiosteal flap revealed a need for modifications in manipulation of the available bone tissue and simultaneous implant placement. Regarding predictability of implant size, only one implant had to be replaced with a smaller-diameter equivalent due to insufficient bone thickness.

Postoperative panoramic radiographs showed that anatomical structures such as the maxillary sinus, mandibular canal, mental foramen, and neighboring teeth were spared as planned. Comparison of postoperative radiographs and panoramic reconstructions created by the planning software revealed substantial differences in implant angle in nine cases.

The authors concluded that virtual plans based on cone-beam CT scans can be reproduced during implant placement surgery, and constitute a reliable method for defining implant position and size, preventing anatomical complications, and enabling wider use of flapless surgery (Nickenig & Eitner, 2007).

The minor variations between planned and actual implant placement in the aforementioned studies show that computer-based treatment plans can be reliably transferred to the operative environment by means of the guided surgery technique.

Furthermore, another key advantage of this procedure is the possibility of immediate loading of functional prostheses. Implant planning and positioning should not only take into account successful intraosseous implant placement, but also ensure that the future prosthesis is passively and securely seated on its fixtures. Prosthetic options for offsetting deviations in implant position vary according to the chosen guided surgery system. Even so, the current literature reveals a concern with the longevity of these implants.

Sanna, Molly, and Van Steenberghe (2007) evaluated the survival of 183 implants (30 patients) placed for rehabilitation of fully edentulous arches with the guided surgery technique, using cone-beam CT scanning, tissue-borne guides, and immediate loading. The results showed that guided placement of dental implants followed by immediate loading of fixed prostheses was associated with survival rates similar to those obtained with the same mode of rehabilitation on implants reopened after the osseointegration period.

Schneider et al. (2009) conducted a systematic review to assess the accuracy and clinical applications of guided implant surgery. A literature search yielded 3120 titles, eight of which met the inclusion criteria in terms of accuracy and 10 in terms the clinical performance. Meta-regression analysis revealed a mean deviation of 1.07 mm at the entry point (95% CI, 0.76 - 1.22 mm) and 1.63 mm at the apex (95% CI, 1.26 - 2 mm). No significant differences between the studies were found regarding method of template production or template support and stabilization. Early surgical complications occurred in 9.1% of cases. Limited access for instrumentation and fracture of the surgical guide were the sole technique-related complications observed—all others were equally possible during conventional implant placement procedures. Early prosthetic complications occurred in 18.8% and late prosthetic complications in 12% of cases. Noteworthy prosthesis-related complications included misfit of abutment to bridge, extensive adjustments of the occlusion, and incomplete seating of the prosthesis. The most common delayed complications were screw loosening and prosthesis fracture.

Implant survival rates, assessed in six clinical studies with a total of 537 implants—most loaded immediately after flapless implantation procedures—ranged between 91 and 100%.

Studies such as these related justify the relevance of investigations that seek improvement toward increasingly accurate and safe methods that are beneficial to patients and dentists alike, such as virtual planning and guided surgery.

5. References

Almog, D. M., Benson, B. W., Wolfgang, L., Frederiksen, N. L. & Brooks, S. L. (2006). Computerized tomography-based imaging and surgical guidance in oral implantology. *J Oral Implantol,* Vol. 32, No. 1, pp. 14-18, ISSN 0160-6972

Balshi, S. F., Wolfinger, G. J. & Balshi, T. J. (2006). Surgical planning and prosthesis construction using computed tomography, CAD/CAM technology, and the Internet for immediate loading of dental implants. *J Esthet Restor Dent,* Vol. 18, No. 6, pp. 312-323; discussion 324-315, ISSN 1496-4155

Choi, J. Y., Choi, J. H., Kim, N. K., Kim, Y., Lee, J. K., Kim, M. K., Lee, J. H. & Kim, M. J. (2002). Analysis of errors in medical rapid prototyping models. *Int J Oral Maxillofac Surg,* Vol. 31, No. 1, (February 2002), pp. 23-32, ISSN 0901-5027

Erben, C., Vitt, K. & Wulf, J. (2002). The Phidias validation study of reported benefits from use of stereolithographic models. *Phidias Newsletter,* Vol. [S.I.], No. 8, (March 2002), pp. 15-16, ISSN

Erickson, D. M., Chance, D., Schmitt, S. & Mathis, J. (1999). An opinion survey of reported benefits from the use of stereolithographic models. *J Oral Maxillofac Surg,* Vol. 57, No. 9, (September), pp. 1040-1043, ISSN 0278-2391

Ganz, S. D. (2003). Use of stereolithographic models as diagnostic and restorative aids for predictable immediate loading of implants. *Pract Proced Aesthet Dent,* Vol. 15, No. 10, (November-December 2003), pp. 763-771; quiz 772, ISSN 1534-6846

Garg, A. K. (2006). Surgical templates in implant dentistry. *Dent Implantol Update,* Vol. 17, No. 6, (June 2006), pp. 41-44, ISSN 1062-0346

Gateno, J., Xia, J., Teichgraeber, J. F., Rosen, A., Hultgren, B. & Vadnais, T. (2003). The precision of computer-generated surgical splints. *J Oral Maxillofac Surg,* Vol. 61, No. 7, (July 2006), pp. 814-817, ISSN 0278-2391

Jacobs, R., Adriansens, A., Naert, I., Quirynen, M., Hermans, R. & Van Steenberghe, D. (1999). Predictability of reformatted computed tomography for pre-operative planning of endosseous implants. *Dentomaxillofac Radiol,* Vol. 28, No. 1, (January 1999), pp. 37-41, ISSN 0250-832X

James, W. J., Slabbekoorn, M. A., Edgin, W. A. & Hardin, C. K. (1998). Correction of congenital malar hypoplasia using stereolithography for presurgical planning. *J Oral Maxillofac Surg,* Vol. 56, No. 4, (April 1998), pp. 512-517, ISSN 0278-2391

Lal, K., White, G. S., Morea, D. N. & Wright, R. F. (2006). Use of stereolithographic templates for surgical and prosthodontic implant planning and placement. Part I. The concept. *J Prosthodont,* Vol. 15, No. 1, (January-February 2006), pp. 51-58, ISSN 1059-941X

Loubele, M., Guerrero, M. E., Jacobs, R., Suetens, P. & van Steenberghe, D. (2007). A comparison of jaw dimensional and quality assessments of bone characteristics with cone-beam CT, spiral tomography, and multi-slice spiral CT. *Int J Oral Maxillofac Implants,* Vol. 22, No. 3, (May-June 2007), pp. 446-454, ISSN 0882-2786

Marchack, C. B. (2007). CAD/CAM-guided implant surgery and fabrication of an immediately loaded prosthesis for a partially edentulous patient. *J Prosthet Dent,* Vol. 97, No. 6, (June 2007), pp. 389-394, ISSN 0022-3913

Meurer, M. I., Meurer, E., Silva, J. V. L. d., Bárbara, A. S., Nobre, L. F., Oliveira, M. G. d. & Silva, D. N. (2008). [Acquisition and manipulation of computed tomography images of the maxillofacial region for biomedical prototyping]. *Radiol. bras,* Vol. 41, No. 1, (January-February 2008), pp. 49-54, ISSN 0100-3984

Nickenig, H. J. & Eitner, S. (2007). Reliability of implant placement after virtual planning of implant positions using cone beam CT data and surgical (guide) templates. *J*

Craniomaxillofac Surg, Vol. 35, No. 4-5, (June-July 2007), pp. 207-211, ISSN 1010-5182

Parel, S. M. & Triplett, R. G. (2004). Interactive imaging for implant planning, placement, and prosthesis construction. *J Oral Maxillofac Surg,* Vol. 62, No. 9 Suppl 2, (September 2004), pp. 41-47, ISSN 0278-2391

Peltola, S. M., Melchels, F. P., Grijpma, D. W. & Kellomaki, M. (2008). A review of rapid prototyping techniques for tissue engineering purposes. *Ann Med,* Vol. 40, No. 4, pp. 268-280, ISSN 1365-2060

Rosenfeld, A. L., Mandelaris, G. A. & Tardieu, P. B. (2006). Prosthetically directed implant placement using computer software to ensure precise placement and predictable prosthetic outcomes. Part 1: diagnostics, imaging, and collaborative accountability. *Int J Periodontics Restorative Dent,* Vol. 26, No. 3, (June 2006), pp. 215-221, ISSN 0198-7569

Sanna, A. M., Molly, L. & van Steenberghe, D. (2007). Immediately loaded CAD-CAM manufactured fixed complete dentures using flapless implant placement procedures: a cohort study of consecutive patients. *J Prosthet Dent,* Vol. 97, No. 6, (June 2007), pp. 331-339, ISSN 0022-3913

Sarment, D. P., Al-Shammari, K. & Kazor, C. E. (2003a). Stereolithographic surgical templates for placement of dental implants in complex cases. *Int J Periodontics Restorative Dent,* Vol. 23, No. 3, (June 2003), pp. 287-295, ISSN 0198-7569

Sarment, D. P., Sukovic, P. & Clinthorne, N. (2003b). Accuracy of implant placement with a stereolithographic surgical guide. *Int J Oral Maxillofac Implants,* Vol. 18, No. 4, (July-August 2003), pp. 571-577, ISSN 0882-2786

Schneider, D., Marquardt, P., Zwahlen, M. & Jung, R. E. (2009). A systematic review on the accuracy and the clinical outcome of computer-guided template-based implant dentistry. *Clin Oral Implants Res,* Vol. 20 No. Suppl 4, (September 2009), pp. 73-86, ISSN 1600-0501

Souza, M. A. d., Centeno, T. M. & Pedrini, H. (2003). [Integrating 3D reconstruction of tomographic images and rapid prototyping for fabrication of medical models]. *Rev. bras. eng. biomed,* Vol. 19, No. 2, (Augoust 2003), pp. 103-115, ISSN 1517-3151

Suomalainen, A., Vehmas, T., Kortesniemi, M., Robinson, S. & Peltola, J. (2008). Accuracy of linear measurements using dental cone beam and conventional multislice computed tomography. *Dentomaxillofac Radiol,* Vol. 37, No. 1, (January 2008), pp. 10-17, ISSN 0250-832X

Tardieu, P. B., Vrielinck, L. & Escolano, E. (2003). Computer-assisted implant placement. A case report: treatment of the mandible. *Int J Oral Maxillofac Implants,* Vol. 18, No. 4, (July-August 2003), pp. 599-604, ISSN 0882-2786

Van Assche, N., van Steenberghe, D., Guerrero, M. E., Hirsch, E., Schutyser, F., Quirynen, M. & Jacobs, R. (2007). Accuracy of implant placement based on pre-surgical planning of three-dimensional cone-beam images: a pilot study. *J Clin Periodontol,* Vol. 34, No. 9, (September 2007), pp. 816-821, ISSN 0303-6979

Viegas, V. N., Dutra, V., Pagnoncelli, R. M. & de Oliveira, M. G. (2010). Transference of virtual planning and planning over biomedical prototypes for dental implant placement using guided surgery. *Clin Oral Implants Res,* Vol. 21, No. 3, (March 2010), pp. 290-295, ISSN 1600-0501

Wulf, J., Vitt, K. D., Erben, C. M., Bill, J. S. & Busch, L. C. (2003). Medical biomodelling in surgical applications: results of a multicentric European validation of 466 cases. *Stud Health Technol Inform,* Vol. 94, No. pp. 404-406, ISSN 0926-9630

2

Changes in Bone Metabolism Around Osseointegrated Implants Under Loading

Shigeto Koyama[1], Hiroto Sasaki[2], Masayoshi Yokoyama[2], Miou Yamamoto[2], Naoko Sato[2], David Reisberg[3] and Keiichi Sasaki[2]
[1]*Maxillofacial prosthetics Clinic, Tohoku University Hospital Dental Center*
[2]*Division of Advanced Prosthetic Dentistry, Tohoku University Graduate School of Dentistry*
[3]*The Craniofacial Center, Department of Surgery, The University of Illinois College of Medicine*
[1,2]*Japan*
[3]*USA*

1. Introduction

The use of osseointgrated dental implants to replace missing teeth is a highly predictable procedure. The scientific lierature is replete with reports of high success rates over long periods of time. Since the phenomenon of osseointegration was first introduced by Brånemark, this procedure has gained great popularity.

One of the measurements for success of an osseointegrated implant is that it be load-bearing and transmit these occlusal forces directly to the adjacent bone. Controlling this load is considered a determinant factor in the long term success of the implant. A related consideration is how this load or mechanical stress influences bone metabolism around the osseointegated implant.

Mechanical stress may lead to an alteration in bone quality and architecture and a distinct reaction within the bone cells at the bone-implant interface. However, there is little published data to support this theory. A few studies have suggested that occlusal overload may contribute to bone loss around an implant and/or loss of integration of a successfully integrated implant. (Rangert et al.,1995; Miyata et al., 2000; Piattelli et al., 2003). Isidor reported implant mobility caused by progressive peri-implant bone loss after the implant were expose to mechanical occlusal trauma for 18 month (Isidor, 1997, 1998). Others report that peri-implant bone loss and/or loss of osseointegration is associated with biological complications such as peri-implant infection (Lang at al., 2000).

A certain level of mechanical loading is required for normal, healthy bone remodeling (Frost, 1989). Misch observed that the change in bone strength from loading and mineralization after one year alters the stress-strain relationship and reduces the risk of microfracture during following years. Mechanical stress might induce a metabolic turnover of the bone based on the changes in osteocyte responses around the implant, resulting in bone remodeling (Misch, 1999).

This chapter is to investigate the dynamic changes in bone metabolism around osseointegrated implants under mechanical loading.

2. Basic information

2.1 Bone formation

Bone forms by either endochondral or intramembranous ossification. In endochondral ossification or long bone formation, there is an intermediate cartilage phase. All craniofacial bones are formed by intramembranous ossification. Wong and Rabie showed that demineralized intramembranous bone matrix induces bone without an intermediate cartilage stage, mesenchymal stem cells differentiate directly into bone cells (Wong & Rabie, 1999). The mesenchymal stem cells differentiate into osteoblasts and form osteoid in a collagen matrix (Palacci et al., 2001). Mineralization of osteoid occurs and the osteoblasts become trapped in mineralized bone and become osteocytes.

Appositional bone formation occurs when osteoblasts produce bone on existing bone surfaces. Examples of appositional bone formation occur in the periosteal enlargement of bones during growth and remodeling. Histological studies show woven bone formation by appositional growth may only begin to form the second week after implant insertion, at a rate of 30 to 50 microns per day. The bone to implant contact is weakest and at the highest risk of overload at approximately 3 to 5 weeks after implant placement (Strid, 1985).

2.2 Osseointegration process

Osseointegration is defined as direct bone deposition on an implant surfaces at the light microscopic level (Brånemark et al., 1997). It generally follows three stages: (1) incorporation by woven bone formation, (2) adaptation of bone mass to load (lamellar and parallel-fibered deposition) and (3) adaptation of bone structure to load (bone remodeling) (Schenk & Buser, 1998). During the third stage, when functional loading has been initiated, the bony structures adapt to the load by improving the quality of the bone; replacing pre-existing, necrotic and/or initially formed more primitive woven bone with mature, viable lamellar bone. This leads to functional adaptation of the bony structures to the load. The dimensions and orientation of the supporting elements change. *In vitro* studies have illustrated the importance of loading forces on the nature of the interface between an implant and the surrounding tissues (Brunski, 1988). Even if implants were initially integrated, the application of excessive loading can create microfractures and mobility which may promote bone resorption around the implant and may promote repair by the undesirable growth of fibrous tissue (Roberts et al., 1989). An undisturbed healing period along with adequate quality and quantity of bone available at the implant site are essential for proper osseointegration. (Wood, 2004). In addition, primary implant stability is determined by bone quality and quantity, implant design, and surgical technique (Sennerby et al., 1998).

2.3 Implant mechano-biology

Factors that influence mechano-implant studies are mechanical loading and detachment of cells. Previous *in vivo* data have demonstrated that optimal mechanical loading led to more favorable bone quality and quantity than situations with no loading. The testing equipment used for most of these studies were stretching devices borrowed from orthopedic stress-strain research measuring elastic stress relative to joint prostheses. Their application in dental implant research is not optimal as there is mostly shear stress and little elastic stress.

More recently, *in vitro* studies of osteoblastic behavior on titanium following loading have been developed. Movement seems to generate negative effects on osteointegration in terms of decreased Alkaline Phosphatase (ALP) activity and osteocalcin, which is consistent with the results in mechano-cell studies. The supressed ALP activity may be attributed to PGE2 production (Bannister et al., 2002). With respect to osteoblast maturation following stimuli, biphasic ALP activity and triphasi osteocalcin level in a 3D study differed from 2D cultures characterized by typical gene expression pattern with time (early up-regulation of collagen and ALP) and osteocalcin production (Akhouayri et al., 1999). It was assumed that actin cables and collagen fibers would be aligned to amplify the mechanical forces and to supply bone maximum strength with little amount of material. This research has demonstrated that number of complex elements exist in the human body environment and it is still necessary to improve experimental designs in order to provide reliable *in vivo* implant data.

2.4 Implant under loading

It is clear that successful osseointegration depends on unfavorable loading. Other factors to consider are the timing of initiation, magnitude, and duration of the load or stress. Excessive occlusal loading will lead to disintegration while adequate loading leads to adaptive remodeling of the bone around the implant (Quirynen, 1992). However, there are some differences in data reported among rearchers.

Gotfredsen et al. demonstrated that implants subjected to a static lateral expansion load showed increased bone density and mineralized bone-to-implant contact compared with control implants (Gotfredsen et al., 2001a, 2001b, 2001c, 2002). Melsen and Lang reported that there was significantly higher bone apposition around loaded implants than unloaded implants but the dimensions of the applied load did not affect the turnover characteristics of the peri-implant alveolar bone (Melsen & Lang, 2001). Vandamme et al. also indicated significantly more osteoid in contact with the implant was found for the loaded conditions compared with no loading. Well-controlled micromovement favorably influenced bone formation at the interface of an implant (Vandamme et al., 2007). In an animal model, Berglundth et al. described osteoclastic activity as early as four days following implant placement and new bone was noted at one week post placement (Berglundth et al., 2003). These results suggest that bone metabolic activity is changed by mechanical stress and that it depends on the loading conditions.

These reports indicate that functinal loading does promote osseointegatein and that overloading or favorable loading may contribute to implant failure. Occlusal overload could result in progressive marginal bone loss or loss of osseointegration. Long ago, Adell recognized that early implant failure may be associated with overload (Adell et al., 1981). In a more recent study, Miyata et al. reported the outcome of occlusal overloading at three different occlusal heights (100μm, 180μm, 250μm) on implant prostheses for four weeks. Bone destruction was observed in the 180μm and 250μm excess occlusal height groups (Miyata et al., 2000).

Bruxism, a non-physiological parafunctional habit is more significant than the forces associated with normal mastication. Excessive micromovement creates stress or occlusal overload and leads to soft tissue encapsulation and prevents osseointegration, thus causing implant failure (Brunski et al., 1979). The occlusal scheme may jeopardize the success rates of immediately loaded implants; they found that 75% of failures in immediately loaded implants occurred in patients with bruxism (Balshi &Wolfinger, 1997). To avoid fibrous encapsulation and subsequent implant failure, implants must withstand functional load with less than 150 microns (Schincalglia et al., 2007). It is the excess of micromotion caused by excessive loading during the healing phase that interferes with bone repair. A threshold of tolerated micromotion exists, that is somewhere between 50 μm and 150 μm in human case. Therefore, keeping the amount of micromotion beneath the threshold of deleterious micromotion might enable the loading protocols to be shortened (Szmukler-Moncler et al., 2010).

2.5 Immediate and early loading

Immediate and early loading of dental implants are concepts introduced to shorten treatment time and further improve a patient's quality of life (Barone, 2003). Linked to this is the fact that appropriate mechanical stimulation is a positive factor for bone formation. In fact, several studies have demonstrated that early functional loading is helpful in preventing marginal bone resorption and enhancement of osteointegration at the implant surface. In a human clinical case report, Ganeles et al. demonstrated that Straumann® implants placed in the posterior mandible and maxilla are safe and predictable when used with immediate and early loading procedures (Ganeles et al., 2008; Esposito et al., 2009). In poor quality bone, survival rates were comparable with those from conventional or delayed loading. The mean bone level change was not deemed to be clinically significant and compared well with the typical bone resorption observed in conventional implant loading (Kinsel & Liss, 2007; Fischer et al., 2008). Several animal studies also reported favorable results when using immediate and early loading principles.

In a study of radiographic evaluation in dogs, Corso et al. showed that immediate masticatory loading of single-standing dental implants did not jeopardize tissue integration, provided the implants had excellent primary stability (Corso et al., 1999). Cha et al. asserted that immediate loading of mini-implants in the dog model is possible for orthodontic applications with a high bone-implant contact and 100% survival rate (Cha et al., 2009). Some immediate loading studies involving the biting stress of mastication showed the potential to increase bone density and prevent crestal bone loss. With respect to histological bone implant contacts, no significant difference between immediately loaded implants and those of delayed loaded or those of unloaded was observed. It was postulated that mechanical stimulation quite possibly enhanced bone formation (Romanos et al., 2002, 2003) Kawahara et al. studied the effect of immediate loading at the implant interface in dogs and concluded that micromotion of less than 30μm did not impede bone ingrowth (Kawahara et al., 2003). For an immediate loading model with varying degrees of implant displacement, micromotion had a positive effect on bone formation around a roughened implant surface and a negative effect on a turned implant surface (Vandamme et al., 2007). De Smet reported that early loading enhanced bone reaction around implant and contributed to stability of the implant (De Smet et al., 2005, 2006). At the same time, it has been reported that excessive loading leads to creater-like bone defects around implants, indicating bone resorption (Duyck et al., 2001).

The benefit of immediate loading was futher borne out by clinical and histological studies indicating that immediately loaded implants had a higher bone-to-implant contact (BIC) value than non-immediately loaded implants. In one case report, the BIC was 64.2% greater with immediately loaded Osseotite® implants (Testori et al., 2002). In another study, histological comparison of non-submerged unloaded and early-loaded implants in a monkey model found a tight contact with new bone to implant surfaces in both study groups (Piattelli et al., 1997, 1998). But the authors found that the bone of the loaded implants had a more compact appearance than non-loaded controls and the mean BIC of immediate-loaded implants was 67.2% in the maxilla and 80.7% mandible.

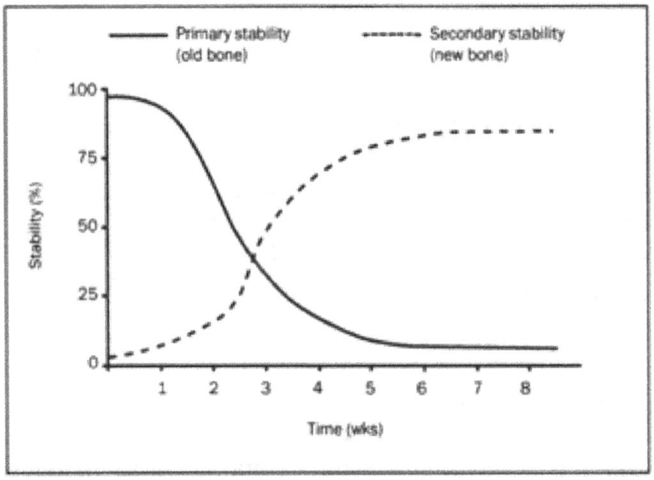

Fig. 1. Changeover from priomary stability created at the time of implant placement to secondary stability created by deposition of new bone (osseointegration) in humans. (Raghavendra et al., 2005)

They felt that the most critical factor in successful osseointegration of an implant is the stability in the bone at the time of placement since a static condition was thought to be a prerequisite during the early healing period. This initial mechanical stability is later replaced by biologic stability as the bone remodels and osseointegartion occurs (Raghavendra et al., 2005). This reportedly occurs during a 2 to 3 week transition phase following implant placement. Ostman listed requirements for long-term success with immediate-loaded implants as high primary implant stability, moderately rough implant surface, prolonged implant stabilization by splinting, controlled occlusion, and biocompatible prosthetic material (Ostman et al., 2008).

The actual type of bone healing around unloaded and loaded implants was investigated by Slaets et al. (Slaets et al., 2006, 2007). These studies showed that the manifestation and duration of the biological processes including the osseointegration of the implant were dependent on the type of bone, cortical or trabecular. Furthermore, the immediate loading protocol caused no differences in the sequential events leading to osseointegration in cortical bone (Slaets et al., 2009). In an unpublished study using bone scintigraphy, the current authors reproted on both immediate and early of loading of implants. The bone metabolic activity increased for the firts seven days after load application and then decreased gradually until returning to the baseline level despite continuous load-application with same magnitude. These results suggest that this change may be attributed to adaptive bone remodeling and immediate and early loading might not prolong the period until achievement of osseointegration.

3. Nuclear medicine approach with bone scintigraphy

Regarding bone metabolic activity, such as bone remodeling and adaptation, histological studies can merely depict static and cross-sectional aspects of the bone activity and phenomena in the remodeling process. In contrast, a nuclear medicine approach with radionuclide bone scanning, including scintigraphy, is widely used to evaluate the dynamic and longitudinal processes in biological response and to help in comprehending the condition of osseointegration (Bambini et al., 2004). Areas with an observed accumulation of radiopharmaceutical isotopes show an increased level of bone metabolic activity, suggesting that this method enables measurement of the changes in bone metabolic activity around implants *in vivo* (Fleisch, 1998; Chisin et al., 1988). *In vivo* scintigraphic imaging using Tc99m-MDP enables the same region to be observed numerous times without sacrificing the host animal. Although the specific binding location of Tc99m-MDP remains unknown, it is associated with areas of bone growth and osteoblast activity (Lysell & Rohlin 1985; Kanishi,1993; Schwartz et al., 1993; Okamoto,1997). Furthermore, bone scintigraphy makes it possible to observe the accumulations with more sensitivity and higher reactivity over time than with conventional radiology (Bijvoet et al., 1995).

3.1 Materials and methods

3.1.1 Animals and insertion of Implants

Thirty-two 12-week-postnatal male Wistar rats were used. Nine rats were used to investigate the biological process of the osseointegration after implant insertion; and twenty-three rats addition to those nine rats were used to investigate the bone metabolic activity under loading. The rats were anesthetized with sodium pentobarbital (50 mg/kg) intraperitoneally with supplemental ether inhalation. Two titanium implants (Orthoanchor®, Dentsply-Sankin, Japan), 1.2 mm in diameter and 9.25 mm in length, were installed in the tibiae perpendicular to the bone surface; the implant heads were exposed about 5 mm. In each rat, one implant was installed 10 mm from the knee joint. The other was installed 13 mm from the first and in the distal aspect.

3.1.2 Loading with coil spring

Healing and osseointegration had gained at eight weeks after insertion. To clarify the biological responses around the implants under continuous loading, closed coil springs (Sentalloy®, Tomy International, Japan) with 0.5 N were attached to the implant heads of nine rats for seven weeks to apply a continuous mechanical stress (Fig 2a). Closed coil springs with 1.0, 2.0, or 4.0 N were also attached to the implant heads of eight, seven, and eight, respectively. The group of rats with two 2.0-N springs is defined as the 4.0-N loading group (Fig 2b). It comprised a tension coil and a hook attachment. The effective length of the tension coil was 12 mm. The springs thus applied the same magnitude of loading continuously within their effective length (10 to 22 mm).

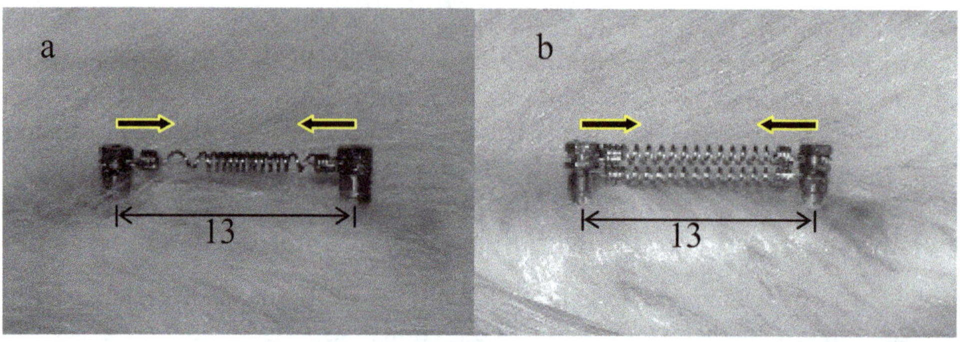

Fig. 2. Attached closed coil springs. Eight weeks after implant insertion, closed coil springs were attached to implant heads. With loading of 0.5, 1.0, or 2.0 N, closed coil spring was set prospectively (a). Two closed coil springs with loading of 2.0 N each were set in parallel for total loading of 4.0 N (b). Arrows show loading directions.

3.1.3 Scintigraphic imaging

Scintigraphic images of the bone were taken using a gamma camera (ZLC7500, Siemens, Japan) with a modified high-resolution pinhole collimator (pinhole diameter: 2 mm). Technetium-99m methylene diphosphonate was used as a radioisotope tracer. Sodium pertechnetate ($Na^{99m}Tc\text{-}O_4$) was eluted from a generator (Ultra-Techne Kow®, Daiichi Radioisotope Laboratories, Japan) and mixed with methylene diphosphonate (Techne® MDP injection solution, Daiichi Radioisotope Laboratories, Japan). The Tc99m-MDP was injected into a vein of a tail of each rat (74 MBq/rat). Static-planar acquisition was initiated two hours after the injection and finished at 50,000 counts with a 512×512 matrix size. The rats were fixed on an exclusive table in the dorsal position, with the implant heads turned to vertical. The images were taken from the backside direction of the rat.

To clarify the bone metabolic activity around the implants during osseointegration, images were taken at 1, 4, 7, and 10 days and 2, 3, 4, 7, and 8 weeks post-implantation. To clarify the bone metabolic activity around the implants under continuous loading, images were taken at three days and every week up to seven weeks after loading with the coil springs.

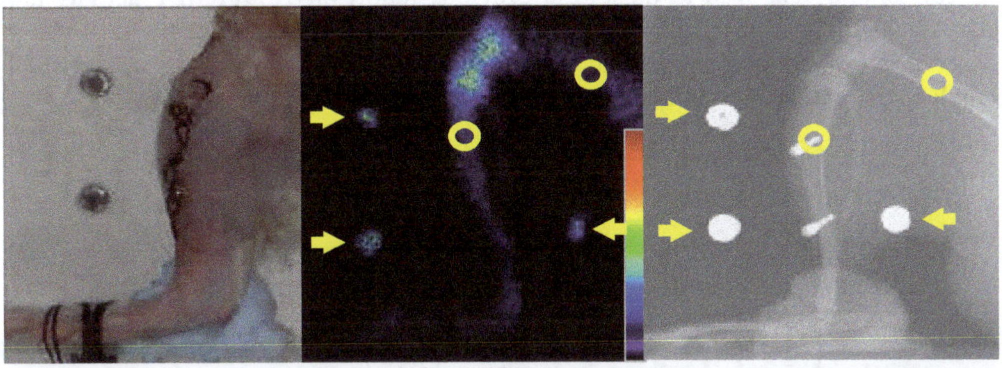

Fig. 3. Image analysis. Photograph on left shows tibia fixation on exclusive table. Device fixes tibia horizontally to equalize distance of implants from pinhole collimator. Scintigram in center and x-ray image on right show planar image. Guide tubes (arrows) were used to overlap two images and to define region of interest (open circles).

3.1.4 X-rayimaging

To identify the region of the reference site and the installed implants, an x-ray image was taken of each rat on the table using an imaging plate (IP; BAS-SR2505, Fuji Film, Japan). Each IP was then scanned with an imaging analyzer (BAS5000, Fuji Film, Japan). The exclusive table had three markers. Before the scintigraphic imaging, Tc99m-MDP was placed in each tube, resulting in an accumulation of Tc99m-MDP in the tube regions on the scintigrams for each rat. These markers indicate the points of overlap with the lead regions in the x-ray images, enabling identification of the implant and reference sites (Fig 3).

3.1.5 Data processing

The scintigrams were translated into TIFF format (16 bits) with a data processing unit (Scintipac 700, Shimazu, Japan) and conversion software (picMAO, Shimazu, Japan). Analysis processing was conducted with image analysis software (Osiris, Geneva University Hospital, Italy). After identification of the implant and reference sites by the overlapping the x-ray images and scintigrams, a round ROI (region of interest, 161 pixels) was defined around both sites and the accumulations of Tc99m-MDP in both regions were measured. As a metric, the ratio of the metabolic activity around the implants to that around the reference site (uptake ratio) was used. The collected data were analyzed using Friedman, Steel, and Tukey tests with statistical software (SPSS 11.0, SPSS Inc., Chicago, IL, USA.). P-values <0.05 were deemed statistically significant.

3.2 Results

3.2.1 Metabolic changes after insertion of Implants

The uptake ratio increased during the first week after implant insertion and then decreased gradually. It was significantly higher than baseline on days 4, 7, and 10 and during the second and third weeks. However, it was not significantly higher on 4 weeks and 7 weeks, in other words, metabolic activity had returned to the baseline level (Fig 4). No clinical mobility of the implants was observed during the healing period. These results suggest that osseointegration is obtained about four weeks after implant insertion. In addition, the timing of the peak level of and subsequent decrease in bone metabolic activity found in this study correspond very well to those of a previous report on Tc99m-MDP activity around implants using bone scintigraphy (McCracken et al., 2001). Therefore, it should be possible to observe in real time the osseointegration process and the degrees and stages of bone metabolism using this method longitudinally.

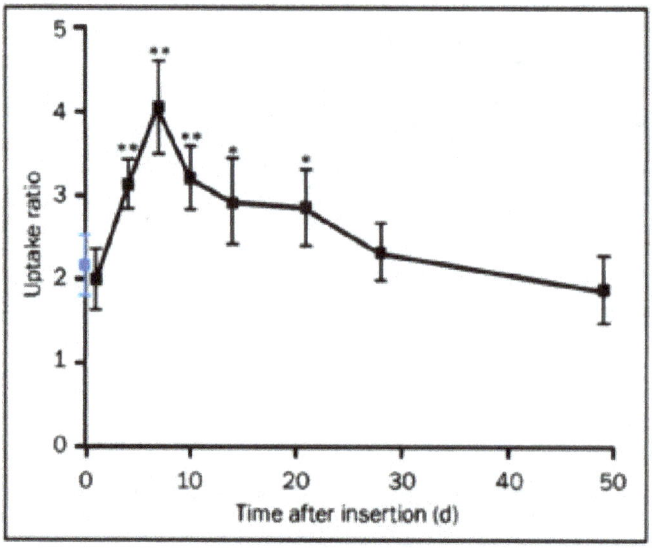

Fig. 4. Change in uptake ratio after insertion of implants using 9 rats.There were significant differences at days 4, 7, and 10 and second and third weeks after insertion. Blue = control. (* p<0.05, **p<0.01) (Sasaki et al., 2008).

3.2.2 Effect of loading period

The uptake ratio changed with the loading. With 2.0- and 4.0-N loading, both changes of activities over the seven-week experimental period were almost the same in terms of magnitude and timing. The ratio reached a maximum during the first week (more than twice that without loading) and then decreased a little. Metabolic activity had returned to the baseline level. The ratio then returned to baseline level of about two on seven weeks after loading. The ratio from three days to six weeks after loading was significantly higher than without loading. There was no significant difference seven weeks after loading.

The results for the 0.5- and 1.0-N loading groups were similar but differed from those for the 2.0- and 4.0-N loading groups. With the smaller loadings, the uptake ratio gradually increased after loading and returned to the baseline level at seven days. It then decreased, reaching about two on seven weeks after loading. With 1.0-N loading, the uptake ratio did not differ among measurement points.

3.2.3 Effect of loading magnitude

The uptake ratios with the 2.0- and 4.0-N loadings were significantly higher than those with the 0.5- and 1.0-N loadings (Tukey test, $p < 0.05$) (Fig 5). This indicates that the metabolic activities are affected by the magnitude of the mechanical loading on the implant. The uptake ratio showed dynamic changes, and the peak levels were similar in the heavy loading group, i.e., there was no difference between 2.0- and 4.0-N loading. It is conceivable that the bone metabolic activity may have an upper limit as far as the loading does not exceed the physiologic threshold of bone adaptation (Frost, 1994). On the other hand, it is possible that the bone metabolic activity increases remarkably when excessive loading is applied to the implant, causing implant disintegration.

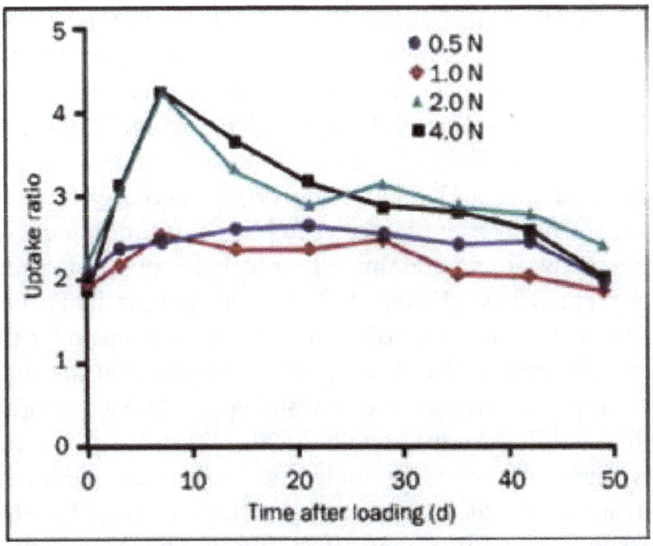

Fig. 5. Change in uptake ratio after loading with coil springs using 32 rats. There were significant differences between 2.0- and 4.0-N loadings and 0.5- and 1.0-N loadings. With 2.0- and 4.0-N loading, the ratio from 3 days to 6 weeks after loading was significantly higher than without loading (Sasaki et al., 2008).

3.3 Discussion

The bone metabolic activity gradually decreased from the peak level despite a static force being applied to the implants and it eventually returned to the pre-loading level. This change can be attributed to an adaptive bone remodeling process similar to those previously reported. Saxon et al. demonstrated that mechanical loading on the rat ulna greatly improved bone formation during the first five weeks of loading, while continual loading reduced the osteogenic response. Moreover, restoring the same level of loading after a period of no loading increased bone formation again (Saxon et al., 2005). Warden et al. investigated the use of mechanical loading with rat ulna to induce bone adaptation and found that fatigue resistance was advanced than control because the structural properties changed due to loading (Warden et al., 2005). Mechanical loading is thus an important factor in the formation and maintenance of skeletal architecture. Bone morphology adapts to the functional loading patterns by responding to the size and distribution of strains that loading engenders in the bone tissue (Lanyon, 1987, 1992). It is concluded that the bone around the implants adapted to the mechanical stress of long-term loading by structurally changing and that the responsiveness to the loading diminished over time.

Mobility normally occurs during the osseous remodeling process (Ganeles et al., 2002). Remodeling is a variable process with balanced osteoclastic and osteoblastic activity, so that a stable implant is preserved during osseointegration (Schnitman et al., 1997). However, clinically stable implants may exhibit mobility on the micro-level when loaded. Sennerby and Meredith revealed that all implants display varying degrees of stability or resistance to load (Sennerby & Meredith, 2008). That is, functional adaptation and maintenance of the bony structures around implants would be caused by cells (i.e., osteocyte, osteoblast, or osteoclast) in active response to environmental biophysical stimuli, in other word, mechanical stress. Microstrain levels 100 times less than the ultimate strength of bone may be responsible for remodeling rates within the structure, since the bone sell membrance are able to act as a mechanosensory system in bone (Cowin & Moss-Salentyin ,1991). In other words, the cellular behavior of bone cells is largely determined by the mechanical environment of strain or deformation of the bone cell (Jones et al., 1991).

At the interface of implant, osteoblasts and osteocytes play roles of transducers of received strain, leading bone modeling and remodeling phase. Verborgt et al. found that fatigue loading produced a large number of osteocytes in bone surrounding microcracks, and stated a strong association between microdamages, osteocyte apotosis, and subsequent bone remodeling (Verborgt et al., 2000). Noble et al. showed that mechanical loading of the bone can be used to regulate osteocyte apoptosis, which has a mechanism for the precise targeting of osteoclasts for bone adaptation (Noble et al., 2003). Miyata et al. speculated that long-term occlusal stress on implants within the physiologic tolerance might stimulate blood circulation, which has an intraosseous bone-inducing factor that promotes bone metabolism and, consequently, enhances bone remodeling to obtain the width needed to counter occlusal stress (Miyata et al., 2000). Futhermore, Isidor indicated that depending on the properties of the tissue, a given force may affect different bones or bone tissues differently, but mechanically loaded bones adapt to the load. If the strain in the bone surrounding an oral implant is in the mild overload range, apposition of bone seems to be the biological response. On the other hand, strain in the bone beyond this range will at some point result in fatigue fracture and bone resorption (Isidor, 2006).

4. Conclusion

Changes in bone metabolic activity around dental implants are dependent on mechanical stress relative to timing, direction, quality, and duration of loading conditions.

The mechanical stress induces metabolic bone remodeling and adptation around osseointegrated implants with structurally changing.

5. Acknowledgment

This work was supported by grants-in-Aid for scientific research (grant no. 14370626, 19592226), from the Ministry of Education, Science, and Culture of Japan.

6. References

Adell R, Ericsson B, Lekholm U, Bolender C et al. (1990). Long-term follow-up study of osseointegrated implants in the treatment of totally edentulous jaws. Int J Oral Maxillofac Implants, Vol.5, No.4, pp. 347-359.

Akhouayri O, Lafage-Proust MH, Rattner A, Laroche N, Caillot-Augusseau A, Alexandre C, Vico L. (1999). Effects of static or dynamic mechanical stresses on osteoblast phenotype expression in three-dimensional contractile collagen gels. *J Cell Biochem*, Vol.76, No.2, (Decenber 1999), pp.217-230.

Balshi TJ, Wolfinger GJ. (1997). Immediate loading of Brånemark implants in edentulous mandibles: a preliminary report. *Implant Dent*, Vol.6, No.2, pp. 83–88.

Bambini F, Meme L, Procaccini M, Rossi B, Lo Muzio L. (2004). Bone scintigraphy and SPECT in the evaluation of the osseointegrative response to immediate prosthetic loading of endosseous implants: a pilot study. *Int J Oral Maxillofac Implants*, Vol.19, No.1, (January-Februry 2004), pp. 80-86.

Bannister SR, Lohmann CH, Liu Y, Sylvia VL, Cochran DL, Dean DD, Boyan BD, Schwartz Z. (2002). Shear force modulates osteoblast response to surface roughness. *J Biomed Mater Res*, Vol.60, No. 1, pp. 167-74.

Barone A, Covani U, Cornelini R, Gherlone E. (2003). Radiographic bone density around immediately loaded oral implants. *Clin Oral Implants Res*, Vol.14, No.5, (October 2003), pp. 610-615.

Berglundh T, Abrahamsson I, Lang NP, Lindhe J. (2003). De novo alveolar bone formation adjacent to endosseous implants. *Clin Oral Implants Res*, Vol.14, No.3, (January 2003), pp. 251-262.

Berglundh T, Abrahamsson I, Welander M, Lang NP, Lindhe J. (2007). Morphogenesis of the peri-implant mucosa: an experimental study in dogs. *Clin Oral Implants Res*, Vol.18, No.1, (January 2007), pp. 1–8.

Bijvoet OLM, Fleisch HA, Canfield RE, Russel RGG. (1995).*Bisphosphonate on bones*, ELSEVIER, pp.87–107, ISBN 978-0-12-260371-6, Vienna, Netherlands

Brånemark PI, Hansson BO, Adell R, Breine U, Lindstrom J, Hallen O, Ohman A.(1997). Osseointegrated implants in the treatment of the edentulous jaw. Experience from a 10-year period. *Scand J Plast Reconstr Surg Suppl.* , Vol.16, No.4, pp. 1-132

Brunski JB, Moccia AFJ, Pollack SR, Korostoff E, Trachtenberg DI. (1979). The influence of f unctional use of endosseous dental implant son the tissue-implant interface. I. Histological aspects. *J Dent Rest*, Vol.58, No.10, (October 1979), pp. 1953-1969.

Brunski JB. (1988).Biomaterials and biomechanics in dental implant design. *Int J Oral Maxillofac Implants* , Vol.3, No.2, pp. 85-97.

Cha JY, Lim JK, Song JW, Sato D, Kenmotsu M, Inoue T, Park YC. (2009). Influence of the length of the loading period after placement of orthodontic mini-implants on changes in bone histomorphology: microcomputed tomographic and histologic analysis. *Int J Oral Maxillofac Implants*, Vol.24, No.5, (September- October 2009) pp. 842-849.

Chisin R, Gazit D, Ulmansky M, Laron A, Atlan H, Sela J. (1988). ^{99m}Tc-MDP uptake and histological changes during rat bone marrow regeneration. *Int J Rad Appl Instrum B,* Vol.15, No.4, pp. 469–476.

Corso M, Sirota C, Fiorellini J, Rasool F, Szmukler-Moncler S, Weber HP. (1999). Clinical and radiographic evaluation of early loaded free-standing dental implants with various coatings in beagle dogs. *J Prosthet Dent,* Vol. 82, No.4, (October 1999), pp. 428–435.

Cowin SC, Moss-Salentyin L. (1991). Candidates for mechanosensory system in bone. *J Biomech Engineer,* Vol.113, No.2, (May 1991), pp. 191-197.

De Smet E, Jaecques SV, Wevers M, Jansen JA, Jacobs R, Sloten JV, Naert IE. (2006). Effect of controlled early implant loading on bone healing and bone mass in guinea pigs, as assessed by micro-CT and histology. *Eur J Oral Sci,* Vol.114, No.3, (June 2006), pp. 232-242.

De Smet E, Jaecques S, Vandamme K, Vander Sloten J, Naert I. (2005). Positive effect of early loading on implant stability in the bi-cortical guinea-pig model. *Clin Oral Implants Res,*PMID:16117763 Vol.16, No.4, (August 2005), pp. 402-407.

Duyck J, Van Oosterwyck H, Vander Sloten J, De Cooman M, Puers R, Naert I. (2001). Pre-load on oral implants after screw tightening fixed full prostheses: an in vivo study. *J Oral Rehabil,* Vol.28, No.3, (March 2001), pp. 226-233.

Esposito M, Grusovin MG, Achille H, Coulthard P, Worthington HV. (2009). Interventions for replacing missing teeth: different times for loading dental implants. Cochrane Database Syst Rev, Vol.21, No.1, (January 2009), CD003878.

Fischer K, Stenberg T, Hedin M, Sennerby L. (2008). Five-year results from a randomized, controlled trial on early and delayed loading of implants supporting full-arch prosthesis in the edentulous maxilla. *Clin Oral Implants Res,* Vol.19, No.5, (May 2008), pp. 433-441.

Fleisch H. (1998). Bisphosphonates: mechanisms of action. *Endocr Rev,* Vol.19, No.1, (February 1998), pp. 80–100.

Frost HM.(1989). *Mechanical adaptation. Frost's mechanostat theory. In: Martin RB, Burr DB, eds. Structure, Function and Adaption of Compact Bone,* pp. 179-181. ISBN 978-08816750096, New York: Raven Press, USA.

Frost HM. (1994). Wolff's Law and bone's structural adaptations to mechanical usage: an overview for clinicians. *Angle Orthod,* Vol.64, No.4, pp. 175–188.

Ganeles J, Rosenberg MM, Holt RL, Reichman LH. (2002). Immediate loading of implants with fixed restorations in the completely edentulous mandible: report of 27 patients from a private practice. *Int J Oral Maxillofac Implants,* Vol.16, No.3, (May-June 2002), pp. 418–426.

Ganeles J, Zöllner A, Jackowski J, ten Bruggenkate C, Beagle J, Guerra F. (2008). Immediate and early loading of Straumann implants with a chemically modified surface (SLActive) in the posterior mandible and maxilla: 1-year results from a prospective multicenter study. *Clin Oral Implants Res,* Vol.19, No.11, (November 2008), pp. 1119-1128.

Gotfredsen K, Berglundh T, Lindhe J. (2001). Bone reactions adjacent to titanium implants subjected to static load. A study in the dog (I). *Clin Oral Implant Res,* Vol.12, No.1, (February 2001), pp. 1-8.

Gotfredsen K, Berglundh T, Lindhe J. (2001). Bone reactions adjacent to titanium implants with different surface characteristics subjected to static load. A study in the dog (II) *Clin Oral Implant Res*, Vol.12, No.3, (June 2001), pp. 196–201.

Gotfredsen K, Berglundh T, Lindhe J. (2001). Bone reactions adjacent to titanium implants subjected to static load of different duration. A study in the dog (III) *Clin Oral Implant Res*, Vol.12, No.6, (December 2001), pp. 552–558.

Gotfredsen K, Berglundh T, Lindhe J. (2002). Bone reactions at implants subjected to experimental peri-implantitis and static load. A study in the dog. *J Clin Periodontol*, Vol.29, No.2, (February 2002), pp. 144–151.

Isidor F. (1997). Histological evaluation of peri-implant bone at implants subjected to occlusal overload or plaque accumulation. *Clinical Oral Implants Research*, Vol.8, No.1, (February 1997), pp. 1-9.

Isidor F. (1998). Mobility assessment with the Periotest system in relation to histologic findings of oral implants. *International Journal of Oral & Maxillofacial Implants*, Vol.13, No.3, (May-June 1998), pp. 377-383.

Isidor F. (2006). Influence of forces on peri-implant bone. *Clin Oral Implants Res*, Vol.17, No. 2, (October 2006), pp. 8-18.

Jones DB, Nolte H, Scholubbers JG, Turner E, Veltel D. (1991). Biochemical signal transduction of mechanical strain in osteoblast-like cells. *Biomateriales*, Vol.12, No.2, (March 1991), pp. 101-110.

Kanishi D. (1993). 99mTc-MDP accumulation mechanisms in bone. *Oral Surg Oral Med Oral Pathol*, Vol.75, No.2, (February 1993), pp. 239-246.

Kawahara H, Kawahara D, Hayakawa M, Tamai Y, Kuremoto T, Matsuda S. (2003). Osseointegration under immediate loading: biomechanical stress-strain and bone formation--resorption. *Implant Dent*, Vol.12, No.1, pp. 61-68.

Kinsel RP, Liss M. (2007). Retrospective analysis of 56 edentulous dental arches restored with 344 single-stage implants using an immediate loading fixed provisional protocol: statistical predictors on implant failure. *Int J Oral Maxillofac Implants*, Vol.22, No.5, (September-October 2007), pp. 823-830.

Lang N.P., Wilson, T.G., Corbet, E.F. (2000). Biological complications with dental implants: their prevention, diagnosis and treatment. *Clinical Oral Implants Research*, II Vol.8, (Suppl.), pp. 146-155.

Lanyon LE. (1992). Control of bone architecture by functional load bearing. *J Bone Miner Res*, Vol.7, (Suppl 2), pp. 369–375.

Lanyon LE. (1987). Functional strain in bone tissue as an objective, and controlling stimulus for adaptive bone remodeling. *J Biomech*, Vol.20, No.11-12, pp. 1083–1093.

Lysell L, Rohlin M. (1985). Initial Tc-99m diphosphonate uptake in mineralized and demineralized bone implants in rats. Int J Oral Surg, Vol.14, No.4, (August 1987), pp. 371-375.

McCracken M, Zinn K, Lemons JE, Thompson JA, Feldman D. (2001). Radioimaging of implants in rats using Tc-99m-MDP. *Clin Oral Implant Res*, Vol.12, No.4, (August 2001), pp. 372-378.

Melsen B, Lang NP. (2001). Biological reactions of alveolar bone to orthodontic loading of oral implants. *Clin Oral Implants Res*, Vol.12, No.2, (April 2001), pp. 144–152.

Misch CE.(1999). Dental evaluation: *Factors of stress.* In Misch CE, ed. Contemporary Implant Dentistry, "2nd ed, pp.122-123. ISBN 0-8151-7059-9 St. Louis: Mosby, USA.

Miyata T, Kobayashi Y, Araki H, Ohto T, Shin K.(2000). The influence of controlled occlusal overload on peri-implant tissue. Part 3: A histologic study in monkeys. *International Journal of Oral & Maxillofacial Implants*, Vol.15, No.3, (May-June 2000), pp. 425-431.

Noble BS, Peet N, Stevens HY, Brabbs A, Mosley JR, Reilly GC, Reeve J, Skerry TM, Lanyon LE. (2003). Mechanical loading: biphasic osteocyte survival and targeting of osteoclasts for bone destruction in rat cortical bone. *Am J Physiol Cell Physiol*, Vol.284, No.4, (April 2002), pp. 934–943.

Okamoto YM. (1997). Mechanism of accumulation of ^{99m}Tc-MDP to bone: correlation of in vivo data with in vitro data. *Radiat Med*, Vol.15 , No.4, (July-August 1997), pp. 209-215.

Ostman PO, Hellman M, Sennerby L. (2008) Immediate Occlusal loading of implants in the partially edentate mandible: a prospective 1-year radiographic and 4-year clinical study. *Int J Oral Maxillofac Implants*, Vol.23, No.2, (March-April 2008), pp.315-322.

Palacci P, Ericsson I. (2001). Esthetic Implant Dentistry: Soft and Hard Tissue Management. Carl Stream; pp.15-31. ISBN 0-86715-382-2, Illinois: Quintessence Pub Co.

Piattelli A, Corigliano M, Scarano A, Quaranta M. (1997). Bone reactions to early occlusal loading of two-stage titanium plasma-sprayed implants: a pilot study in monkeys. *Int J Periodontics Restorative Dent*, Vol.17, No.2, (April 1997), pp. 162–169.

Piatelli A, Corigliano M, Scarano A, Costigliola G, Paolantonio M. (1998). Immediate loading of titanium plasma-sprayed implants: An histologic analysis in monkeys. *J Periodontol*, Vol.69, No.3, (March 1998), pp. 321-327.

Piattelli A, Scarano A, Favero L, Iezzi G, Petrone G, Favero GA. (2003). Clinical and histologic aspects of dental implants removed due to mobility. *Journal of Periodontology*, Vol.74, No.3, (March 2003), pp. 385-390.

Quirynen M, Naert I, van Steenberghe D. (1992). Fixture design and overload influence marginal bone loss and fixture success in the Brånemark system. *Clin Oral Implants Res*, Vol.3, No.3, (September 1992), pp.104–111.

Rangert B, Krogh PH, Langer B, Van Roekel N. (1995). Bending overload and implant fracture: a retrospective clinical analysis. *International Journal of Oral & Maxillofacial Implants*, Vol.10, No.3, (May-June 1995), pp. 326-334.

Raghavendra S, Wood MC, Taylor TD. (2005). Early wound healing around endosseous implants: a review of the literature. *Int J Oral maxillofac implants*, Vol.20, No.3, (May-June 2005), pp. 425-431.

Roberts WE, Garetto LP, De Castro RA. (1989). Remodeling of devitalized bone threatens periosteal margin integrity of endosseous titanium implants with treated or smooth surfaces: indications for provisional loading and axillary directed occlusion. *J Indiana Dental Association*, Vol.68, No.4, (July-August 1989), pp. 19-24.

Romanos GE, Toh CG, Siar CH, Swaminathan D. (2002). Histologic and histomorphometric evaluation of peri-implant bone subjected to immediate loading: an experimental study with Macaca fascicularis. *Int J Oral Maxillofac Implants*, Vol.17, No.1, (January-February 2002), pp. 44-51.

Romanos GE, Toh CG, Siar CH, Wicht H, Yacoob H, Nentwig GH. (2003). Bone-implant interface around titanium implants under different loading conditions: a histomorphometrical analysis in the Macaca fascicularis monkey. *J Periodontol*, Vol.74, No.10, (October 2003), pp. 1483-1490.

Sasaki H, Koyama S, Yokoyama M, Yamaguchi K, Itoh M, Sasaki K. (2008). Bone Metabolic Activity Around Dental implants Under Loading Observed Using bone

Scintigraphy. *Intl J Oral and Maxillofac Implants*, Vol.23, No.5, (September-October 2008), pp. 827-834.

Saxon LK, Robling AG, Alam I, Turner CH. (2005). Mechanosensitivity of the rat skeleton decreases after a long period of loading, but is improved with time off. *Bone*, Vol.36, No.3, (March 2005), pp. 454–464.

Schenk RK, Buser D. Osseointegration: a reality. (1998). *Periodontology 2000*, Vol.17, pp. 22-35.

Schincalglia G, Marzola R, Scapioli C, Scotti R. (2007). Immediate Loading of Dental Implants Supporting Fixed Partial Dentures in the Posterior Mandible: A Randomized Controlled Split-Mouth Study-Machined Versus Titanium Oxide Implant Surface. *Int J Oral Maxilllofac Implants*, Vol.22, No.1, (January- February 2007), pp.35-46.

Schnitman PA, Wohrle PS, Rubenstein JE, DaSilva JD, Wang NH. (1997). Ten-year results for Branemark implants immediately loaded with fixed prostheses at implant placement. *Int J Oral Maxillofac Implants*, Vol.12, No.4, (July- August 1997), pp.495–503.

Schwartz Z, Shani J, Soskolne WA, Touma H, Amir D, Sela J. (1993). Uptake and biodistribution of technetium-99m-MD32P during rat tibial bone repair. *J Nucl Med* , Vol.34, No.1, (January 1993), pp.104-108.

Sennerby L, Meredith N. (2008). Implant stability measurements using resonance frequency analysis: biological and biomechanical aspects and clinical implications. *Periodontol 2000*, Vol.47, pp. 51- 66.

Slaets E, Carmeliet G, Naert I, Duyck J. (2006). Early cellular responses in cortical bone healing around unloaded titanium implants: an animal study. *Journal of Periodontology*, Vol.77, No.6, (June 2006), pp. 1015–1024.

Slaets E, Carmeliet G, Naert I, Duyck J. (2007). Early trabecular bone healing around titanium implants: a histological study in the rabbit. *Journal of Periodontology*, Vol.78, No.3, March 2007), pp. 510–517.

Slaets E, Naert I, Carmeliet G, Duyck J. (2009). Early cortical bone healing around loaded titanium implants: a histological study in the rabbit. *Clin Oral Impl Res*, Vol.20, No.2, (February 2009), pp. 126-134.

Strid KG. (1985). *Tissue-Integrated Prostheses: Osseointegration in Clinical Dentistry.Radiographic results.* In: Branemark PI, Zarb GA, Albrektsson T, eds. pp. 187–191. Quintessence: Chicago

Szmukler-Moncler S, Piattelli A, Favero GA, Dubruille JH. (2000). Considerations preliminary to the application of early and immediate loading protocols in dental implantology. *Clin Oral Implants Res*, Vol.11, No.1, (February 2000), pp. 12-25.

Testori T, Szmukler-Moncler S, Francetti L, Del Fabbro M, Trisi P, Weinstein RL. (2002). Healing of Osseotite implants under submerged and immediate loading conditions in a single patient: a case report and interface analysis after 2 months. *Int J Periodontics Restorative Dent*, Vol.22, No.4, (August 2002), pp.345–353.

Vandamme K, Naert I, Geris L, Vander Sloten J, Puers R, Duyck J. (2007). The effect of micro-motion on the tissue response around immediately loaded roughened titanium implants in the rabbit. *Eur J Oral Sci*, Vol.115, No.1, (February 2007), pp. 21-29.

Verborgt O, Gibson GJ, Schaffler MB. (2000). Loss of osteocyte integrity in association with microdamage and bone remodeling after fatigue in vivo. *J Bone Miner Res*, Vol.15, No.1, (January 2000), pp. 60-67.

Warden SJ, Hurst JA, Sanders MS, Turner CH, Burr DB, Li J. (2005). Bone adaptation to a mechanical loading program significantly increases skeletal fatigue resistance. *J Bone Miner Res*, Vol.20, No.5, (December 2005), pp. 809–816.

Wong RW, Rabie AB. (1999). A quantitative assessment of the healing of intramembranous and endochondral autogenous bone grafts. *Eur J Orthod*, Vol.21, No.2, (April 1999), pp. 119-126.

3

n-SiO_2 Embedded HA/TiO_2 Composite Coatings Deposited on Pure Titanium Substrate by Micro-Arc Oxidation

Feng-ying Yan, Yu-long Shi and Jia-hua Ni
School of Material Science and Engineering,
Qingdao University of Science and Technology
China

1. Introduction

As orthopaedic and dental metallic implant materials, titanium and titanium alloys are widely used due to their relatively low modulus, good fracture toughness, excellent strenth-to-weight ration, and superior biocompatibility and corrosion resistance (Long and Rack, 1998). They have become the first choice above all other candidate metallic implant materials such as Co-Cr-Mo alloys, stainless steel in recent years. But smooth titanium or titanium alloy implants are considered to have weak bioactivity and bone-bonding in vivo (Li et al., 2004; Sul, 2003; Xie et al., 2000). Therefore, a composite system including an hydroxyapatite (HA) film on the titanium or titanium alloy implant, which combines the mechanical benefits of metal alloys with the biological properties of HA, has generated widespread interest because of the HA has excellent biocompatibility and tissue bioactivity (Tkalcec et al., 2001; Weng et al., 1997). Many techniques including plasma-spraying, pulsed laser deposition and electrophoretic deposition have been studied to produce HA films over the last 20 years, and plasma-spraying was the only one that achieved commercial success (Yang et al., 2005; Cotell et al., 1992; ZHITOMIRSKY, 1997; Liu, et al., 2002; Wen et al., 2002; Gu et al., 2003; Clèries et al., 2000; Koike & Fujii, 2001). But the film formed by plasma-spraying was easily separated from the surfaces or resorbed in the body environment because of the unstable characteristics through its rapid solidification, inhomogeneous composition, melted and decomposed phases, etc (Xu et al., 2006). The other methods such as electrophoretic deposition may produce highly crystalline coatings, which are difficult to resorb in the body (Gross & Berndt, 1994).

Recently, it was reported that hydroxyapatite-containing titania coating on titanium or titanium alloy was prepared by micro-arc oxidation (MAO) technique (Barrere et al., 2002; Chen et al., 2006; Fu et al., 2002; Han et al., 2003; Wei et al., 2009; Ni et al., 2008). The obtained coating has a porous surface and exhibits perfect biocompatibility and biological activity, which is essential for orthopaedic and dental metallic implant materials. This technique is very suitable for the bioactive surface modification of titanium and its alloy implants.

2. Micro-arc oxidation technique

Micro-arc oxidation (MAO) technique, also named plasma electrolytic oxidation , micro-plasma oxidation, or anodic spark deposition developed from anodic oxidation from the

1970s. MAO is an electrochemical, plasma chemical technology in an electrolyte to obtain ceramic coating on valve-metal surfaces such as aluminium, titamium, magnesium, et al. and their alloys. During MAO treatment, the valve metal substrate is used as anode and a stainless steel plate was used as a cathode in an electrolyte cell. Sometimes, the cathode can be the stainless cell which hold the electrolyte simultaneously. When the applied voltage to the substrate immersed in electrolyte is increased to a certain point, a micro-arc occurs on the surface and a ceramic layer is formed. The method makes it possible to obtain a new coating strongly adhering to the surface and characterized by high mechanical, heat-resistant, wear resistance and other functional properties.

2.1 Micro arc oxidation of aluminium

At its earlier development stage, MAO technique was mainly studied to enhanced friction, wearing and corrosion resistance of aluminium and its alloys. It was first reported depositing oxide coating on aluminium anode by Markov and co-work, Van and co-work in 1970s (Markov et al., 1976; Van et al., 1977). Subsequently, Dittrich et al., Krysmann et al., Kurze et al.(Dittrich et al., 1984; Krysmann et al., 1984; Kurze et al., 1987) in the 1980s, and Wirtz et al (Wirtz et al., 1991) in the early 1990s contributed to the development of the MAO process. However, the MAO process gained worldwide recognition as an eco-friendly technology for deposition the tribologically superior ceramic coatings on aluminum and its alloy by the pioneering research contribution made by Yerokhin et al. of Tula State University (Russia) in the 1990s (Voevodin et al., 1996; Yerokhin et al., 1998; Yerokhin et al., 1999). After that, more researchers from United States, United kingdom, China, et al. have contributed to the further research on the Formation and Mechanism of Ceramic Coating and its properties (Krishna et al., 2007; Lukiyanchuk et al., 2002; Mertsalo et al., 2003; Rudnev et al., Shi et al., 2004; Tianet al., 2002; 2004;Xue et al., 2001).

2.2 Micro arc oxidation of titanium

MAO technique used to modify the surface of titanium and its alloys began with 2000's on the base of research development of that on aluminium. The main purposes at incipient stage were wear resistance and corrosion resistance, and quickly turned to biomaterial modification. Micro-arc oxidation can produce a porous, relatively rough and firmly adherent titanium oxide coating on titanium surface, which is beneficial for the biological performance of the titanium implants. The obtained MAO films on titanium can be used for such applications as orthopaedic or dental implants. A large number of scientists have investigated this technology and have obtained their results.

2.3 Microstructure of MAO coating on titanium

It was reported by almost all investigators that the oxide film formed using MAO on titanium surface exhibited a porous microstructure with SEM. The holes which were regarded as discharge channels of micro-arc in electrolyte were relatively well separated and homogrneously distributed over the surface (Chen et al., 2006; Han et al., 2002a, 2002b, 2003; Li et al., 2004; Ni et al., 2008). Theoretically speaking (Akin et at., 2001; Dunn et al., 1993), this micro-porous morphology of the implant surface is beneficial to bone tissue growth and enhanced anchorage of implant to bone; furthermore, a porous surface may be valuable for bioactive constituents such as growth factors or bone morphogenic proteins and has the function of an enhanced cell proliferation. The cross-sections of the oxide layers formed with different oxidation time showed that there was no obvious discontinuity between the film and the underlying substrate, which indicated that the film could be tightly adhered to the substrate (Han et al., 2002a, 2002b, 2003; Ni et al., 2008). The morphological difference such as diameter of the pores and the thickness of the film associated with electrolyte concentration, discharge voltage and treatment time, have been found by many investigators (Li et al., 2004; Han et al., 2002a, 2003; Kuromoto et al., 2007; Yao et al. 2008).

Ti and O are two primary elements in the MAO coating analyzed by EDX analysis, which came from substrate and component or water of electrolyte respectively. In addition, the elemental component in electrolyte can incorporate into the coating too. The contents of the elements in the coating are different with the change of oxidation time, electrolyte concentration, and so on. (Chen et al., 2006; Han et al., 2002a, 2003; Li et al., 2004; Ni et al., 2008).

XRD patterns prove that the MAO coating formed by MAO is mainly composed of anatase and rutile, the peaks of which are strongly depending on the electrolyte concentration and parameter such as oxidation time, applied voltage et al (Han et al., 2003; Ni et al., 2008). The diffraction peaks of some other materials such as $CaTiO_3$, β-$Ca_2P_2O_7$ and α-$Ca_3(PO_4)_2$, which related to electrolyte composition can be detected at the same time, and this is also decided by electrolyte concentration, oxidation time, and applied voltage et al. (Chen et al., 2006; Fu et al., 2002; Ni et al., 2008, Han et al., 2003).

2.4 Properties of MAO coating on titanium

One main purpose of using MAO technique on titanium and its alloys implants is to improved its biological behavior by modifying the composition and morphology of the implant surface. So some biological and mechanical properties were measured to evaluate MAO process (Akin et al., 2001; Han et al., 2002a, 2002b, 2003; Ishizawa & Ogino, 1995; Li et al., 2004; Lim et al., 1996; Song et al., 2004 ; Sul, 2003; Wang et al., 2000; Wu et al., 2003). It also has been found that the biological behavior of the MAO samples closely related to the morphology, Elemental and phase composition, roughness, and so on.

2.4.1 Bioactivity of MAO coating on titanium-apatite-induced ability in SBF solution

The bioactivity of the MAO film can be studied by immersing the coated samples in simulated body fluid (SBF) for a period of time (Han et al., 2003; Song et al., 2004). The aim is to evaluate the apatite induction of the film in a body-analogous solution by analyzing the changes in chemistry, corrosion resistance, apatite-induced ability, and crystallinity of the coating.

In vitro bioactivity of the MAO titania-based films on titanium surface was evaluated in simulated body fluid (SBF) by Han et al. (Han et al., 2003). They found that only the film containing $CaTiO_3$, β-$Ca_2P_2O_7$ and α-$Ca_3(PO_4)_2$ could induce an apatite layer on its surface, exhibiting bioactivity. $CaTiO_3$ combined with β -$Ca_2P_2O_7$ and α-$Ca_3(PO_4)_2$ seems to be the key structural factor for MAO-formed titania-based films to be of bioactivity. Han et al. analysed the morphologies of the sample which has the apatiteinduced ability in SBF solution immersed in SBF for 40 and 50 days (Han et al., 2003). They found that after 40 days immersion, the surface of the sample exhibits the decrease of pore size and porosity, and starts to be covered with the mineralized apatite. When immersed for 50 days, original porous characterization of the sample disappears and its surface is fully covered with a dense layer of apatite. When observed at high magnification, the apatite layer is in fact composed of network structure, and the diameter of the net pores is less than 100 nm. similar results can be found in the work of others (Song et al., 2004).

Some literatures suggested that TiO_2, regardless of anatase or rutile in the MAO-formed film on titanium seems to be bioactive (Li et al., 2004; Wu et al., 2003). While others hold the view that the in vitro bioactivity is ascribed to Ti-OH group or negatively charged surface as well as to an epitaxial effect of the anatase structure (Lim et al., 1996; Wang et al., 2000; Wu et al., 2003).

2.4.2 Biocompatibility of MAO coating on titanium

Biocompatibility can be evaluated by in vitro cell tests which comprise proliferation and differentiation behavior of the cells and in vivo tests (Akin et al., 2001; Li et al., 2004). Evaluation parameters can be proliferation and differentiation behaviors (alkaline phosphatase (ALP) activity) of the cells of in vitro cell tests and the bond strength between the bone and the implant in of vivo tests.

Akin et al. found that the in vitro proliferation of human bone-derived cells (HBDC) is similar on three samples with 0.50, 16, and 50 μm diameter pores, respectively. However, higher [3H]thymidine (3H-TdR) incorporation by the HBDC is observed when they are grown on 0.50- and 16-μm pores compared to the 50-μm pores, suggesting an enhanced cell proliferation for the smaller pores(Akin et al., 2001).

In the work of Li and co-work (Li et al., 2004), the proliferation and differentiation behaviors of MAO specimens were evaluated by in vitro cell tests using MG63 and human osteosarcoma (HOS) cell lines, respectively. In their works, the proliferation behavior was determined by counting the number of cells after culturing them for 7 days. The differentiation behavior was estimated by measuring the alkaline phosphatase (ALP) activity of the HOS cells after culturing them for 10 days. The results showed Even though the proliferation rate was highest when the specimen was oxidized at the relatively low voltage of 190 V and decreased steadily with increasing voltage, the number of cells increased more than 10 times compared to the originally plated cells. However, The ALP activities of the HOS cells was not much affected by the MAO process when the applied voltage was lower than 300 V, but increased rapidly when the voltage was higher than 300 V. the result shows that the roughness and the amount of Ca and P ions incorporated into the titanium oxide layer strongly affect the cell response. Especially, the ALP activity significantly increased at higher voltages, which is deemed to be closely related to the increase in surface roughness and the increased amount of Ca and P contained in the oxide layer.

In the work of Li et al., the bond strength between the bone and the MAO-treated specimens was measured with a torque measurement device by in vivo tests on female, New Zealand white rabbits (Li et al., 2004). The removal torque of the MAO-treated Ti implants was more than three times higher than that of the as-machined Ti implant. The results showed a considerable improvement in osseointegration capability of MAO-treated specimens as compared to the pure titanium implant. This enhancement is attributable to the increase of surface roughness and to the presence of the Ca and P ions, which were incorporated into oxide layer during the MAO process.

2.4.3 Mechanical properties of MAO coating on titanium

Mechanical properties, including hardness, elastic modulus, and adhesion strength were some other important properties and were tested in some investigations (Han et al., 2002a, 2002b; Sul, 2003; Ishizawa & Ogino, 1995).

According to research results of Han et al. (Han et al., 2002a), The film prepared at 350 V exhibited a low hardness and Young's modulus which were 0.9±0.2 GPa and 32±4 GPa, respectively. The film exhibited a significant plasticity and ductility compared to the conventional coarse-grained titania ceramics which were 9 and 230 GPa, respectively. However, the adhesion of the film to the substrates was fairly strong, as high as approximately 37±3 MPa when the film prepared at 350 V (Han et al., 2002a) . Another research received by the same authors revealed that the bond strength of the films prepared at 350 V was approximately 30±2 MPa and fracture occurred inside the films but not at the interface (Han et al., 2002b). They pointed out that this adhesive strength is much higher than that of sol-gel derived titania films, which is usually less than 10 MPa.

In study of Sul (Sul, 2003), multifactorial biocompatibility of the surface of oxidized implants by MAO method resulted in significantly improved bone reactions as evaluated by biomechanical and histomorphometrical techniques after 6 weeks of implant insertion. Mechanical interlocking and biochemical interaction, separately or together, explain the primary modes of the forces acting over the bone to implant interface. The results of the P and Ca implants point to the possibility of biochemical bonding between bone and oxidized titanium implant. Another literature, wrote by Ishizawa and co-work, proved that the sample with low contents of Ca and P had a high adhesive strength after soaking in a simulated body fluid for 300 days (Ishizawa & Ogino, 1995)

2.5 Influencing factors on MAO film of titanium

The surface morphology, elemental composition, phase components and properties of the MAO coatings on the titanium and its alloys' surface are influence largely by treatment conditions. To find the relationship between them and control them freely are always the purpose of researchers. The main influencing factors are often regarded as electrolyte factors such as its composition and concentration and operation parameters as treatment time, applied voltage, current density et al.

2.5.1 Electrolyte composition and concentration

An advantage of MAO technic is the possibility of incorporating of element in the electrolyte (e.g. Ca, P ions) into the coating by changing the composition and concentration of the electrolyte (Han et al., 2002b; Ishizawa & Ogino, 1995; Li et al., 2004; Song et al., 2004; Ni et al., 2008). The salts have been used in studies include acetate monohydrate ($(CH_3COO)_2Ca \cdot H_2O$), sodium dihydrogenphosphate ($NaH_2PO_4 \cdot 2H_2O$), sodium phosphate (Na_3PO_4), sodium carbonate (Na_2CO_3), β-glycerophosphate disodium salt pentahydrate ($C_3H_7Na_2O_6P \cdot 5H_2O$, e.g. β-GP), and calcium acetate monohydrate (CA), et.al. (Chen et al.,2006; Han et al., 2002a, 2002b, 2003 ; Ni et al., 2008; Song et al., 2004). For example, EDS spectrum of the films formed in solution containing 0.2 M calcium acetate monohydrate ($Ca(CH_3COO)_2 \cdot H_2O$) by Han et al (Han et al., 2002b) proved that Ca can incorporated into the film during the MAO process and the atomic concentration was estimated to be ~3.2%.

However, there are also some opposite results emerged by Han et al (Han et al., 2002a, 2003) that the film didn't contain element in the eletrolyte which containing sodium carbonate (Na_2CO_3). The reasons for this difference may relate to other factors such as concentration of salt, applied voltage, oxidation time, et al. which have not yet been clearly studied by investigators.

As studied by EDX analysis in our previous work (Ni et al., 2008), The films contained Ca and P as well as Ti and O. Ca and P came from electrolyte composition $(CH_3COO)_2Ca \cdot H_2O$

and $NaH_2PO_4 \cdot 2H_2O$) and the content of which increased with increase of electrolyte concentration. The conclusion is that the increase of the electrolyte concentration was in favor of the increase of relative content of Ca and P compounded into the films. The same result was obtained by Ishizawa & Ogino (Ishizawa & Ogino, 1995) too.

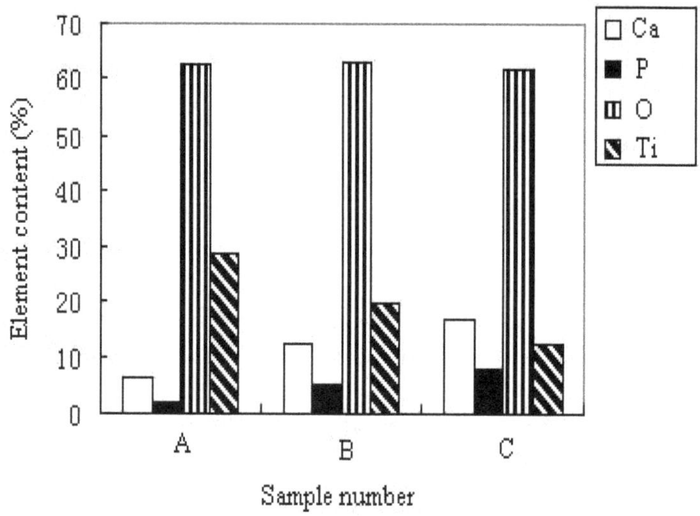

Fig. 1. The element content in coatings subjected to sample A, B, C obtained in different electrolyte concentration (A) $(CH_3COO)_2Ca.H_2O$ 0.13mol/L; $(NaH_2PO_4.2H_2O)$ 0.06mol/L (B) $(CH_3COO)_2Ca.H_2O$ 0.26mol/L ; $(NaH_2PO_4.2H_2O)$ 0.12mol/L; (C) $(CH_3COO)_2Ca.H_2O$ 0.39mol/L; $(NaH_2PO_4.2H_2O)$ 0.18mol/L (Ni et al., 2008)

Another effect of electrolyte composition and concentration to the obtained MAO film is the surface morphology of the surface (Han et al., 2003; Ni et al., 2008). According to Han et al. (Han et al., 2003), at the same voltage, the films formed in CA- and b-GP-containing electrolytic solution become more rough compared with the films formed in Na_2CO_3- and Na_3PO_4-containing solutions, and exhibit similar roughness to the films formed in CA-containing solution. It was observed in Fig.2 obtained in our previous work (Ni et al., 2008) that the discharge pores changed from clearer and bigger to unsharp and smaller when the electrolyte concentration increased gradually. The possible reason that the diameters of the pores tend to reduce with increasing of the electrolyte concentration may be incorporating of electrolyte concentration. The more the electrolyte concentration was, the more electrolyte deposited by sintering on the surface of the film and covered the edge of pores.

Apparently, because of changing of elements composition in the MAO coating on Ti substrate with altering of electrolyte concentration, the phase components of the coating would changed too. Fig.3 (Ni et al., 2008) affirmed this deduction using XRD patterns of MAO coatings formed in different concentration of electrolyte in our previous work. Except for Ti, anatase and rutile, the peak of hydroxyapatite was gradually appeared with increase of electrolyte concentration. The result imply us that hydroxyapatite can be prepared by controlling of electrolyte used in MAO process.

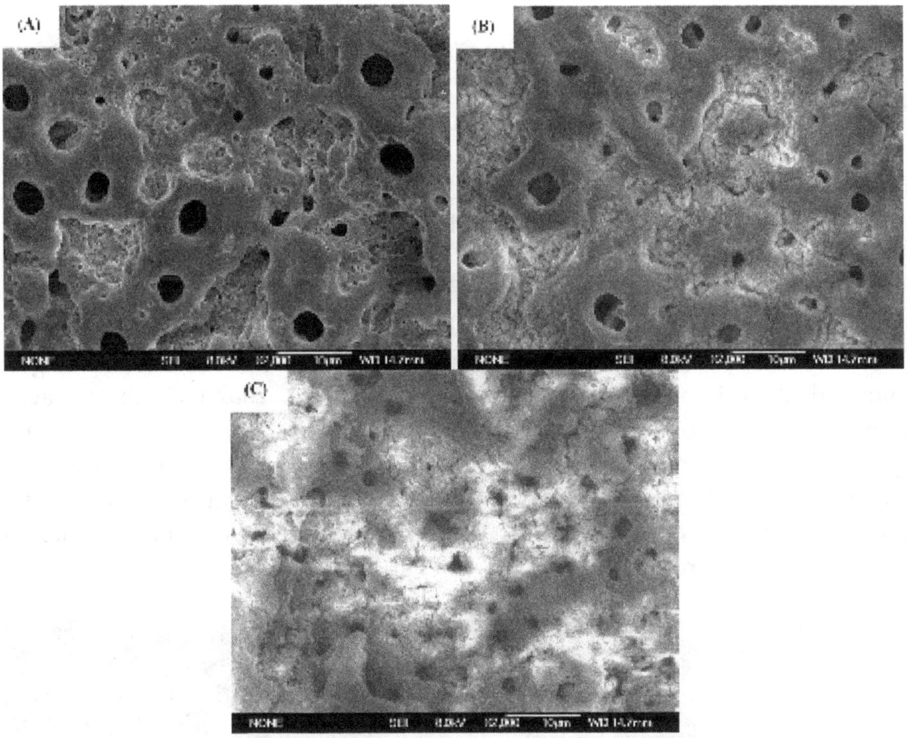

Fig. 2. SEM surface morphologies of micro-arc oxidation coatings formed in different electrolyte concentration: (A) $(CH_3COO)_2Ca.H_2O$ 0.13mol/L, $(NaH_2PO_4.2H_2O)$ 0.06mol/L; (B) $(CH_3COO)_2Ca.H_2O$ 0.26mol/L, $(NaH_2PO_4.2H_2O)$ 0.12mol/L; (C) $(CH_3COO)_2Ca.H_2O$ 0.39mol/L, $(NaH_2PO_4.2H_2O)$ 0.18mol/L (Ni et al., 2008)

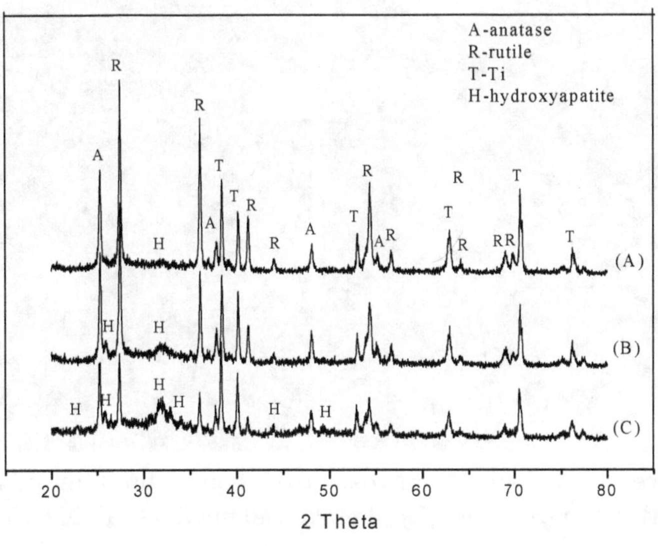

Fig. 3. XRD patterns of the MAO samples formed in different electrolyte concentration for 10min. (A) $(CH_3COO)_2Ca.H_2O$ 0.13mol/L, $(NaH_2PO_4.2H_2O)$ 0.06mol/L ;(B) $(CH_3COO)_2Ca.H_2O$ 0.26mol/L ,$(NaH_2PO_4.2H_2O)$ 0.12mol/L ; (C) $(CH_3COO)_2Ca.H_2O$ 0.39mol/L , $(NaH_2PO_4.2H_2O)$ 0.18mol/L (Ni et al., 2008)

2.5.2 Process parameters

Beside influence of electrolyte to the MAO film, process parameters such as oxidation time, applied voltage, power supply mode, and current density et al. are other factors that should not be ignored. The uppermost process parameters are oxidation time and applied voltage which can be controlled from several min to several quarters and from dozens volts to several hundred volts, respectively (Han et al. 2002a, 2002b, 2003; Ishizawa & Ogino, 1995; Kuromoto et al., 2007; Li et al., 2004; Ni et al. 2008; Song et al., 2004; Sul et al., 2002). The phase, element content, morphology, and thickness of the films were strongly dependent on the treatment time and applied voltage.

The morphological difference associated with treatment time and discharge voltage have been found by many investigators (Han et al. 2002a, 2003; Ishizawa & Ogino, 1995; Kuromoto et al., 2007; Li et al., 2004; Ni et al. 2008;; Sul et al., 2002). On the surface of MAO coating on titanium, the diameters of discharge pores tend to increase with treatment time prolonged within certain period time, and it will not increase in the time that upon the time bucket. The periods of time are not stationary because it is influenced by others process of MAO and sometimes it would not appear. The roughness of the coating also increased with increasing of voltage (Kuromoto et al., 2007; Li et al., 2004).

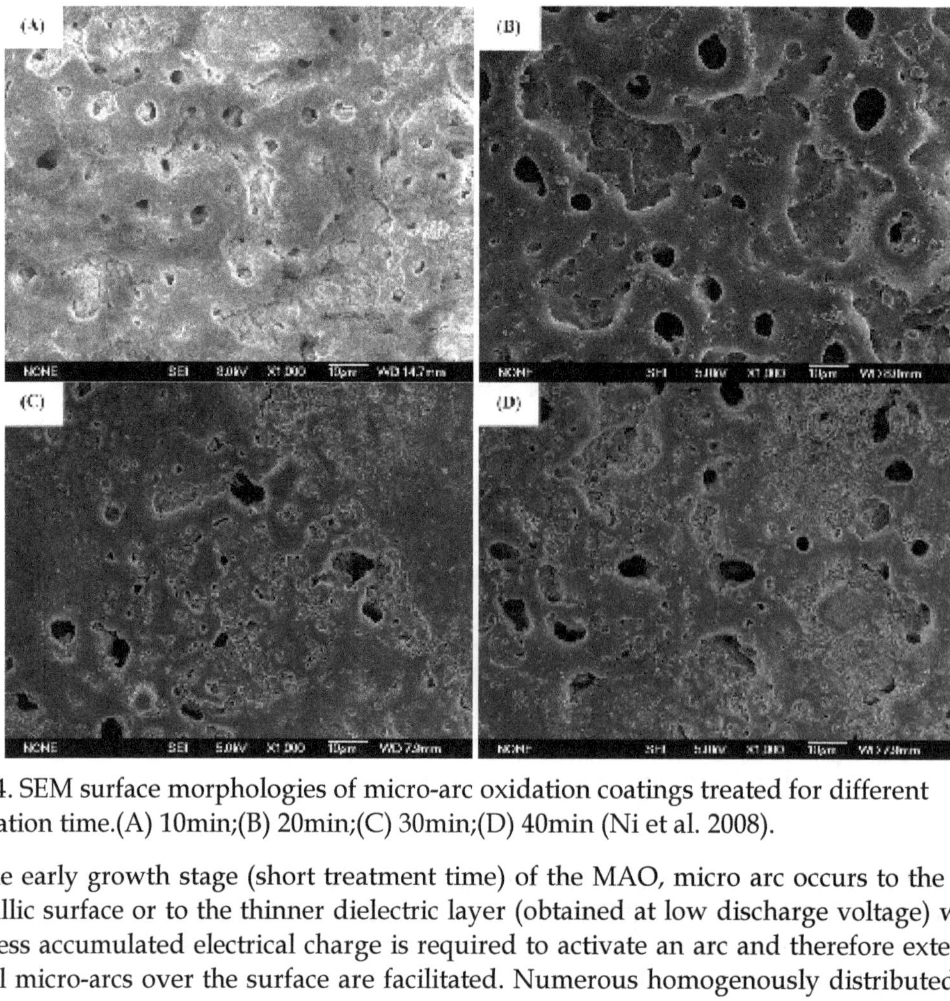

Fig. 4. SEM surface morphologies of micro-arc oxidation coatings treated for different oxidation time.(A) 10min;(B) 20min;(C) 30min;(D) 40min (Ni et al. 2008).

In the early growth stage (short treatment time) of the MAO, micro arc occurs to the fresh metallic surface or to the thinner dielectric layer (obtained at low discharge voltage) where the less accumulated electrical charge is required to activate an arc and therefore extensive small micro-arcs over the surface are facilitated. Numerous homogenously distributed tiny pores with thin layer thickness were thus found for the specimens, as opposed to those specimens prepared at high discharge voltages or extended treatment times, where less but large arc events occur. Fig.4 demonstrated the morphological difference between coatings obtained for different treatment time in our previous work (Ni et al. 2008).

The phases of the oxide layers formed by MAO process characterized by XRD analysis are dependent on oxidation time and applied voltage, too. Generally, with increase of oxidation time, the crystal of TiO_2 become better and diffraction peaks of hydroxyapatite in the coatings were stronger. In other words, a shorter treatment time favor the growth of anatase in the MAO film. Anatase formation requires much lower activation energy than the rutile polymorphism as had been reported (Shibata et al., 1993). Under a short treatment time, the available energy is only sufficient to overcome the activation energy for the formation of anatase and the film is thus exclusively composed of this form. A longer treatment time thermodynamically favors the stable rutile phase. Fig.5 showed this tend for us by work of our previous work (Ni et al. 2008). And it agrees well with the results revealed by Lie et al (Li et al., 2004).

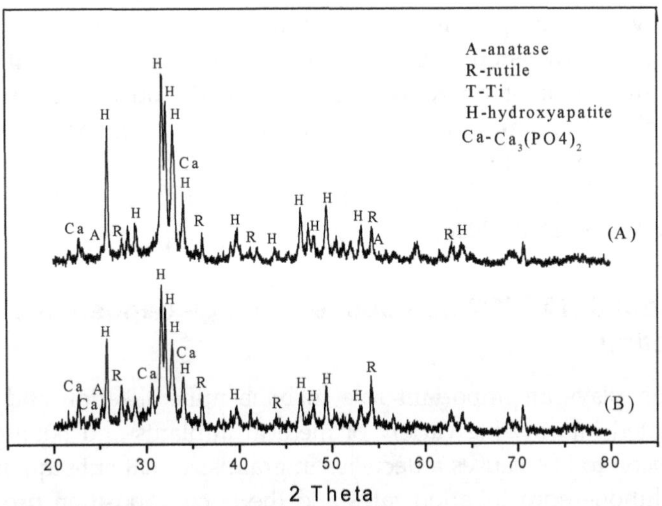

Fig. 5. XRD patterns of the MAO samples treated for (A) 30 min and (B) 40 min (Ni et al., 2008)

The same trend as treatment time was seen in discharge voltage, and the reasons can be same too (Han et al., 2003; Li et al., 2004; Shibata et al., 1993). XRD patterns of the films obtained by Han et al (Han et al., 2002a) showed that at low applied voltage, the film was composed of rutile and a small amount of anatase and with increasing the applied voltage, anatase phase gradually disappeared and rutile phase gradually increased. Sometimes, other Ca- and P-containing compounds such as $Ca_3(PO_4)_2$, $CaTiO_3$, b-$Ca_2P_2O_7$ and a-$Ca_3(PO_4)_2$ could be observed also (Ni et al., 2008; Han et al., 2003; Song et al., 2004). The possible reason for which may be higher applied voltage used (Han et al., 2003; Song et al., 2004).

As discussed above, the thickness, pore size and the content of Ca and P tended to increase with the applied voltage. And the morphology of the oxide layer was dependent on the treatment time and voltage applied during the oxidation treatment. On the other hand, the thickness and elements content changes of the MAO coating with oxidation time are not same with each other in different investigators' works. Sometimes, the thickness sostenuto thickened with the time increase (chen et al., 2006), and sometimes it thickened first and then decreased at a certain value time (Ni et al., 2008). The tendency may be influenced by some other factors. The same condition can be seen in element content of the coating (chen et al., 2006; Ni et al., 2008).

There are also many other factors than affect the MAO film on titanium surface, such as power mode, current density, electrolyte temperature, substrate material, and so on. They all influence the microstructure, properties and of course application of the MAO coating formed on titanium and its alloy.

2.6 Summary of MAO on titanium

In a word, MAO is a simple, controllable, and cost-effective method of forming a porous TiO_2 layer on the titanium implant surface. The microstructure of the oxide layer such as amount and diameter of the pores, thickness, and roughness are easily controllable by adjusting the electrolyte concentration, voltage, processing time, current during the MAO process. Moreover, the element concentration in the coating such as Ti, O, Ca and P can also be regulated by above factors. Thus, phase composition of coating will regulate with it regulately to meet biological performance of the materials. In order to obtain HA in the coating to improve biocompatibility and biological activity of the sample, many investigators employed two-step approach such as Microarc Oxidization-Hydrothermal synthesis, hybrid treatment of micro-arc discharge oxidation (MDO) and electrophoretic deposition (Fu et al., 2002; Han et al., 2002b; Wei & Yang, 2009; Xie et al., 2000; Xu et al., 2006). Whereas, a composite film of HA and TiO_2 also can be prepared directly by MAO in Ca- and P- containing electrolyte by regulating process parameter (Chen et al., 2006; Han et al., 2003; Li et al., 2004; Ni et al., 2008).

3. n-SiO2 embedded HA/TiO2 composite coatings deposited on titanium by micro-arc oxidation

As reported, silicon plays an important role in bone mineralization and formation and is therefore incorporated into a wide variety of medical implants and bone grafts used today. The addition of silicon to HA causes a decrease in grain size that subsequently affects surface topography, dissolution-reprecipitation rates and the bone apposition process (Porter, 2006; Porter et al., 2004). In our present work, based on our preliminary works (Chen et al., 2006; Ni et al., 2008) and the function of silicon in bone mineralization and formation, a novel thought that nano-silicon dioxide particles are added to the composite coating of HA/TiO_2 formed by MAO is produced, and the primary experiment was carried out.

3.1 Experimental procedure

The material oxidized was commercially pure titanium (TA_2), the element composition of which was shown in Table 1.

The titanium plates (30×15×2 mm^3) were polished progressively using 200, 400, 800, and 1000-grit silican carbon paper and ultrasonicly cleaned with acetone and deionized water respectively. The cleaned Ti plate was oxidized as an anode in an electrolyte containing sodium phosphate monobasic dehydrate ($NaH_2PO_4.2H_2O$, AR), calcium acetate monohydrate ($(CH_3COO)_2Ca.H_2O$, AR), a little ethylene glycol ($C_2H_6O_2$, AR) as dispersant and a small quantity of SiO_2 nano-particles. The electrolyte was treated with ultrasonic in order that the solute was dissolved sufficiently and the n-SiO_2 particles were dispersed in the electrolyte uniformly. While a stainless steel plate was used as a cathode in an electrolytic cell. After the MAO treatment, the sample was washed with water and dried with a blower.

TA_2	Fe	O	C	N	H	Ti
Contents of impurities (<wt%)	0.30	0.20	0.10	0.05	0.015	remains

Table 1. Element composition of the pure commercial titanium

For the MAO treatment, a pulse power supply was employed. The pulse parameters (e.g. voltage, current, and duty cycle) can be adjusted independently. In this study, MAO was carried out at current density of 22~25A/dm^2 for different oxidation time as 10 min and 20 min at room temperature, and the duty cycle was 15%. The final voltage was 450V and 500V.

The surface and cross-sectional morphologies of the films were observed by scanning electron microscopy (SEM, JSM-6700F, Japan). The elemental composition was examined with energy dispersive X-ray spectrometer (EDX, INCA, Oxford) incorporated into the scanning electron microscope. The phase components of the coatings were analyzed using X-ray diffraction (XRD, D/max-γB, Japan) using CuKα radiation at 40 KV and 150mA with a scanning speed of 9°/min and a step size of 0.02^{o}.

According to ISO7405:1997(E)standard (ISO 7405:1997(E)), 3-[4,5-dimethylthiazol-2-yl]-2-5-diphenyl-tetrazolium bromide (MTT) assay method was used to preliminarily evaluate the cylotoxicity of the films on L-929 mouse fibroblast. After sterilization of the samples, the extracted liquid of the films, pure titanium substrates was prepared respectively by adding the samples together with DMEM with 10% fetal bovine serum in aseptic test tube and then cultivated at 37℃ in CO_2 standing-temperature incubator for 24 h. L-929 cell suspension of 5×10^3 cells/ml was made by diluting the cells with DMEM with 10% fetal bovine serum. Aliquots of 200 uL of the cell suspension were seeded into each well of 96-well plate and cultivated at 37℃ in CO_2 standing-temperature incubator for 24 h. And then, the extracted liquid was added into the well with 200μl per well after removing the previous culture medium and washing twice with PBS. DMEM with 10% fetal bovine serum was added for negative group and 1% solution of phenol was added for positive group. After the 96-well plate was cultured at 37℃ in CO_2 standing-temperature incubator for 2d, 4d and 7d respectively, about 20μl MTT solution (5mg/ml) was added in each well for 4h at 37℃ in the CO_2 standing-temperature incubator. After washing with PBS twice, about 150μl dimethyl sulfoxide (DMSO) was added to dissolve crystals. After shaking at room temperature for 10 min and appearing of bluish violet crystals, absorbance (Optical density - OD) of each well was determined at 490 nm using a microplate reader. Cylotoxicity grade of the samples was converted by relative growth rate (RGR) according to table 2.

$$RGR = \frac{\text{average value of the samples}}{\text{average value of the negative group}} \times 100\% \qquad (1)$$

RGR(%)	≥100	75~99	50~74	25~49	1~24	0
cytotoxicity grade	0	1	2	3	4	5

Table 2. Relation between cytotoxicity grade and RGR

3.2 Results and discussion

3.2.1 Morphology of the coatings

Fig.6 showed SEM micrographs of the surfaces of the MAO coatings formed at different oxidation time. In Fig.6 (A), there were micro-pores and snaky apertures on the surface of the film when the treated time was 10min. The higher magnification images indicated that there was a reticular structure at the edge of the pores while the network structure was not observed on the other area of the surface (in Fig.6 (B) and Fig.6 (C)). When the treated time extended to 20 min, the pores and the snaky apertures on the surface disappeared and the surface was covered by many micron-sized globules whose size was about 5~10μm.(in Fig.6 (D)). In the higher magnification the coating was a coralloid structure on the surface of the micro-sized globules (in Fig.6 (E) and Fig.6 (F)).

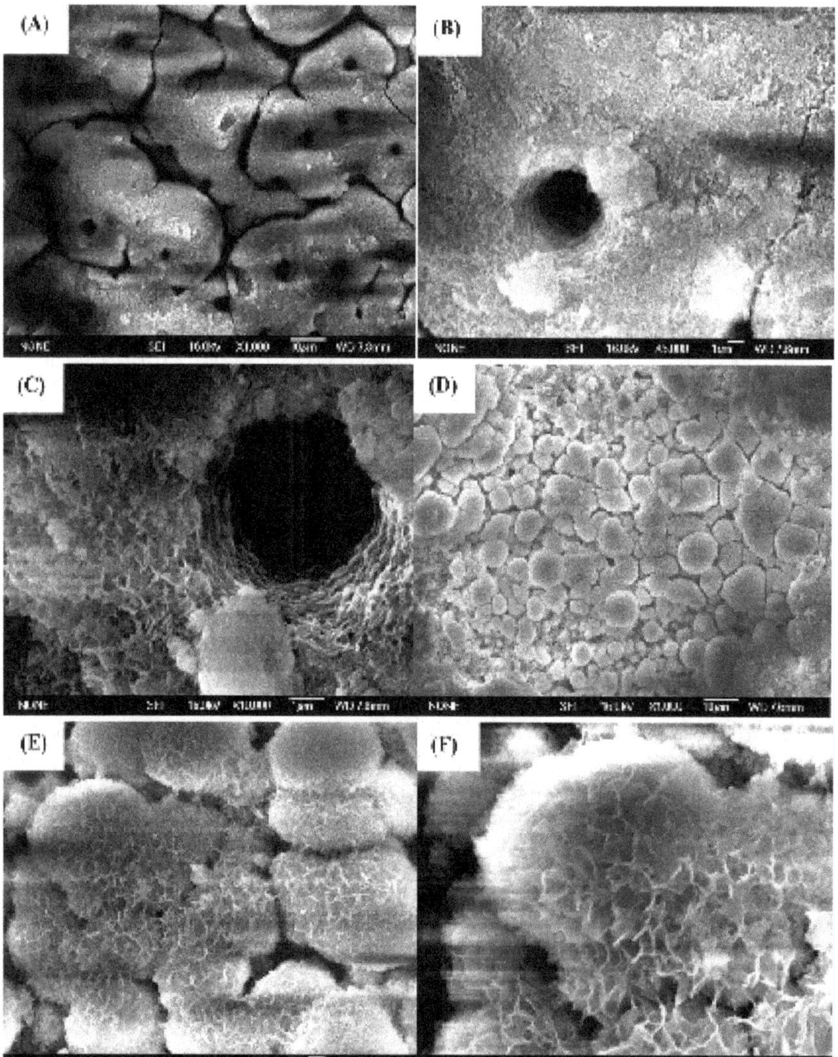

Fig. 6. SEM surface morphologies of micro-arc oxidation coatings treated for 10min (A) low magnification (×1000); (B) local magnification of (A) (×5000); (C) local magnification of (B) (×10000) and for 20min (D) low magnification (×1000); (E) local magnification (D) (×5000); (F) local magnification of (E) (×10000)

The cross-sections of the typical coating were shown in Fig.7 When the oxidation time was 10min, the thickness was about 25μm. The thickness of the film increased with the oxidation time increasing. The thickness was nearly 40μm when the oxidation time reached 20min. There was no obvious discontinuity between the deposited film and the substrate. That indicated that the film can be tightly adhered to the substrate.

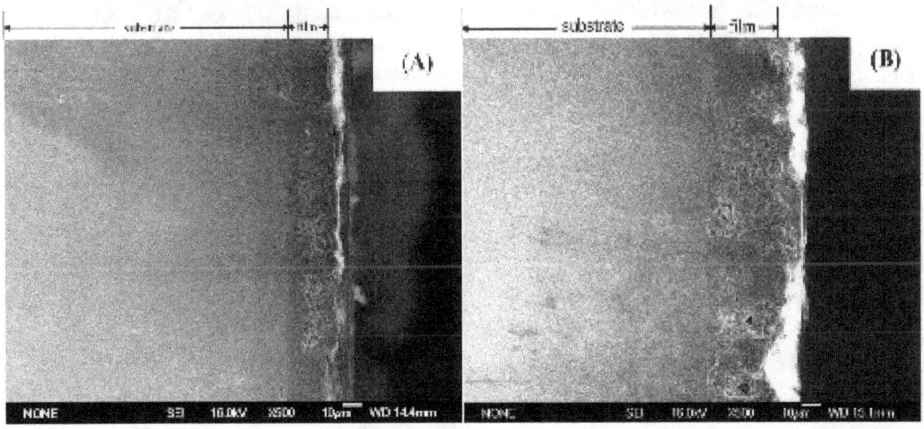

Fig. 7. SEM cross-sectional views of micro-arc oxidation coatings treated for (A) 10min and (B) 20min

3.2.2 Elemental composition of MAO coatings

The coating formed by MAO contained Ca, P, and Si as well as Ti and O, as shown in Fig.8 and in Fig.9. The atomic content of silicon was 0.74% and 1.31% respectively in films treated for 10min and 20min. It was suggested that the elemental compositions in an electrolytic solution could be compounded into the coating during MAO process. As shown in Fig.9 the content of Ca, P, Si and O were gradually reduced from the surface of the coating to the titanium substrate, while the content of Ti was gradually increased.

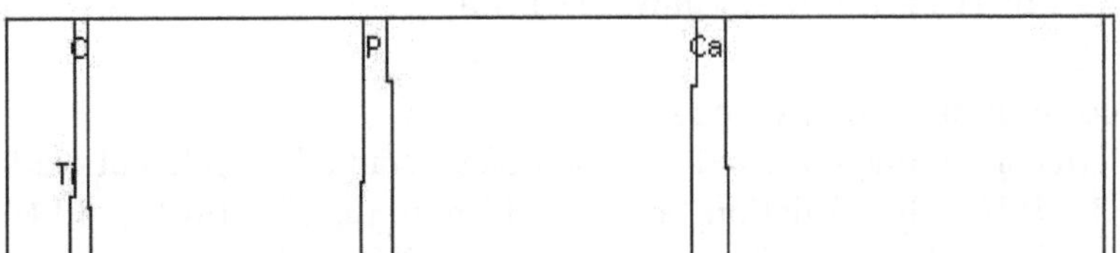

Fig. 8. EDX spectrum of Ti specimens treated with MAO

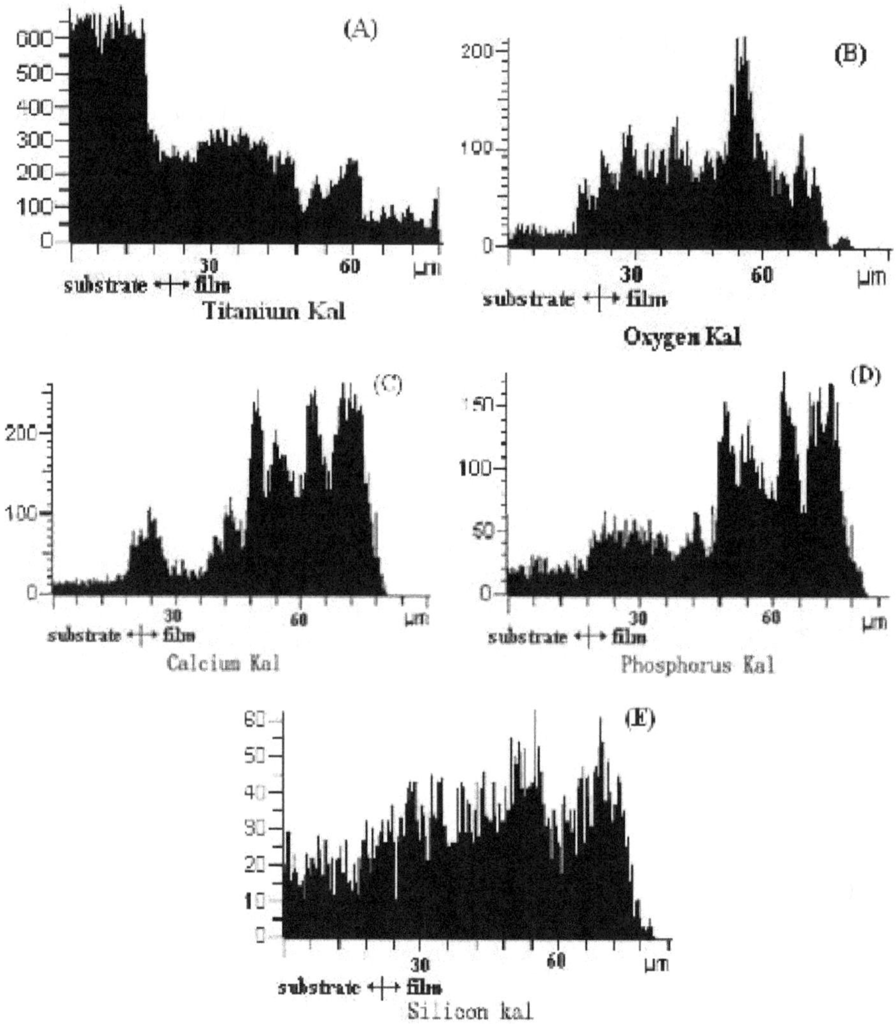

Fig. 9. Depth profiles of the elements in the oxidized coating of titanium (A) titanium; (B) oxygen; (C) calcium; (D) phosphorus and (E) silicon

3.2.3 Phase components of MAO coatings

The XRD patterns of the micro-arc oxidized samples obtained at different oxidation time was shown in Fig.10. When the oxidation time was 10 min, the film (in Fig. 10 (A)) was mainly composed of rutile, anatase and Ti, especially the peaks of rutile were strong. The peaks of hydroxyapatite could be observed, but the peaks were broad and weak, which implied that the crystallization of the formed hydroxyapatite was poor. When the treatment time was 20 min (in Fig. 10 (B)), the diffraction peaks of hydroxyapatite in the coatings were strong and became a predominant component in the films. It is shown that in the experiment with increasing treatment time, the applied voltage increased, the working energy increased, the HA coating formed under the effects of thermochemistry, electrochemistry and plasma-chemistry. On the contrary, the peaks of rutile weakened and the peaks of anatase and Ti were hardly observed. But the diffraction peaks of silicon or silicon oxide was not observed. It could be inferred that silicon in the coating by MAO was little.

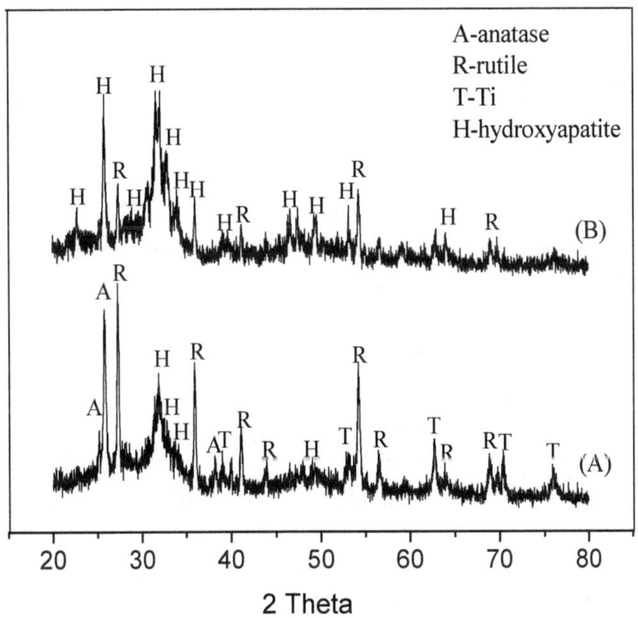

Fig. 10. XRD patterns of the MAO samples treated for (A) 10 min and (B) 20 min

3.2.4 Cytotoxicity of MAO films

The average OD-value, RGR and cytotoxicity grade of each tested group for different cultivation days were listed in table3, table 4 and table 5 respectively. The OD value increased with the increase of the cultivation time and presented its dependence on ultivation time. The cytotoxicity grade of each MAO sample was 0 and the cytotoxicity grade of titanium substrates was 0 or 1. But every cytotoxicity grade for that of the positive groups was 4. The biocompatibility of MAO films is better then that of the titanium substrate because there are HA, rutile and anatase in the film. The OD—value of each tested group were similar to the negative group and significantly different from positive group which indicated that the materials tested were safe to L-929 cells.

groups	MAO samples		titanium substrates	negative groups	positive groups
	treated for 10 min	treated for 20 min			
OD	0.275±0.026	0.281±0.028	0.256±0.031	0.235±0.025	0.055±0.007
RGR(%)	117.02	119.57	108.94	100	23.40
cytotoxicity grade	0	0	0		4

Table 3. Average values of OD, RGR and cytotoxidty grade for the tested groups at 2 days

groups	MAO samples treated for 10 min	MAO samples treated for 20 min	titanium substrates	negative groups	positive groups
OD	0.393±0.039	0.409±0.028	0.379±0.037	0.383±0.031	0.050±0.004
RGR(%)	102.61	106.79	98.95	100	13.05
cytotoxicity grade	0	0	1		4

Table 4. Average values of OD, RGR and cytotoxidty grade for the tested groups at 4 days

groups	MAO samples treated for 10 min	MAO samples treated for 20 min	titanium substrates	negative groups	positive groups
OD	0.835±0.023	0.852±0.021	0.817±0.022	0.832±0.024	0.072±0.005
RGR(%)	100.36	102.40	98.20	100	8.65
cytotoxicity grade	0	0	1		4

Table 5. Average values of OD，RGR and cytotoxidty grade for the tested groups at 7 days

4. Conclusion and remarks

According to above study, nano-silicon embedded HA/TiO_2 composite coatings can be prepared by micro-arc oxidation in Ca- and P- containing electrolyte by adding a little n-SiO_2 nano-particles in it. The surface of the coatings on titanium substrate produced a network structure without apparent interface to the titanium substrates. The thickness of the film could reach about 40μm. The film contained Ca, P, and Si along with Ti and O. As the treatment time increased, the hydroxyapatite became a predominant component in the film when the treatment time was 20min. the cytotoxicity grade of the coatings was 0 according to the MTT test and that of titanium substrate was 0 or 1, meaning that the films and substrate all had no cytotoxicity. The coatings' biocompatibility became better with increase of treatment time and were better than biocompatibility of substrate.

Based on the preparation of the composite coating of HA and TiO_2, the new work introduced a novel idea adding silicon to the composite coating in order to improve the bioactivity of the coating, and the results also proved the realizability. But, there are also many works needed to be done in depth. Although the EDS spectrum of the films revealed that the deposited coatings were composed of Ti, O, Ca, P and Si, but no siliceous crystalline was detected by XRD. The chemical status and location of the silicon are not clearly understood yet. Does silicon existe as an ion, atom, or other valence state in the HA and TiO2 coating? Or, does it constitute the structure of Si-HA? Further studies are needed to answer these questions. Primary cylotoxicity of the films on L-929 cell was evaluated and the results were perfect. However, detailed mechanical behavior and bioactivity of the coating such as apatite induction and corrosion resisting of the film in simulated body fluid (SBF), in vitro cell tests, and in vivo tests need to be researched. Furthermore, more efforts needed to pay for the optimization and mechanism study of MAO technique on titanium.

5. Acknowledgements

The work was supported by the Natural Science Foundation of Shan dong Province of China (Y2006F07) and the Youth Foundation of Natural Science Foundation of Shan dong Province of China (ZR2010HQ025)

6. References

Akin, F.A., Zreiqat, H. & Jordan, S. (2001). Preparation and analysis of macroporous TiO2 films on Ti surfaces for bone-tissue implants, *Journal of Biomedical Materials Research*, Vol. 57, No 4, pp. 588-596

Barrere, F. C., Blitterswijk, A . & Groot, K. (2002). Influence of ionic strength and carbonate on the Ca-P coating formation from SBF×5 solution, *Biomaterials*, Vol. 23, No. 9, pp. 1921-1930, ISSN 0142-9612

Chen, J-Z., Shi, Y-L. & Wang, L., et al. (2006). Preparation and properties of hydroxyapatite-containing titania coating by micro-arc oxidation, *Materials Letters*, Vol. 60, No. 20, pp. 2538-2543

Clèries, L., Fernández-Pradas, J. M. & Morenza, J. L. (2000). Behavior in simulated body fluid of calcium phosphate coatings obtained by laser ablation, *Biomaterials*, Vol. 21, No. 18, pp. 1861-1865, ISSN 0142-9612

Cotell, C. M., Chrisey, D. B. & Grabowski, K. S. et al. (1992). Pulsed laser deposition of hydroxylapatite thin films on Ti-6Al-4V, *Journal of Applied Biomaterials*, Vol. 3, No. 2, pp. 87-93

Dittrich, K. H., Krysmann, W. & Kurze, P., et al. (1984). Structure and properties of ANOF Layers, *Crystal Research and Technology*, Vol. 19, No.1, pp. 93-99

Dunn, D.S., Raghavan, S. & Volz, R.G. (1993). Gentamicin sulfate attachment and release from anodized Ti-6Al-4V orthopedic materials, *Journal of Biomedical Materials Research*, Vol. 27, No 7, pp. 895-900

Fu, T., Han, Y. & Huang, P., et al. (2002). Structure and Properties of Bioactive Titania Layer by Microarc Oxidization-Hydrothermal Synthesis, *Raremetal Materials and Engineering*, Vol. 31, No. 2, pp. 115-117

Gross, K. A., & Berndt, C. C. (1994). In vitro testing of plasma-sprayed hydroxyapatite coatings, *Journal of materials science: materials in medicine*, Vol. 5, No4, pp. 219-224

Gu, Y. W., Khor, K. A. & Cheang, P. (2003). In vitro studies of plasma-sprayed hydroxyapatite /Ti-6Al-4V composite coatings in simulated body fluid (SBF), *Biomaterials*, Vol. 24, No. 9, pp. 1603-1611, ISSN 0142-9612

Han, Y., Hong, S.H. & Xu, K.W. (2002). Porous nanocrystalline titania films by plasma electrolytic oxidation, *Surface and Coating Technology*, Vol. 154, No 2-3, pp. 314-318

Han, Y., Hong, S.H. & Xu, K.W. (2002). Synthesis of nanocrystalline titania films by micro-arc oxidation, *Materials Letters*, Vol. 56, pp. 744-747

Han, Y., Hong, S. H. & Xu, K.W. (2003). Structure and in vitro bioactivity of titania-based films by micro-arc oxidation, *surface and coating technology*, Vol. 168, No. 2-3, pp. 249-258

Ishizawa, H. & Ogino, M. (1995). Formation and characterization of anodic titanium oxide films containing Ca and P, *Journal of Biomedical Materials Research*, Vol. 29, No 1, pp. 65-72

ISO 7405:1997(E). Dentistry preclinical evaluation of biocompatibility of medical devices used in dentistry test methods for dental materials.

Koike, M. & Fujii, H. (2001). The corrosion resistance of pure titanium in organic acids, *Biomaterials*, Vol. 22, No. 21, pp. 2931-2936, ISSN 0142-9612

Krishna, L. M., Purnima, A.s. & Wasekar, N. P. (2007). Kinetics and properties of micro arc oxidation coatings deposited on commercial Al alloys, *Metallurgical and materials transaction A*, Vol. 38A, pp. 370-378

Krysmann, W., Kurze, P. & Dittrich, K. H., et al. (1984). Process Characteristics and Parameters of Anodic Oxidation by Spark Discharge(ANOF), *Crystal Research and Technology*, Vol. 18, No.7, pp. 973-979

Kuromoto, N. K., Simão, R. A. & Soares, G. A. (2007). Titanium oxide films produced on commercially pure titanium by anodic oxidation with different voltages, *Materials Characterizatiion*, Vol. 58, No 2, pp. 114-121

Kurze, P., Krysmann, W. & Schreckenbach J., et al. (1987). Coloured ANOF Layers on Aluminiu m, *Crystal Research and Technology*, Vol. 22, No.1, pp. 53-58

Li, L-H., Young, M-K., & Kim, H-W., et al. (2004). Improved biological performance of Ti implants due to surface modification by micro-arc oxidation, *Biomaterials*, Vol. 25, No. 14, pp. 2867-2875, ISSN 0142-9612

Lim, H. M., Miyaji, F. & Kokubo, T. et al. (1996). Preparation of bioactive Ti and its alloys via simple chemical surface treatment, *Journal of biomedical materials research.* Part A, Vol. 32, No 3, pp. 409-417

Liu, D-M., Yang, Q. Z. & Troczynski, T. (2002). Sol–gel hydroxyapatite coatings on stainless steel substrates, *Biomaterials*, Vol. 23, No. 3, pp. 691-698, ISSN 0142-9612

Long, M. & Rack, H. J. (1998). Titanium alloys in total joint replacement-a materials science perspective, *Biomaterials*, Vol. 19, No. 18, pp. 1621-1639, ISSN 0142-9612

Lukiyanchuk, I. V., Rudnev, V. S. & Tyrina, L. M. et al. (2002). Anodic-Spark Layers Formed on Aluminum Alloy in Tungstate-Borate Electrolytes, *Russian Journal of Applied Chemistry*, Vol.75, No. 12, pp. 1972-1978

Markov G. A. & Markova G. V. (1976). A method of forming anodes of electrolytic condensers, *Bull. Inventions*, vol. 32. 2., Inventor's Certificate No. 526961 (USSR)

Mertsalo, I. P., Yavors'kyi, V. T. & Klapkiv, M. D., et al. (2003). Wear Resistance of Anodic-Spark Coatings on Aluminum Alloys, *Materials Science*, Vol. 39, No. 1, pp. 136-139

Ni, J-H., Shi, Y-L. & Yan, F-Y. (2008) Preparation of hydroxyapatite-containing titania coating on titanium substrate by micro-arc oxidation, *Materials Research Bulletin*, Vol. 43, No. 1, pp. 45-53

Porter, A. E . (2006) Nanoscale characterization of the interface between bone and hydroxyapatite implants and the effect of silicon on bone apposition, *Micron* , Vol. 37, No 8, pp. 681-688, ISSN 0968-4328

Porter, A. E., Patel, N. & Skepper, J. N., et al. (2004). Effect of sintered silicate-substituted hydroxyapatite on remodelling processes at the bone–implant interface, *Biomaterials*, Vol. 25, No. 16, pp. 3303-3314, ISSN 0142-9612

Rudnev, V. S., Vasil'eva, M. S. & Lukiyanchuk, I. V., et al. (2004). On the Surface Structure of Coatings Formed by Anodic Spark Method, *Protection of Metals*, Vol. 40, No. 4, pp. 352-357

Shi, Y. L., Yan F. Y. & Xie G. W. (2005). Effect of pulse duty cycle on micro-plasma oxidation of aluminum alloy, Materials Letter, Vol. 59, No. 22, pp. 2725-2728

Shibata, A., Okimura, K. & Yamamoto, Y., et al. (1993). Effect of Heating Probe on Reactively Sputtered TiO_2 Film Growth, *Japanese journal of applied physics*, Vol. 32, pp. 5666-5670

Song, W.H., Jun, Y.K. & Han, Y. (2004). Biomimetic apatite coatings on micro-arc oxidized titania, *Biomaterials*, Vol. 25, No 17, pp. 3341-3349, ISSN 0142-9612

Sul, Y-T. (2003). The significance of the surface properties of oxidized titanium to the bone response: special emphasis on potential biochemical bonding of oxidized titanium implant, *Biomaterials*, Vol. 24, No. 22, pp. 3893-3907, ISSN 0142-9612

Sul, Y.T., Johansson, C.B. & Petronis, S., et al. (2002). Characteristics of the surface oxides on turned and electrochemically oxidized pure titanium implants up to dielectric breakdown: : the oxide thickness, micropore configurations, surface roughness, crystal structure and chemical composition, *Biomaterials*, Vol. 23, No. 2, pp. 491-501, ISSN 0142-9612

Tian, J., Luo, Z. Z., & Qi, S. K., et al. (2002). Structure and antiwear behavior of micro-arc oxidized coatings on aluminum alloy, *Surface and Coating Technology*, Vol.154, No. 1, pp. 1-7

Tkalcec, E., Sauer, M., & Nonninger, R., et al. (2001). Sol-gel-derived hydroxyapatite powders and coatings, *Journal of materials science*, Vol. 36, No. 21, pp. 5253-5263

Van, T. B., Brown S. D. & Wirtz G. P. (1977). Mechanism of anodic spark deposition, *Am. Ceram. Soc. Bull.*, Vol. 56, No. 6, pp. 563-566.

Voevodin, A. A., Yerokhin, A. L. & Lyubimov, V. V. (1996). Characterization of wear protective Al---Si---O coatings formed on Al-based alloys by micro-arc discharge treatment, *Surface and Coatings Technology*, Vol. 86-87, No. 2, pp. 516-521

Wang, X.X., Hayakawa, S. & Tsuru, K. et al. (2000). A comparative study of in vitro apatite deposition on heat-, H_2O_2-, and NaOH-treated titanium surfaces, *Journal of materials science: materials in medicine*, Vol. 54, No 2, pp. 172-178

Wei, D. Q., Zhou, Y. & Yang, C.H. (2009). Characteristic and microstructure of the microarc oxidized TiO2-based film containing P before and after chemical- and heat treatment, *Applied Surface Science*, Vol. 225, No. 18, pp. 7851-7857

Wen, C. E., Yamad, Y. & Shimojima, K, et al. (2002), Novel titanium foam for bone tissue engineering, *Journal of Materials Research*, Vol. 17, pp. 2633-2639

Weng, J., Liu, Q., Wolke, J. G. C., et al. (1997). Formation and characteristics of the apatite layer on plasma-sprayed hydroxyapatite coatings in simulated body fluid, *Biomaterials*, Vol. 18, No. 15, pp. 1027-1035, ISSN 0142-9612

Wirtz, G. P, Brown, S. D, & Kriven, W. M. (1991). Ceramics coatings by anodic spark deposition, Materials & Manufacturing Processes, Vol. 6, No.1, pp. 87-115

Wu. J. M., Xiao, F. & Hayakawa, S. (2003). Bioactivity of metallic biomaterials with anatase layers deposited in acidic titanium tetrafluoride solution, *Journal of materials science: materials in medicine*, Vol. 14, pp. 1027-1032

Xie, N., Leyland, A. & Matthews, M. (2000). Deposition of layered bioceramic hydroxyapatite/TiO_2 coatings on titanium alloys using a hybrid technique of micro-arc oxidation and electrophoresis, *Surface Technology*, Vol. 125, No. 1-3, pp. 407-414

Xu, W., Hu, W.Y. & Li, M. H. (2006). Sol-gel derived HA/TiO_2 double coatings on Ti scaffolds for orthopaedic applications, *Transactions of Nonferrous Mrtals Society of China*, Vol. 16, Supplement 18, pp. s209-s216

Xue, W.B., Deng, Z.W., & Chen, R.Y. (2001). Microstructure and properties of ceramic coatings produced on 2024 aluminum alloy by microarc oxidation, *Journal of Materials Science*, Vol.36, No. 11, pp. 2615-2619

Yang, Y. Z., Kim, K-H, & Ong, J. L. (2005). A review on calcium phosphate coatings produced using a sputtering process-an alternative to plasma spraying, *Biomaterials*, Vol. 26, No. 3, pp. 327-337, ISSN 0142-9612

Yao, Z. P., Jiang, Y. L. & Jiang, Z. H., et al. (2008). Preparation and structure of ceramic coatings containing zirconium oxide on Ti alloy by plasma electrolytic oxidation, *Journal Materials Processing Technology*, Vol. 205, No 1-3, pp. 303-307

Yerokhin, A. L., Lyubimov, V. V. & Ashitkov, R. V. (1998). Phase formation in ceramic coatings during plasma electrolytic oxidation of aluminium alloys, *Ceramics International,* Vol. 24, No. 1, pp. 1-6

Yerokhin, A. L., Nie, X. & Leyland, A., et al. (1999). Plasma electrolysis for surface engineering, *Surface and Coatings Technology,* Vol. 122, No. 2-3, pp. 73-93

ZHITOMIRSKY, L. GAL-OR. (1997). Electrophoretic deposition of hydroxyapatite, *Journal of materials science: materials in medicine*, Vol. 8, pp. 213-219, ISSN 0957-4530

4

The Current Knowledge of Genetic Susceptibility Influencing Dental Implant Outcomes

Fabiano Alvim-Pereira[1], Claudia Cristina Alvim-Pereira[2] and Paula Cristina Trevilatto [3]
[1]*Federal University of Sergipe (UFS), Lagarto-SE,*
[2]*Federal University of Pernambuco (UFPE), Recife-PE,*
[3]*Pontifical Catholic University of Paraná (PUCPR), Curitiba-PR, Brazil*

1. Introduction

Oral diseases are still a major global health burden, in spite of big efforts in research and dental services, where disbursement on treatment may exceed that for other diseases, including major illnesses such as cancer, heart disease, stroke, and dementia (Williams, 2011). In this context, tooth loss is a topic of public health concern, since it is the final result of the first and second most prevalent diseases in dentistry: caries and periodontitis (Pihlstrom et al., 2005; Pitts et al., 2011). Although the prevalence of edentulism has decreased over the last decades, there will be a relevant proportion of edentulous individuals worldwide (Polzer et al., 2010a).

Tooth loss is a problem complex to be solved all over the world which affects children, adults and elderly. Complete edentulism prior 65 years old was associated with all-cause mortality, an evidence supporting the notion that poor oral health is an important public health issue across the lifespan (Brown, 2009). Although edentulism is not a life threatening condition, tooth loss impairs several orofacial structures, such as bony tissues, nerves, receptors and muscles. Consequently, most orofacial functions are diminished in edentate subjects (Polzer et al., 2010a). Regarding partially edentulous people, tooth loss is found in 5-20% of most adult populations all over the world (Petersen et al., 2005). Quality life levels were reported to be direct related to the number of remaining teeth (Polzer et al., 2010a). Thus, edentulism was found to be a global problem, with estimates for an increasing demand for oral rehabilitation in the future (Felton, 2009). In this context, oral health restoration should aim to restore function and esthetics. Dentistry has the challenge of improving the access and quality of oral rehabilitation (Tilman, 1985), although oral health care is still being conducted without a solid research evidence base (Pang et al., 2011).

2. Oral rehabilitation

A wide variety of treatments is available to replace tooth loss. Osseointegrated dental implant is the gold standard treatment modality to replace missing teeth in terms of

function and aesthetics (Davarpanah et al., 2002; Fugazzotto, 2005). It is estimated that over 10 million implants are installed all over the world annually (Hospitalar, 2007).
The term osseointegration was coined by Branemark to define a structural and functional contact between titanium surface and bone (Albrektsson et al., 1981; Branemark et al., 1969). Since 1982 in the Toronto Conference in Clinical Dentistry, when the guidelines for Implantology were proposed, they remain mainly unaltered. The main protocol change was regarding different times for loading (immediate and early load), which seem to be positive if patients present high degree of primary implant stability (high value of insertion torque) (Esposito et al., 2009). Other treatment differences regarding modification of implant macro and microstructure have limited evidence of clinical improvement supported by longitudinal studies (Esposito et al., 2007).
Dental implants are considered a very predictable rehabilitation procedure in dentistry, with a success rate above 90% showed in longitudinal studies (Adell et al., 1990). In spite of the high success rate, the absolute number of dental implant failure becomes significant and causes economic and social impact for patients and dental professionals. Dental implant failure has been extensively studied during the last years (Esposito et al., 1998a; b). The comprehension of the implant failure process may provide novel insights into the mechanisms underlying osseointegration (Mengatto et al., 2011).

3. The challenges of implantology

Dental implant failure could include surgical complications, patient aesthetic concerning or implant functional disability. A significant reduction in the bone-implant contact may jeopardize the osseointegration process and lead to implant loss. Implant loss is considered a complex, multifactorial trait, investigated by several clinical follow-up and retrospective studies (Esposito et al., 2004; Fugazzotto, 2005; Graziani et al., 2004).
The process is divided into early and late events: early failure occurs before implant load, and late failure takes place after the implant has received occlusal load (Esposito et al., 1999). Early failures have been related to smoking (Ganeles and Wismeijer, 2004), aging (Moy et al., 2005), systemic diseases (Quirynen and Teughels, 2003; Weyant and Burt, 1993), bone quantity and quality (Degidi and Piattelli, 2005; Rosenberg et al., 2004; Stanford, 2003), surgical trauma (Gruica et al., 2004), and contamination during surgical procedure (Kuttenberger et al., 2005; van Steenberghe et al., 1990). Late failures have been related to peri-implantitis (Rosenberg et al., 2004), and occlusal overload (Misch et al., 2004).
Although many studies have provided an important contribution to the understanding of the implant failure process, in some situations, clinical factors alone do not explain why some present implant loss (Deas et al., 2002; Montes et al., 2007). The goal that should be achieved by modern implantology research is developing tools able to predict the patient biological response to treatment before implant surgery intervention.

4. Physiopathology of dental implant loss

Inflammation surrounding implant placement area is a crucial physiopathological process that permits the elimination of local tissue damage and substitution for a viable tissue; process termed regeneration. An augmentation of this inflammatory process is directly related to the quantity of tissue that may be substituted (Thomas and Puleo, 2011).

A complete stabilization between implant pins and surrounding bone is required to achieve a successful implant osseointegration. Primary stability is a mechanical feature achieved during surgical implant placement, which helps stabilization at early phases, leading to a desirable outcome (Szmukler-Moncler et al., 1998). When the process is developing in the post-surgery timeline, implant stability in relation to surrounding bone tends to decline, with the lowest implant stability quotient values being reached at 3 weeks (Han et al., 2010). After the bone regeneration process, stability reaches the maximum value when the osseointegration is achieved.

The two of the main factors for achieving predictable success of osseointegrated oral implants are lack of stability and micromovements (Albrektsson et al., 1981; Turkyilmaz et al., 2009). An abnormal exacerbated inflammatory process may lead to an abnormal decline in implant stability. Micromovements of implants in this crucial phase may result in the formation of a conjunctive tissue between implant and surrounding bone, process known as implant encapsulation (Lioubavina-Hack et al., 2006). Encapsulated dental implants do not become integrated to the bone, not reaching sufficient stability, and sometimes causing patient local pain. Those implants cannot be used as support for a tooth prosthesis and need to be removed, representing the major cause of implant failure.

4.1 Interleukin (IL)-1 as a key inflammatory cytokine

Implant surface biological aggregates interact with the cell membrane-bound proteins or receptors, eventually initiating cell attachment to the implant surface (Kasemo and Gold, 1999). Studies have shown that the coating material of the implants, considered innocuous, can stimulate cells to produce immunogenic inflammatory mediators in vitro (Harada et al., 1996; Perala et al., 1992).

Interleukin-1 (IL-1) is considered a pro-inflammatory mediator with central importance in the initiation and maintenance of acute inflammatory responses (Hoffman and Brydges, 2011). Its name as an interleukin, which means "between leukocytes", is misleading because IL-1 is synthesized not only by leukocytes but by other cell lineages as well. Besides acting as a mediator of local inflammation, IL-1 can produce systemic effects (Dinarello, 2007). IL-1 is the term for two polypeptides: IL-1α and IL-1β that possess a wide spectrum of inflammatory, metabolic, physiologic, hematopoietic, and immunologic properties (Pelegrin, 2008). IL-1β has been particularly studied as a critical determinant of tissue destruction due to its proinflammatory and bone resorptive properties and increased levels of IL-1β in gingival crevicular fluid were correlated with the severity of periodontal disease (Bloemen et al., 2011; Goutoudi et al., 2004; Hellmig et al., 2005; Stashenko et al., 1991). Although both forms of IL-1 are distinct gene products, they recognize the same cell surface receptors and share the various biologic activities. The IL-1 natural occurring inhibitor, the interleukin 1 receptor antagonist (IL-1ra), acts by binding the IL-1 receptors (IL-1R) inhibiting biological responses (Lennard, 1995). Produced and secreted by almost all cells expressing IL-1, IL-1ra functions as a competitive receptor antagonist, binding to IL-1 receptors, but not activating target cells (Molto and Olive, 2010). Today, IL-1 family is recognized to include 11 total members (Smith, 2011), which play particular roles in immune-inflammatory aspects of the host response. IL-1 is thus a "cytokine" and this term is used to connote that the sources and actions of IL-1 and related polypeptides include several different cell types. Moreover, IL-1 belongs to a group of cytokines with overlapping biologic properties such as tumor necrosis factor (TNF). IL-1 and TNF share the ability to stimulate T and B lymphocytes, augment cell proliferation, and initiate or suppress gene expression for several proteins (Laurincova, 2000). IL-1α, IL-1β, and TNF-α were observed to signal fibroblasts to produce matrix metalloproteinases (MMPs) that induce connective tissue degradation (Kornman, 2006; Takashiba et al., 2003). Circulating levels of IL-1 are elevated in a variety of clinical situations and, together with elevated levels of TNF, correlate with the severity of some diseases, suggesting that these cytokines participate in the host response to or development of illnesses.

There is a dramatic increase in IL-1 production by a variety of cells in response to infection, microbial toxins, inflammatory agents, products of activated lymphocytes, complement, and clotting components. At the site of inflammation, IL-1 acts on macrophages, further increasing the production of IL-1 and inducing the synthesis of IL-6. In endothelial cells, increases the expression of surface molecules that mediate leukocyte adhesion (Abbas et al., 1998). This cytokine also acts on fibroblasts, stimulating their proliferation and transcription of collagen type I, III and IV. Thus, the development of fibrosis appears to be partly mediated by IL-1 (Dinarello, 1988). Indeed, production of IL-1 in tissues is thought to contribute to local effects such as fibrosis and tissue matrix breakdown, besides the influx of inflammatory cells (Stevens et al., 2009). IL-1 has also significant effects on bone, increasing constitutive receptor activator of NF-kappa-B ligand (RANKL)/osteoprotegerin (OPG) ratios (Stein et al., 2011). In vivo experiments indicated that IL-1 cytokine plays potent activity in bone resorption (Polzer et al., 2010b). Osteoclasts possess surface receptors for IL-1, which, when activated, stimulate the production of prostaglandins and IL-1 itself, modulating gene expression of several other cytokines. Thus, it is suggested that IL-1 participates in the pathogenesis of diseases involving bone tissue (Masada et al., 1990; Tatakis, 1993).

Many studies have investigated tissues surrounding unsuccessful dental implants in order to clarify the implant failure mechanisms (Aboyoussef et al., 1998; Ruhling et al., 1999). The bone-implant interface area is first occupied by red blood and inflammatory cells, degenerating cellular elements, then is gradually replaced with spindle-shaped or flattened cells, with initiation of host bone surface osteolysis (Futami et al., 2000). An abnormal immune-inflammatory response involving different cell types such as macrophages, polymorphonuclear neutrophils, T and B lymphocytes, endothelial cells, fibroblasts, keratinocytes, osteoclasts, and osteoblasts can impair periodontal and peri-implant tissues (Seymour et al., 1989). If activated, these cells can synthesize and release cytokines such as IL-1, which mediates both inflammatory and bone resorption processes (Gainet et al., 1998).

Searching for diagnostic markers to monitoring implant health status, levels of interleukins have been measured in diseased implant sites (Boynuegri et al., 2011). Higher levels of IL-1β were found in diseased implant sites when compared with healthy ones (Aboyoussef et al., 1998), suggesting that such inflammatory mediator is associated with implant failure (Salcetti et al., 1997). Higher levels of TNF-α also showed association with unfavorable clinical outcomes at 2 and 14 days after implant placement, being proposed that TNF-α gene expression may predict clinical complications (Slotte et al., 2010). The association between implant surface modification and inflammation molecular markers has been investigated and suggested as an additional indicator of implant clinical outcome (Monjo et al., 2008).

4.2 Extracellular matrix (ECM) on the osseointegration process

Osseointegration has been considered not the result of an advantageous tissue response but rather the lack of a negative tissue response (Mavrogenis et al., 2009). Some research has been progressed in order to better understand the implant-bone tissue interface and the kinds of matrix produced on an implant surface (Wierzchos et al., 2008), although those events have only been characterized at a morphological level, using several histological approaches (Linder et al., 1983; McKibbin, 1978; Schenk and Perren, 1977; Winet and Albrektsson, 1988). Extracellular matrix (ECM) appears to vary morphologically between different material surfaces, suggesting that the extracellular response can be affected by the implant surface. However, ECM investigations, valuable in determining the vascular and morphological changes occurring in the healing site, suffer from the inability to biochemically evaluate the cellular response around a fixture (Winet and Albrektsson, 1988). Only more recently, studies aiming to characterize ECM at a molecular level start dissecting the structural components during implant osseointegration process and a cartilage ECM gene was found to be expressed (Mengatto et al., 2011). Patient individual response to implant treatment, in terms of the interfacial response of cells in contact with the implant surface, seems to impact clinical outcomes (Huang et al., 2004).

4.2.1 Matrix metaloproteinases (MMPs) and other mediators involved in ECM remodeling

Matrix metalloproteinases (MMPs) represent the major class of enzymes responsible for ECM metabolism (Kerrigan et al., 2000). They are metal-dependent proteolytic enzymes that contribute to the degradation and removal of collagen from damaged tissue. MMPs are secreted by inflammatory cells in response to stimuli such as lipopolysaccharide and cytokines (Birkedal-Hansen, 1993). Specific enzymes of this family can function beneficially during tissue remodeling and during formation of the ECM (Fanchon et al., 2004). However, MMPs may increase the adverse effects of cardiovascular disease (Kukacka et al., 2005), cancer metastasis (Nemeth et al., 2002), caries process (Sulkala et al., 2001) and periodontal disease (Liu et al., 2006) by destruction of collagen and other proteins of the ECM.

Previous studies have also shown that MMPs (e.g. collagenases, gelatinases) are present in peri-implant sulcular fluid (Apse et al., 1989; Ingman et al., 1994; Ma et al., 2000; Teronen et al., 1997) and may play a pathologic role in peri-implant bone loss (Golub et al., 1997).

Matrix metalloproteinase-1 (MMP-1), also known as collagenase-1, is a key mediator of the degradation of collagen, which is abundant in connective tissue and bone matrix (Yamada et al., 2002). MMP-1 degrades types I, II, III, and IX collagen, which are the most abundant protein components of extracellular matrices (de Souza et al., 2003; Dunleavey et al., 2000). An enhanced secretion of MMP-1 was verified in peri-implantitis fibroblasts compared to healthy and periodontitis sites (Bordin et al., 2009). Gelatinase B (MMP-9) is particularly active against gelatins, denaturing type I collagen, and type IV collagen, a major component of the basement membrane. It also acts proteolytically against proteoglycan core protein and elastin, which are resistant to degradation by some other MMPs (Birkedal-Hansen, 1993). MMP-9 is produced by inflammatory cells as well as by stimulated connective tissue cells (Foda and Zucker, 2001) and has been identified in many human cancers both in neoplastic tissues and in the surrounding stromal and inflammatory cells (Crawford and Matrisian, 1994). Related to dental implants, zymography studies showed increased activities of MMP-9 in cells exposed to titanium particles between 48 to 72 hours (Choi et al., 2005). Transforming growth factor-beta 1 (TGF-β1) is a member of a large family of growth factors and cytokines, which are synthesized by a wide range of cells and therefore are distributed in many different tissues (Massague, 1990). There are at least three homologous TGF-β isoforms in humans: TGF-β1, TGF-β2, and TGF-β3. TGF-β1 is the best characterized TGF-β isoform, and its primary sequence is highly conserved throughout evolution (Syrris et al., 1998). It is synthesized as precursor latent forms, and the active form consists of two identical disulfide linked polypeptide chains (Derynck et al., 1985; Syrris et al., 1998). TGF-β possesses some major activities: it inhibits proliferation of most cells, but can stimulate the growth of some mesenchymal cells; exert immunosuppressive effects and reduction of inflammation; is involved in extracellular matrix deposition, and promotion of wound healing (Lawrence, 1996; Santos et al., 2004a). In the health organism TGF-β is involved in wound repair processes and in starting inflammatory reactions and then in their resolution. The latter effects of the TGF-β derive in part from their chemotactic attraction of inflammatory cells and of fibroblasts (Lawrence, 1996). In periodontal diseases, TGF-β concentration was directly associated with plaque index and probing pocket depth. Moreover, decreases in gingival crevicular fluid concentration levels after surgical treatment of periodontitis sites was also found (Sattari et al., 2011). Cytokines such as TGF-β and MMPs can affect the attachment and synthetic activities of osteoblasts and cause the reduction of bone matrix and mineral deposition (Kwon et al., 2000; Kwon et al., 2001).

4.3 Bone metabolism on implant healing

The properties of bone are directly related to the features of the mineralized ECM adjacent to implants in two ways. First, the implant geometry and the insertion approach (surgery technique) determine the principal bone–implant relation. Second, the properties of bone homeostasis and turnover have a major impact on the load-related characteristics of the microenvironment adjacent to implants (Joos et al., 2006). The cortical part of bone provides the mechanical and protective functions, whereas cancellous bone is also involved in metabolic functions (e.g. calcium homeostasis). Both aspects (structural and metabolic) are closely related to the features of the mineralized extracellular matrix at implant surfaces. Trabecular bone fills the initial gap and arranges in a three-dimensional network at day 14 (Franchi et al., 2005). The de novo formation of primary bone spongiosa offers not only a biological fixation to ensure secondary implant stability (Ferguson et al., 2006) but also a biological scaffold for cell attachment and bone deposition (Franchi et al., 2005). After 28 days, delineated bone marrow space and thickened bone trabeculae with parallel-fibered and lamellar bone can be found within the interfacial area. After 8 to 12 weeks, the interfacial area appears histologically to be completely replaced by mature lamellar bone in direct contact with titanium (Berglundh et al., 2003).

Osseointegration has been defined as the direct structural and functional connection between ordered, living bone and the surface of a load-carrying implant (Branemark et al., 1969). Since Branemark's initial observations, the concept of osseointegration has been defined at multiple levels such as clinically (Adell et al., 1981), anatomically (Branemark et al., 1977), histologically, and ultrastructurally (Linder et al., 1983). When an implant is placed, the space between the fixture and bony crypt will heal with new bone by reparative osteogenesis resulting in clinical fixation of the implant. The bone turnover is also evidenced by bone changes during the first 6-year period *in vivo*, resulting in an increased thickness (up to 200 nm), which contain increased levels of organic and inorganic (Ca, P, S) material. This may suggest the potential for a surface reactivity not usually associated with titanium and supports the concept of a dynamic definition of osseointegration (Stanford and Keller, 1991).

Patients have a mean time to repair an implant surgery in terms of bone, and create new mineralized tissue around implants. The meantime repair does not have to apply to all patients because they present different bone turnover rate (Chang et al., 2010; Courbebaisse and Souberbielle, 2011). This issue is not clinically measured and may have an impact on implant osseointegration. Quality and quantity differences in proteins that are classically involved in bone metabolism may modulate bone remodeling (Alvim-Pereira et al., 2008b). Guidelines taking into account bone tissue repair and turnover rate are desirable to ensure a successful osseointegration. These characteristics are nowadays based only clinically, considering medical and dental history. In this way, it cannot be established a clear cutline across patients that are suitable or have an increased risk for dental implant therapy in terms of host response. Therefore, it has been proposed that progression of osseointegration may be accelerated by growth factors and modification of implant surface, and functional integration of peri-implant structure may be feasible to predict the implant function during osseointegration (Chang et al., 2010). Although it is important to study extrinsic factors which could impair or accelerate osseointegration, there is still a lack of understanding over inter-individual differences on host physiologic response.

4.3.1 Bone metabolism proteins

Bone is one of the classical target tissues for vitamin D action. Vitamin D regulates calcium homeostasis by influencing intestinal calcium absorption, renal calcium reabsorption, and bone calcium metabolism (Binkley, 2006). Vitamin D is ingested or cutaneously produced upon exposure to ultraviolet B radiation in an inactive form. To be activated, vitamin D is transported in the blood bound to a vitamin D-binding protein, hydroxylated in the liver and the resulting metabolite is further hydroxylated mainly at the kidney, resulting in the active form called 1,25-dihydroxyvitamin D3 (Panda et al., 2004). In target tissues, 1,25-$(OH)_2D3$ is believed to exert most of its actions by binding to the vitamin D receptor (VDR), a member of the nuclear steroid hormone receptor superfamily, and by regulating the transcription of vitamin D target genes (Haussler et al., 1998). VDR also plays a complex role in the control of bone homeostasis and recruits co-regulators, which may have activating or repressing effects. In VDR knockout growing mice, the primary defect of calcium metabolism is at the intestine; loss of VDR causes calcium malabsorption and rickets that can be prevented by a high-calcium diet. Additionally, VDR knockout mice reveal that VDR plays a role in suppression of bone formation (Fleet, 2006). Functionally, in experimental model, vitamin D analogs dramatically increase bone mass, size and strength in rodents (Slatopolsky et al., 2003). Observations suggest that bone integration around implants may be critically impaired by vitamin D deficiency (Mengatto et al., 2011).

Bone morphogenetic protein (BMP) family, as a member of the TGF-β superfamily, has a variety of functions in the development and reparation of bone tissue (Rider and Mulloy, 2010). The hallmark of the BMPs is their ability to induce bone formation *in vivo* by promoting osteoblast differentiation (Rider and Mulloy, 2010). BMP-2 has been shown to stimulate bone ingrowth, gap healing, and implant fixation in several animal studies (Cochran et al., 1999; Sumner et al., 2004). BMP-2 recombinant protein application showed a good potential in terms of regeneration and decreased morbidity as compared with bone autografts (Tonetti and Hammerle, 2008), also suggesting an important role on bone regulation in oral reparation sites.

Calcitonin is a peptide hormone that rapidly, transiently, and reversibly inhibits osteoclast-mediated bone resorption and also modulates calcium ion excretion by the kidney (Pondel, 2000). The physiological effects of calcitonin are specifically mediated by high affinity calcitonin receptors (CTRs), which belong to the class B subfamily of seven-transmembrane domain G protein-coupled receptors. The effect of calcitonin drugs during the period of bone maturation around titanium implants was investigated in animal model, and a positive time effect was verified improving bone mass (Januario et al., 2001). Moreover, it was shown that implant surface modifications might alter the expression of calcitonin receptor gene in osteoclasts (Monjo et al., 2008).

The system RANK/RANKL/OPG has been described as a central regulator of bone metabolism. RANKL was shown to bind its receptor, RANK, on osteoclast lineage cells to induce osteoclastogenesis. The molecule blocked by the soluble receptor OPG was identified as the key mediator of osteoclastogenesis in both a membrane-bound form expressed on preosteoblastic/stromal cells as well as a soluble form. The RANK/RANKL/OPG regulatory axis is also involved in inflammatory bone destruction induced by pro-inflammatory cytokines such prostaglandin E_2 (PGE_2), IL-1β, IL-6, and TNF-α (Boyle et al., 2003). In addition, a number of other mediators of bone metabolism, such as TGF-β (Takai et al., 1998), parathormone (PTH) (Lee and Lorenzo, 1999), 1,25-dihydroxyvitamin D3 (Kitazawa et al., 1999), glucocorticoids (Hofbauer et al., 1999), and estrogen (Hofbauer et al., 1999; Saika et al., 2001) exert their effects on osteoclastogenesis by regulating osteoblastic/stromal cell production of OPG and RANKL. RANKL and OPG concentrations were significantly higher at the crevicular fluid sampling sites of patients presenting peri-implantitis, suggesting an increased risk of alveolar bone loss around dental implants (Arikan et al., 2011).

5. A research focus on the host genetic susceptibility

The knowledge that implant loss i) is not totally explained by clinical conditions and ii) tends to cluster in subsets of individuals (Montes et al., 2007; Weyant and Burt, 1993) may indicate that specific host response characteristics, that disturb the osseointegration process, are influenced by genetic factors (Alvim-Pereira et al., 2008a).

Gene polymorphisms are a mechanism by which individuals may exhibit variations in DNA sequence. These variations may impact specific protein production and/or function (Hu et al., 2005) that in turn could alter host response modulating disease susceptibility or implant treatment outcome. Most polymorphisms are single nucleotide exchanges (SNPs) that occur in a high frequency in the human genome (Venter et al., 2001). Functional polymorphisms may account for variation in the production or function of proteins (Hu et al., 2005; Pociot et al., 1992). Those resultant slight changes in the immunoinflammatory response modulation might influence implant loss (Lachmann et al., 2007; Laine et al., 2006).

The focus of studies investigating genetic susceptibility to dental implant failure has been limited to candidate gene, population-based association analysis (Alvim-Pereira et al., 2008a). In this approach the physiology and involved metabolic pathways of healing and osseointegration process are the basis to search for candidate genes underlying host susceptibility to implant failure. But, a number of biologic mechanisms is involved in the osseointegration complex process, some of which have not yet been identified (Mengatto et al. 2011; Montes et al., 2007). Although some similarities between osseointegration and tooth extraction socket were seen, different pathways of transcription and growth factors, extracellular matrix molecules, and chemokines were proposed (Lin et al., 2010). A recent study with rats showed a possible network of genes that associated with success and failure of implant osseointegration (Mengatto et al., 2011).

In the PUBMED library available literature, a total of twenty-three original papers analyzing genetic polymorphisms in candidate genes in humans related to implant outcomes were found. The main data and results of each study are summarized in Table 1.

5.1 Genetic polymorphisms and dental implant failure

The most commonly studied polymorphisms in genetics of implant failure are funtional variations in the interleukin-1 (IL-1) gene cluster in several populations. Because of IL-1 proinflammatory and bone resorbing properties, a role has been suggested for this cytokine in controlling genetic risk of implant failure. The association of *IL1A* gene (which codes for IL-1α) polymorphisms with dental implant outcome was investigated in several studies (Campos et al., 2005c; Feloutzis et al., 2003; Gruica et al., 2004; Jansson et al., 2005; Lachmann et al., 2007; Laine et al., 2006; Lin et al., 2007; Rogers et al., 2002; Shimpuku et al., 2003b; Wilson and Nunn, 1999). Since *IL1B* gene (which codes for IL-1β) was seen to be up-regulated at early stages of healing and then down-regulated at later stages (Lin et al., 2010), polymorphisms in *IL1B* gene were also investigated for association with implant failure susceptibility (Campos et al., 2005b; Dirschnabel et al., 2011; Feloutzis et al., 2003; Gruica et al., 2004; Jansson et al., 2005; Lachmann et al., 2007; Laine et al., 2006; Lin et al., 2007; Melo et al., 2011; Montes et al., 2009; Rogers et al., 2002; Shimpuku et al., 2003b; Wilson and Nunn, 1999). Moreover, *IL1RN* gene (which codes for IL-1ra) was also searched for association to implant failure (Campos et al., 2005c; Laine et al., 2006; Montes et al., 2009). Even though *IL1* gene cluster is the most frequent analyzed inflammatory candidate genes, the results are divergent, yet not conclusive and generally not replicated (see table 1 for review). However, genotype 2/2 of *IL1RN* polymorphism was significantly more frequent in patients who presented multiple losses. Some other functional polymorphisms in inflammatory candidate genes were also analyzed: *IL2* (Campos et al., 2005a), *IL6* (Campos et al., 2005a; Melo et al., 2011), and *TNFA* (Campos et al., 2004; Cury et al., 2007; Cury et al., 2009) (Table 1).

Also, genes involved in the regulation of ECM such as *TGFB1* (Santos et al., 2004a), *MMP1* (Leite et al., 2008; Santos et al., 2004b) and *MMP9* (Santos et al., 2004b) have been investigated (Table 1).

It has been suggested that polymorphisms in the *VDR* gene significantly alter expression and/or function of VDR, which may interfere in mineral bone density (Shishkin et al., 2010). So far, only one paper has investigated the association of *VDR* gene polymorphisms with dental implant loss with no association evidenced between a functional polymorphism and implant loss (Alvim-Pereira et al., 2008b) (Table 1).

Bone morphogenetic protein 4 (*BMP4*) gene expression was reported to be slowly increased during osseointegration and the bone healing process (Lin et al., 2010), and a gene polymorphism in this gene was associated with marginal bone loss around dental implants (Shimpuku et al., 2003a) (Table 1). Another polymorphism in the *CTR* gene was also associated with marginal bone loss in the jaw, but not in the maxilla (Nosaka et al., 2002) (Table 1). Polymorphisms in *CTR* gene were also associated with bone metabolism regulation in postmenopausal women (Masi et al., 1998; Nakamura et al., 2001) and severe periodontitis (Suzuki et al., 2004).

Authors	Year	Polymorphisms	Case (n) / Control (n)	Mean age (years)	Smoking Yes / No	Population	Results
Wilson and Nunn	1999	*IL1A* (-889) and *IL1B* (+3953)	17 / 38	57	27 / 35	?	Not associated with implant failure
Nosaka et al.	2002	*CTR* (+1377)	15 / 20	54.8	15 / 20	Asian Japanese	Associated with marginal bone loss in mandible, but not in maxilla
Rogers et al.	2002	*IL1A* (-889) and *IL1B* (+3953)	19 / 31	66	?	Australian Caucasian	Not associated with implant failure
Shimpuku et al.	2003	*IL1A* (-889) and *IL1B* (-511, +3954)	17 / 22	55.1	14 / 25	Asian Japanese	Associated with marginal bone loss
Shimpuku et al.	2003	*BMP4* (+538)	21 / 36	52.6	24 / 38	Asian Japanese	Associated with marginal bone loss
Feloutzis et al.	2003	*IL1A* (+4845) and *IL1B* (+3954)	?	59.5	41 / 39	European Caucasian	Smoking + *IL1* positive genotype associated with marginal bone loss
Campos et al.	2004	*TNFA* (-308)	38 / 38	47.2	0 / 66	Brazilian	Not associated with early implant failure
Santos et al.	2004	*TGFB1* (-509, -800)	28 / 40	46	0 / 68	Brazilian	Not associated with early implant failure
Santos et al.	2004	*MMP1* (-1607) and *MMP9* (-1562)	20 / 26	45.9	0 / 46	Brazilian	*MMP1*: associated, and *MMP9*: not associated with implant failure
Gruica et al.	2004	*IL1A* (+4845) and *IL1B* (+3954)	34 / 176	25 to 90	53 / 127	European Caucasian	Smoking + *IL1* positive genotype associated with late infection
Campos et al.	2005	*IL1A* (-889), *IL1B* (-511, +3953), and *IL1RN* (intron 2 - 86 bp repeats)	28 / 34	47.5	0 / 62	Brazilian	Not associated with early implant failure
Campos et al.	2005	*IL2* (-330) and *IL6* (-174)	34 / 40	46.3	0 / 74	Brazilian	Not associated with early implant failure
Jansson et al.	2005	*IL1A* (-889) and *IL1B* (+3954)	6 /16	54	10 /12	European Caucasian	Smoking + *IL1* positive genotype associated with implant loss
Laine et al.	2006	*IL1A* (-889), *IL1B* (-511, +3953), and *IL1RN* (intron 2 - 86 bp repeats)	71 / 49	67.2	84 / 36	European Caucasian	*IL1RN* associated with peri-implantitis
Lin et al.	2007	*IL1A* (-889), IL1B (-511, +3953)	29 / 30	42.8	32 / 27	Asian Chinese	*IL1B* associated with marginal bone loss
Cury et al.	2007	*TNFA* (-308)	36	46	0 / 36	Brazilian	Not associated with marginal bone loss
Lachmann et al.	2007	*IL1A* (-889), *IL1B* (+3953)	11 / 18	66	?	European Caucasian	Not associated with levels of peri-implant crevicular fluid nor with cytokine concentration
Alvim-Pereira et al.	2008	*VDR* (exon 9, T*aq* I)	80 / 137	51.7	43 / 174	Brazilian	Not associated with implant failure
Leite et al.	2008	*MMP1* (-1607 and -519)	44 / 60	?	0 / 104	Brazilian	*MMP1* associated with early implant failure
Montes et al.	2009	*IL1B* (+3954) and *IL1RN* (intron 2)	90 / 176	51.5	58 / 208	Brazilian	*IL1RN* associated with multiple implant loss
Cury et al.	2009	*TNFA* (-308)	49 / 41	?	?	Brazilian	Not associated with peri-implantitis
Dirschnabel et al.	2011	*IL1B* (-511)	92 / 185	53.6	61 / 216	Brazilian	Not associated with implant loss
Melo et al.	2011	*IL1B* (+3954), *IL1B* (-511), and *IL6* (-174)	31 / 16	?	?	Brazilian	Not associated with peri-implantitis

Table 1. Studies investigating the association between genetic polymorphisms and dental implant failure.

5.2 Future insights in dental implants genetic research

Although candidate gene, association analysis has proved to be a promising tool for the dissection of the nature of the genetic component controlling dental implant failure, the design is limited by the fact that just a small segment of the genome is analyzed. Moreover, the sample sizes are often small; therefore, findings must be replicated in larger populations (Alvim-Pereira et al., 2008a). As a consequence, genetic susceptibility to osseointegrated implant failure remains widely unknown.

Despite these promising advances, the exact number, identity and role of regulatory factors that lead to a successful implant osseointegration and its maintenance are still largely unknown, which limits genetic analysis approaches based on functional candidate genes. The challenge then is to map all the involved genes (Bosse et al., 2004), a considerably difficult task given that the human genome is composed of at least 30,000 genes (Baltimore, 2001), reaching 4.1 million of SNPs catalogued in public databases markers.

Genomewide association scans (GWAS) are a fully automated technology that allows genotyping hundreds of thousands of SNPs in a single experiment (Thomas et al., 2005). This extremely high throughput SNP genotyping technology is making possible the development of association-based case-control design covering the entire genome (Hirschhorn and Daly, 2005). However, some limitations do exist. Those analyzes are still very expensive and need cutting-edge genotyping technology (Detera-Wadleigh and McMahon, 2004) and tremendous amount of raw data demands adequate statistical methods of analysis (Devlin et al., 2001). False-positive results are likely to increase (Marchini et al., 2004), in this context, replication in independent populations becomes mandatory (Neale and Sham, 2004). On the other way around, the great amount of failure in identifying significant associations of complex traits and diseases with common variants across the genome may indicate that those complex phenotypes may possibly be determined by rare gene variants. In this context, the whole genome sequencing of a few individuals, whose phenotype is very well characterized and extreme, may be cheaper and offer more valuable results.

Another development in the genetic field is called next-generation sequencing (NGS) technology, which includes genome sequencing and resequencing, transcriptional profiling (RNA-Seq) and high-throughput survey of DNA-protein interactions (ChIP-Seq) (de Magalhaes et al., 2010). The advantages may change the landscape of genetics by a reasonable cost and high throughput (Mardis, 2008). In spite of giving rise to new challenges, in particular in processing, analyzing and interpreting data, this type of application may clarify and increase knowledge over physiologic pathways of bone remodeling and osseointegration.

6. Conclusion

Despite the difficulties, the motivation to continue applying traditional and new approaches for genetic analysis to the effort towards a better understanding of dental implant physiology and failure mechanisms is clear. For example, genetic studies may shed new light not only upon the physiopathology of dental implant failure, but also upon broader, related processes, such as bone healing. In addition, a direct result of such studies may be the definition of potential targets for effective screening, prevention and maintenance of dental implants.

7. References

Abbas AK, Lichtman A, Pober J (1998). Imunologia cellular e molecular. 2ed ed. Rio de Janeiro: Revinter.

Aboyoussef H, Carter C, Jandinski JJ, Panagakos FS (1998). Detection of prostaglandin E2 and matrix metalloproteinases in implant crevicular fluid. Int J Oral Maxillofac Implants 13(5):689-96.

Adell R, Lekholm U, Rockler B, Branemark PI (1981). A 15-year study of osseointegrated implants in the treatment of the edentulous jaw. Int J Oral Surg 10(6):387-416.

Adell R, Eriksson B, Lekholm U, Branemark PI, Jemt T (1990). Long-term follow-up study of osseointegrated implants in the treatment of totally edentulous jaws. The International Journal of Oral & Maxillofacial Implants 5(4):347-59.

Albrektsson T, Branemark PI, Hansson HA, Lindstrom J (1981). Osseointegrated titanium implants. Requirements for ensuring a long-lasting, direct bone-to-implant anchorage in man. Acta Orthop Scand 52(2):155-70.

Alvim-Pereira F, Montes CC, Mira MT, Trevilatto PC (2008a). Genetic susceptibility to dental implant failure: a critical review. Int J Oral Maxillofac Implants 23(3):409-16.

Alvim-Pereira F, Montes CC, Thome G, Olandoski M, Trevilatto PC (2008b). Analysis of association of clinical aspects and vitamin D receptor gene polymorphism with dental implant loss. Clin Oral Implants Res 19(8):786-95.

Apse P, Ellen RP, Overall CM, Zarb GA (1989). Microbiota and crevicular fluid collagenase activity in the osseointegrated dental implant sulcus: a comparison of sites in edentulous and partially edentulous patients. J Periodontal Res 24(2):96-105.

Arikan F, Buduneli N, Lappin DF (2011). C-Telopeptide Pyridinoline Crosslinks of Type I Collagen, Soluble RANKL, and Osteoprotegerin Levels in Crevicular Fluid of Dental Implants with Peri-implantitis: A Case-Control Study. Int J Oral Maxillofac Implants 26(2):282-9.

Baltimore D (2001). Our genome unveiled. Nature 409(6822):814-6.

Berglundh T, Abrahamsson I, Lang NP, Lindhe J (2003). De novo alveolar bone formation adjacent to endosseous implants. Clin Oral Implants Res 14(3):251-62.

Binkley N (2006). Summary - The role of vitamin D in musculoskeletal health. J Musculoskelet Neuronal Interact 6(4):347-48.

Birkedal-Hansen H (1993). Role of matrix metalloproteinases in human periodontal diseases. J Periodontol 64(5 Suppl):474-84.

Bloemen V, Schoenmaker T, de Vries TJ, Everts V (2011). IL-1beta favors osteoclastogenesis via supporting human periodontal ligament fibroblasts. J Cell Biochem.

Bordin S, Flemmig TF, Verardi S (2009). Role of fibroblast populations in peri-implantitis. Int J Oral Maxillofac Implants 24(2):197-204.

Bosse Y, Chagnon YC, Despres JP, Rice T, Rao DC, Bouchard C, et al. (2004). Compendium of genome-wide scans of lipid-related phenotypes: adding a new genome-wide search of apolipoprotein levels. J Lipid Res 45(12):2174-84.

Boyle WJ, Simonet WS, Lacey DL (2003). Osteoclast differentiation and activation. Nature 423(6937):337-42.

Boynuegri AD, Yalim M, Nemli SK, Erguder BI, Gokalp P (2011). Effect of different localizations of microgap on clinical parameters and inflammatory cytokines in peri-implant crevicular fluid: a prospective comparative study. Clin Oral Investig.

Branemark PI, Adell R, Breine U, Hansson BO, Lindstrom J, Ohlsson A (1969). Intra-osseous anchorage of dental prostheses. I. Experimental studies. Scand J Plast Reconstr Surg 3(2):81-100.

Branemark PI, Hansson BO, Adell R, Breine U, Lindstrom J, Hallen O, et al. (1977). Osseointegrated implants in the treatment of the edentulous jaw. Experience from a 10-year period. Scand J Plast Reconstr Surg Suppl 16(1-132.

Brown DW (2009). Complete edentulism prior to the age of 65 years is associated with all-cause mortality. J Public Health Dent 69(4):260-6.

Campos MI, dos Santos MC, Trevilatto PC, Scarel-Caminaga RM, Bezerra FJ, Line SR (2004). Early failure of dental implants and TNF-alpha (G-308A) gene polymorphism. Implant Dent 13(1):95-101.

Campos MI, Godoy dos Santos MC, Trevilatto PC, Scarel-Caminaga RM, Bezerra FJ, Line SR (2005a). Interleukin-2 and interleukin-6 gene promoter polymorphisms, and early failure of dental implants. Implant Dent 14(4):391-6.

Campos MI, Santos MC, Trevilatto PC, Scarel-Caminaga RM, Bezerra FJ, Line SR (2005b). Evaluation of the relationship between interleukin-1 gene cluster polymorphisms and early implant failure in non-smoking patients. Clin Oral Implants Res 16(2):194-201.

Campos MI, Santos MC, Trevilatto PC, Scarel-Caminaga RM, Bezerra FJ, Line SR (2005c). Evaluation of the relationship between interleukin-1 gene cluster polymorphisms and early implant failure in non-smoking patients. Clinical Oral Implants Research 16(2):194-201.

Chang PC, Lang NP, Giannobile WV (2010). Evaluation of functional dynamics during osseointegration and regeneration associated with oral implants. Clin Oral Implants Res 21(1):1-12.

Choi MG, Koh HS, Kluess D, O'Connor D, Mathur A, Truskey GA, et al. (2005). Effects of titanium particle size on osteoblast functions in vitro and in vivo. Proc Natl Acad Sci U S A 102(12):4578-83.

Cochran DL, Schenk R, Buser D, Wozney JM, Jones AA (1999). Recombinant human bone morphogenetic protein-2 stimulation of bone formation around endosseous dental implants. J Periodontol 70(2):139-50.

Courbebaisse M, Souberbielle JC (2011). [Phosphocalcic metabolism: Regulation and explorations.]. Nephrol Ther.

Crawford HC, Matrisian LM (1994). Tumor and stromal expression of matrix metalloproteinases and their role in tumor progression. Invasion Metastasis 14(1-6):234-45.

Cury PR, Joly JC, Freitas N, Sendyk WR, Nunes FD, de Araujo NS (2007). Effect of tumor necrosis factor-alpha gene polymorphism on peri-implant bone loss following prosthetic reconstruction. Implant Dent 16(1):80-8.

Cury PR, Horewicz VV, Ferrari DS, Brito R, Jr., Sendyk WR, Duarte PM, et al. (2009). Evaluation of the effect of tumor necrosis factor-alpha gene polymorphism on the risk of peri-implantitis: a case-control study. Int J Oral Maxillofac Implants 24(6):1101-5.

Davarpanah M, Martinez H, Etienne D, Zabalegui I, Mattout P, Chiche F, et al. (2002). A prospective multicenter evaluation of 1,583 3i implants: 1- to 5-year data. The International Journal of Oral & Maxillofacial Implants 17(6):820-8.

de Magalhaes JP, Finch CE, Janssens G (2010). Next-generation sequencing in aging research: emerging applications, problems, pitfalls and possible solutions. Ageing Res Rev 9(3):315-23.

de Souza AP, Trevilatto PC, Scarel-Caminaga RM, Brito RB, Line SR (2003). MMP-1 promoter polymorphism: association with chronic periodontitis severity in a Brazilian population. J Clin Periodontol 30(2):154-8.

Deas DE, Mikotowicz JJ, Mackey SA, Moritz AJ (2002). Implant failure with spontaneous rapid exfoliation: case reports. Implant Dent 11(3):235-42.

Degidi M, Piattelli A (2005). 7-year follow-up of 93 immediately loaded titanium dental implants. J Oral Implantol 31(1):25-31.

Derynck R, Jarrett JA, Chen EY, Eaton DH, Bell JR, Assoian RK, et al. (1985). Human transforming growth factor-beta complementary DNA sequence and expression in normal and transformed cells. Nature 316(6030):701-5.

Detera-Wadleigh SD, McMahon FJ (2004). Genetic association studies in mood disorders: issues and promise. Int Rev Psychiatry 16(4):301-10.

Devlin B, Roeder K, Bacanu SA (2001). Unbiased methods for population-based association studies. Genet Epidemiol 21(4):273-84.

Dinarello CA (1988). Biology of interleukin 1. Faseb J 2(2):108-15.

Dinarello CA (2007). Historical insights into cytokines. Eur J Immunol 37 Suppl 1(S34-45.

Dirschnabel AJ, Alvim-Pereira F, Alvim-Pereira CC, Bernardino JF, Rosa EA, Trevilatto PC (2011). Analysis of the association of IL1B(C-511T) polymorphism with dental implant loss and the clusterization phenomenon. Clin Oral Implants Res.

Dunleavey L, Beyzade S, Ye S (2000). Rapid genotype analysis of the matrix metalloproteinase-1 gene 1G/2G polymorphism that is associated with risk of cancer. Matrix Biol 19(2):175-7.

Esposito M, Hirsch JM, Lekholm U, Thomsen P (1998a). Biological factors contributing to failures of osseointegrated oral implants. (I). Success criteria and epidemiology. Eur J Oral Sci 106(1):527-51.

Esposito M, Hirsch JM, Lekholm U, Thomsen P (1998b). Biological factors contributing to failures of osseointegrated oral implants. (II). Etiopathogenesis. Eur J Oral Sci 106(3):721-64.

Esposito M, Hirsch J, Lekholm U, Thomsen P (1999). Differential diagnosis and treatment strategies for biologic complications and failing oral implants: a review of the literature. The International Journal of Oral & Maxillofacial Implants 14(4):473-90.

Esposito M, Worthington HV, Coulthard P (2004). Interventions for replacing missing teeth: treatment of perimplantitis. Cochrane Database Syst Rev 4):CD004970.

Esposito M, Murray-Curtis L, Grusovin MG, Coulthard P, Worthington HV (2007). Interventions for replacing missing teeth: different types of dental implants. Cochrane Database Syst Rev 4):CD003815.

Esposito M, Grusovin MG, Achille H, Coulthard P, Worthington HV (2009). Interventions for replacing missing teeth: different times for loading dental implants. Cochrane Database Syst Rev 1):CD003878.

Fanchon S, Bourd K, Septier D, Everts V, Beertsen W, Menashi S, et al. (2004). Involvement of matrix metalloproteinases in the onset of dentin mineralization. Eur J Oral Sci 112(2):171-6.

Feloutzis A, Lang NP, Tonetti MS, Burgin W, Bragger U, Buser D, et al. (2003). IL-1 gene polymorphism and smoking as risk factors for peri-implant bone loss in a well-maintained population. Clin Oral Implants Res 14(1):10-7.

Felton DA (2009). Edentulism and comorbid factors. J Prosthodont 18(2):88-96.

Ferguson SJ, Broggini N, Wieland M, de Wild M, Rupp F, Geis-Gerstorfer J, et al. (2006). Biomechanical evaluation of the interfacial strength of a chemically modified sandblasted and acid-etched titanium surface. J Biomed Mater Res A 78(2):291-7.

Fleet JC (2006). Molecular regulation of calcium and bone metabolism through the vitamin D receptor. J Musculoskelet Neuronal Interact 6(4):336-7.

Foda HD, Zucker S (2001). Matrix metalloproteinases in cancer invasion, metastasis and angiogenesis. Drug Discov Today 6(9):478-482.

Franchi M, Fini M, Martini D, Orsini E, Leonardi L, Ruggeri A, et al. (2005). Biological fixation of endosseous implants. Micron 36(7-8):665-71.

Fugazzotto PA (2005). Success and failure rates of osseointegrated implants in function in regenerated bone for 72 to 133 months. The International Journal of Oral & Maxillofacial Implants 20(1):77-83.

Futami T, Fujii N, Ohnishi H, Taguchi N, Kusakari H, Ohshima H, et al. (2000). Tissue response to titanium implants in the rat maxilla: ultrastructural and histochemical observations of the bone-titanium interface. J Periodontol 71(2):287-98.

Gainet J, Chollet-Martin S, Brion M, Hakim J, Gougerot-Pocidalo MA, Elbim C (1998). Interleukin-8 production by polymorphonuclear neutrophils in patients with rapidly progressive periodontitis: an amplifying loop of polymorphonuclear neutrophil activation. Lab Invest 78(6):755-62.

Ganeles J, Wismeijer D (2004). Early and immediately restored and loaded dental implants for single-tooth and partial-arch applications. Int J Oral Maxillofac Implants 19 Suppl(92-102.

Golub LM, Lee HM, Greenwald RA, Ryan ME, Sorsa T, Salo T, et al. (1997). A matrix metalloproteinase inhibitor reduces bone-type collagen degradation fragments and specific collagenases in gingival crevicular fluid during adult periodontitis. Inflamm Res 46(8):310-9.

Goutoudi P, Diza E, Arvanitidou M (2004). Effect of periodontal therapy on crevicular fluid interleukin-1beta and interleukin-10 levels in chronic periodontitis. J Dent 32(7):511-20.

Graziani F, Donos N, Needleman I, Gabriele M, Tonetti M (2004). Comparison of implant survival following sinus floor augmentation procedures with implants placed in pristine posterior maxillary bone: a systematic review. Clin Oral Implants Res 15(6):677-82.

Gruica B, Wang HY, Lang NP, Buser D (2004). Impact of IL-1 genotype and smoking status on the prognosis of osseointegrated implants. Clin Oral Implants Res 15(4):393-400.

Han J, Lulic M, Lang NP (2010). Factors influencing resonance frequency analysis assessed by Osstell mentor during implant tissue integration: II. Implant surface modifications and implant diameter. Clin Oral Implants Res 21(6):605-11.

Harada Y, Watanabe S, Yssel H, Arai K (1996). Factors affecting the cytokine production of human T cells stimulated by different modes of activation. J Allergy Clin Immunol 98(6 Pt 2):S161-73.

Haussler MR, Whitfield GK, Haussler CA, Hsieh JC, Thompson PD, Selznick SH, et al. (1998). The nuclear vitamin D receptor: biological and molecular regulatory properties revealed. J Bone Miner Res 13(3):325-49.

Hellmig S, Titz A, Steinel S, Ott S, Folsch UR, Hampe J, et al. (2005). Influence of IL-1 gene cluster polymorphisms on the development of H. pylori associated gastric ulcer. Immunol Lett 100(2):107-12.

Hirschhorn JN, Daly MJ (2005). Genome-wide association studies for common diseases and complex traits. Nat Rev Genet 6(2):95-108.

Hofbauer LC, Gori F, Riggs BL, Lacey DL, Dunstan CR, Spelsberg TC, et al. (1999). Stimulation of osteoprotegerin ligand and inhibition of osteoprotegerin production by glucocorticoids in human osteoblastic lineage cells: potential paracrine mechanisms of glucocorticoid-induced osteoporosis. Endocrinology 140(10):4382-9.

Hoffman HM, Brydges SD (2011). The genetic and molecular basis of inflammasome-mediated disease. J Biol Chem.

Hospitalar (2007). Congresso mundial comemorativo dos 40 anos de osseointegração: http://www.hospitalar.com/noticias/not2331.html.

Hu S, Song QB, Yao PF, Hu QL, Hu PJ, Zeng ZR, et al. (2005). No relationship between IL-1B gene polymorphism and gastric acid secretion in younger healthy volunteers. World J Gastroenterol 11(41):6549-53.

Huang HH, Ho CT, Lee TH, Lee TL, Liao KK, Chen FL (2004). Effect of surface roughness of ground titanium on initial cell adhesion. Biomol Eng 21(3-5):93-7.

Ingman T, Kononen M, Konttinen YT, Siirila HS, Suomalainen K, Sorsa T (1994). Collagenase, gelatinase and elastase activities in sulcular fluid of osseointegrated implants and natural teeth. J Clin Periodontol 21(4):301-7.

Jansson H, Hamberg K, De Bruyn H, Bratthall G (2005). Clinical consequences of IL-1 genotype on early implant failures in patients under periodontal maintenance. Clin Implant Dent Relat Res 7(1):51-9.

Januario AL, Sallum EA, de Toledo S, Sallum AW, Nociti JF, Jr. (2001). Effect of calcitonin on bone formation around titanium implant. A histometric study in rabbits. Braz Dent J 12(3):158-62.

Joos U, Wiesmann HP, Szuwart T, Meyer U (2006). Mineralization at the interface of implants. Int J Oral Maxillofac Surg 35(9):783-90.

Kasemo B, Gold J (1999). Implant surfaces and interface processes. Adv Dent Res 13(8-20.

Kerrigan JJ, Mansell JP, Sandy JR (2000). Matrix turnover. J Orthod 27(3):227-33.

Kitazawa R, Kitazawa S, Maeda S (1999). Promoter structure of mouse RANKL/TRANCE/OPGL/ODF gene. Biochim Biophys Acta 1445(1):134-41.

Kornman KS (2006). Interleukin 1 genetics, inflammatory mechanisms, and nutrigenetic opportunities to modulate diseases of aging. Am J Clin Nutr 83(2):475S-483S.

Kukacka J, Prusa R, Kotaska K, Pelouch V (2005). Matrix metalloproteinases and their function in myocardium. Biomed Pap Med Fac Univ Palacky Olomouc Czech Repub 149(2):225-36.

Kuttenberger JJ, Hardt N, Rutz T, Pfyffer GE (2005). [Bone collected with a bone collector during dental implant surgery]. Mund Kiefer Gesichtschir 9(1):18-23.

Kwon SY, Takei H, Pioletti DP, Lin T, Ma QJ, Akeson WH, et al. (2000). Titanium particles inhibit osteoblast adhesion to fibronectin-coated substrates. J Orthop Res 18(2):203-11.

Kwon SY, Lin T, Takei H, Ma Q, Wood DJ, O'Connor D, et al. (2001). Alterations in the adhesion behavior of osteoblasts by titanium particle loading: inhibition of cell function and gene expression. Biorheology 38(2-3):161-83.

Lachmann S, Kimmerle-Muller E, Axmann D, Scheideler L, Weber H, Haas R (2007). Associations between peri-implant crevicular fluid volume, concentrations of crevicular inflammatory mediators, and composite IL-1A -889 and IL-1B +3954 genotype. A cross-sectional study on implant recall patients with and without clinical signs of peri-implantitis. Clin Oral Implants Res 18(2):212-23.

Laine ML, Leonhardt A, Roos-Jansaker AM, Pena AS, van Winkelhoff AJ, Winkel EG, et al. (2006). IL-1RN gene polymorphism is associated with peri-implantitis. Clin Oral Implants Res 17(4):380-5.

Laurincova B (2000). Interleukin-1 family: from genes to human disease. Acta Univ Palacki Olomuc Fac Med 143(19-29.

Lawrence DA (1996). Transforming growth factor-beta: a general review. Eur Cytokine Netw 7(3):363-74.

Lee SK, Lorenzo JA (1999). Parathyroid hormone stimulates TRANCE and inhibits osteoprotegerin messenger ribonucleic acid expression in murine bone marrow cultures: correlation with osteoclast-like cell formation. Endocrinology 140(8):3552-61.

Leite MF, Santos MC, de Souza AP, Line SR (2008). Osseointegrated implant failure associated with MMP-1 promotor polymorphisms (-1607 and -519). Int J Oral Maxillofac Implants 23(4):653-8.

Lennard AC (1995). Interleukin-1 receptor antagonist. Crit Rev Immunol 15(1):77-105.

Lin YH, Huang P, Lu X, Guan DH, Man Y, Wei N, et al. (2007). The relationship between IL-1 gene polymorphism and marginal bone loss around dental implants. J Oral Maxillofac Surg 65(11):2340-4.

Lin Z, Rios HF, Volk SL, Sugai JV, Jin Q, Giannobile WV (2010). Gene Expression Dynamics During Bone Healing and Osseointegration. J Periodontol.

Linder L, Albrektsson T, Branemark PI, Hansson HA, Ivarsson B, Jonsson U, et al. (1983). Electron microscopic analysis of the bone-titanium interface. Acta Orthop Scand 54(1):45-52.

Lioubavina-Hack N, Lang NP, Karring T (2006). Significance of primary stability for osseointegration of dental implants. Clin Oral Implants Res 17(3):244-50.

Liu KZ, Hynes A, Man A, Alsagheer A, Singer DL, Scott DA (2006). Increased local matrix metalloproteinase-8 expression in the periodontal connective tissues of smokers with periodontal disease. Biochim Biophys Acta 1762(8):775-80.

Ma J, Kitti U, Teronen O, Sorsa T, Husa V, Laine P, et al. (2000). Collagenases in different categories of peri-implant vertical bone loss. J Dent Res 79(11):1870-3.

Marchini J, Cardon LR, Phillips MS, Donnelly P (2004). The effects of human population structure on large genetic association studies. Nat Genet 36(5):512-7.

Mardis ER (2008). The impact of next-generation sequencing technology on genetics. Trends Genet 24(3):133-41.

Masada MP, Persson R, Kenney JS, Lee SW, Page RC, Allison AC (1990). Measurement of interleukin-1 alpha and -1 beta in gingival crevicular fluid: implications for the pathogenesis of periodontal disease. J Periodontal Res 25(3):156-63.

Masi L, Becherini L, Colli E, Gennari L, Mansani R, Falchetti A, et al. (1998). Polymorphisms of the calcitonin receptor gene are associated with bone mineral density in postmenopausal Italian women. Biochem Biophys Res Commun 248(1):190-5.

Massague J (1990). The transforming growth factor-beta family. Annu Rev Cell Biol 6(597-641.

Mavrogenis AF, Dimitriou R, Parvizi J, Babis GC (2009). Biology of implant osseointegration. J Musculoskelet Neuronal Interact 9(2):61-71.

McKibbin B (1978). The biology of fracture healing in long bones. J Bone Joint Surg Br 60-B(2):150-62.

Melo RF, Lopes BM, Shibli JA, Marcantonio Junior E, Marcantonio RA, Galli GM (2011). Interleukin-1beta and Interleukin-6 Expression and Gene Polymorphisms in Subjects with Peri-Implant Disease. Clin Implant Dent Relat Res.

Mengatto CM, Mussano F, Honda Y, Colwell CS, Nishimura I (2011). Circadian rhythm and cartilage extracellular matrix genes in osseointegration: a genome-wide screening of implant failure by vitamin D deficiency. PLoS One 6(1):e15848.

Misch CE, Wang HL, Misch CM, Sharawy M, Lemons J, Judy KW (2004). Rationale for the application of immediate load in implant dentistry: part II. Implant Dent 13(4):310-21.

Molto A, Olive A (2010). Anti-IL-1 molecules: new comers and new indications. Joint Bone Spine 77(2):102-7.

Monjo M, Lamolle SF, Lyngstadaas SP, Ronold HJ, Ellingsen JE (2008). In vivo expression of osteogenic markers and bone mineral density at the surface of fluoride-modified titanium implants. Biomaterials 29(28):3771-80.

Montes CC, Pereira FA, Thomé G, Alves ED, Acedo RV, de Souza JR, Melo AC, Trevilatto PC. Failing factors associated with osseointegrated dental implant loss. Implant Dent. 2007 Dec;16(4):404-12.

Montes CC, Alvim-Pereira F, de Castilhos BB, Sakurai ML, Olandoski M, Trevilatto PC (2009). Analysis of the association of IL1B (C+3954T) and IL1RN (intron 2) polymorphisms with dental implant loss in a Brazilian population. Clin Oral Implants Res 20(2):208-17.

Moy PK, Medina D, Shetty V, Aghaloo TL (2005). Dental implant failure rates and associated risk factors. Int J Oral Maxillofac Implants 20(4):569-77.

Nakamura M, Morimoto S, Zhang Z, Utsunomiya H, Inagami T, Ogihara T, et al. (2001). Calcitonin receptor gene polymorphism in japanese women: correlation with body mass and bone mineral density. Calcif Tissue Int 68(4):211-5.

Neale BM, Sham PC (2004). The future of association studies: gene-based analysis and replication. Am J Hum Genet 75(3):353-62.

Nemeth JA, Yousif R, Herzog M, Che M, Upadhyay J, Shekarriz B, et al. (2002). Matrix metalloproteinase activity, bone matrix turnover, and tumor cell proliferation in prostate cancer bone metastasis. J Natl Cancer Inst 94(1):17-25.

Nosaka Y, Tachi Y, Shimpuku H, Kawamura T, Ohura K (2002). Association of calcitonin receptor gene polymorphism with early marginal bone loss around endosseous implants. Int J Oral Maxillofac Implants 17(1):38-43.

Panda DK, Miao D, Bolivar I, Li J, Huo R, Hendy GN, et al. (2004). Inactivation of the 25-hydroxyvitamin D 1alpha-hydroxylase and vitamin D receptor demonstrates independent and interdependent effects of calcium and vitamin D on skeletal and mineral homeostasis. J Biol Chem 279(16):16754-66.

Pang T, Therry RF, Editors TPm (2011). WHO/PLoS Collection "No Health Without Research": a call for papers. PLoS Med 8:e1001008.

Pelegrin P (2008). Targeting interleukin-1 signaling in chronic inflammation: focus on P2X(7) receptor and Pannexin-1. Drug News Perspect 21(8):424-33.

Perala DG, Chapman RJ, Gelfand JA, Callahan MV, Adams DF, Lie T (1992). Relative production of IL-1 beta and TNF alpha by mononuclear cells after exposure to dental implants. J Periodontol 63(5):426-30.

Petersen PE, Bourgeois D, Bratthall D, Ogawa H (2005). Oral health information systems--towards measuring progress in oral health promotion and disease prevention. Bull World Health Organ 83(9):686-93.

Pihlstrom BL, Michalowicz BS, Johnson NW (2005). Periodontal diseases. Lancet 366(9499):1809-20.

Pitts N, Amaechi B, Niederman R, Acevedo AM, Vianna R, Ganss C, et al. (2011). Global oral health inequalities: dental caries task group--research agenda. Adv Dent Res 23(2):211-20.

Pociot F, Molvig J, Wogensen L, Worsaae H, Nerup J (1992). A TaqI polymorphism in the human interleukin-1 beta (IL-1 beta) gene correlates with IL-1 beta secretion in vitro. Eur J Clin Invest 22(6):396-402.

Polzer I, Schimmel M, Muller F, Biffar R (2010a). Edentulism as part of the general health problems of elderly adults. Int Dent J 60(3):143-55.

Polzer K, Joosten L, Gasser J, Distler JH, Ruiz G, Baum W, et al. (2010b). Interleukin-1 is essential for systemic inflammatory bone loss. Ann Rheum Dis 69(1):284-90.

Pondel M (2000). Calcitonin and calcitonin receptors: bone and beyond. Int J Exp Pathol 81(6):405-22.

Quirynen M, Teughels W (2003). Microbiologically compromised patients and impact on oral implants. Periodontol 2000 33(119-28.

Rider CC, Mulloy B (2010). Bone morphogenetic protein and growth differentiation factor cytokine families and their protein antagonists. Biochem J 429(1):1-12.

Rogers MA, Figliomeni L, Baluchova K, Tan AE, Davies G, Henry PJ, et al. (2002). Do interleukin-1 polymorphisms predict the development of periodontitis or the success of dental implants? J Periodontal Res 37(1):37-41.

Rosenberg ES, Cho SC, Elian N, Jalbout ZN, Froum S, Evian CI (2004). A comparison of characteristics of implant failure and survival in periodontally compromised and periodontally healthy patients: a clinical report. Int J Oral Maxillofac Implants 19(6):873-9.

Ruhling A, Jepsen S, Kocher T, Plagmann HC (1999). Longitudinal evaluation of aspartate aminotransferase in the crevicular fluid of implants with bone loss and signs of progressive disease. Int J Oral Maxillofac Implants 14(3):428-35.

Saika M, Inoue D, Kido S, Matsumoto T (2001). 17beta-estradiol stimulates expression of osteoprotegerin by a mouse stromal cell line, ST-2, via estrogen receptor-alpha. Endocrinology 142(6):2205-12.

Salcetti JM, Moriarty JD, Cooper LF, Smith FW, Collins JG, Socransky SS, et al. (1997). The clinical, microbial, and host response characteristics of the failing implant. Int J Oral Maxillofac Implants 12(1):32-42.

Santos MC, Campos MI, Souza AP, Scarel-Caminaga RM, Mazzonetto R, Line SR (2004a). Analysis of the transforming growth factor-beta 1 gene promoter polymorphisms in early osseointegrated implant failure. Implant Dent 13(3):262-9.

Santos MC, Campos MI, Souza AP, Trevilatto PC, Line SR (2004b). Analysis of MMP-1 and MMP-9 promoter polymorphisms in early osseointegrated implant failure. Int J Oral Maxillofac Implants 19(1):38-43.

Sattari M, Fathiyeh A, Gholami F, Darbandi Tamijani H, Ghatreh Samani M (2011). Effect of Surgical Flap on IL-1beta and TGF-beta Concentrations in the Gingival Crevicular Fluid of Patients with Moderate to Severe Chronic Periodontitis. Iran J Immunol 8(1):20-6.

Schenk RK, Perren SM (1977). [Biology and biomechanics of fracture healing in long bones as a basis for osteosynthesis]. Hefte Unfallheilkd 129):29-41.

Seymour GJ, Gemmell E, Lenz LJ, Henry P, Bower R, Yamazaki K (1989). Immunohistologic analysis of the inflammatory infiltrates associated with osseointegrated implants. Int J Oral Maxillofac Implants 4(3):191-8.

Shimpuku H, Nosaka Y, Kawamura T, Tachi Y, Shinohara M, Ohura K (2003a). Bone morphogenetic protein-4 gene polymorphism and early marginal bone loss around endosseous implants. Int J Oral Maxillofac Implants 18(4):500-4.

Shimpuku H, Nosaka Y, Kawamura T, Tachi Y, Shinohara M, Ohura K (2003b). Genetic polymorphisms of the interleukin-1 gene and early marginal bone loss around endosseous dental implants. Clin Oral Implants Res 14(4):423-9.

Shishkin AN, Mazurenko SO, Aseev MV (2010). [Effect of TT genotype of the vitamin D receptor gene on bone mineral density in dialysis patients]. Ter Arkh 82(6):39-43.

Slatopolsky E, Finch J, Brown A (2003). New vitamin D analogs. Kidney Int Suppl 85):S83-7.

Slotte C, Lenneras M, Gothberg C, Suska F, Zoric N, Thomsen P, et al. (2010). Gene Expression of Inflammation and Bone Healing in Peri-Implant Crevicular Fluid after Placement and Loading of Dental Implants. A Kinetic Clinical Pilot Study Using Quantitative Real-Time PCR. Clin Implant Dent Relat Res.

Smith DE (2011). The biological paths of IL-1 family members IL-18 and IL-33. J Leukoc Biol 89(3):383-92.

Stanford CM, Keller JC (1991). The concept of osseointegration and bone matrix expression. Crit Rev Oral Biol Med 2(1):83-101.

Stanford CM (2003). Bone quantity and quality: are they relevant predictors of implant outcomes? Int J Prosthodont 16 Suppl(43-5; discussion 47-51.

Stashenko P, Fujiyoshi P, Obernesser MS, Prostak L, Haffajee AD, Socransky SS (1991). Levels of interleukin 1 beta in tissue from sites of active periodontal disease. J Clin Periodontol 18(7):548-54.

Stein SH, Dean IN, Rawal SY, Tipton DA (2011). Statins regulate interleukin-1beta-induced RANKL and osteoprotegerin production by human gingival fibroblasts. J Periodontal Res.

Stevens AL, Wishnok JS, White FM, Grodzinsky AJ, Tannenbaum SR (2009). Mechanical injury and cytokines cause loss of cartilage integrity and upregulate proteins associated with catabolism, immunity, inflammation, and repair. Mol Cell Proteomics 8(7):1475-89.

Sulkala M, Wahlgren J, Larmas M, Sorsa T, Teronen O, Salo T, et al. (2001). The effects of MMP inhibitors on human salivary MMP activity and caries progression in rats. J Dent Res 80(6):1545-9.

Sumner DR, Turner TM, Urban RM, Turek T, Seeherman H, Wozney JM (2004). Locally delivered rhBMP-2 enhances bone ingrowth and gap healing in a canine model. J Orthop Res 22(1):58-65.

Suzuki A, Ji G, Numabe Y, Ishii K, Muramatsu M, Kamoi K (2004). Large-scale investigation of genomic markers for severe periodontitis. Odontology 92(1):43-7.

Syrris P, Carter ND, Metcalfe JC, Kemp PR, Grainger DJ, Kaski JC, et al. (1998). Transforming growth factor-beta1 gene polymorphisms and coronary artery disease. Clin Sci (Lond) 95(6):659-67.

Szmukler-Moncler S, Salama H, Reingewirtz Y, Dubruille JH (1998). Timing of loading and effect of micromotion on bone-dental implant interface: review of experimental literature. J Biomed Mater Res 43(2):192-203.

Takai H, Kanematsu M, Yano K, Tsuda E, Higashio K, Ikeda K, et al. (1998). Transforming growth factor-beta stimulates the production of osteoprotegerin/osteoclastogenesis inhibitory factor by bone marrow stromal cells. J Biol Chem 273(42):27091-6.

Takashiba S, Naruishi K, Murayama Y (2003). Perspective of cytokine regulation for periodontal treatment: fibroblast biology. J Periodontol 74(1):103-10.

Tatakis DN (1993). Interleukin-1 and bone metabolism: a review. J Periodontol 64(5 Suppl):416-31.

Teronen O, Konttinen YT, Lindqvist C, Salo T, Ingman T, Lauhio A, et al. (1997). Human neutrophil collagenase MMP-8 in peri-implant sulcus fluid and its inhibition by clodronate. J Dent Res 76(9):1529-37.

Thomas DC, Haile RW, Duggan D (2005). Recent developments in genomewide association scans: a workshop summary and review. Am J Hum Genet 77(3):337-45.

Thomas MV, Puleo DA (2011). Infection, Inflammation, and Bone Regeneration: a Paradoxical Relationship. J Dent Res.

Tilman HH (1985). Oral rehabilitation to maintain independence. Arch Phys Med Rehabil 66(2):117-8.

Tonetti MS, Hammerle CH (2008). Advances in bone augmentation to enable dental implant placement: Consensus Report of the Sixth European Workshop on Periodontology. J Clin Periodontol 35(8 Suppl):168-72.

Turkyilmaz I, Sennerby L, McGlumphy EA, Tozum TF (2009). Biomechanical aspects of primary implant stability: a human cadaver study. Clin Implant Dent Relat Res 11(2):113-9.

van Steenberghe D, Lekholm U, Bolender C, Folmer T, Henry P, Herrmann I, et al. (1990). Applicability of osseointegrated oral implants in the rehabilitation of partial edentulism: a prospective multicenter study on 558 fixtures. Int J Oral Maxillofac Implants 5(3):272-81.

Venter JC, Adams MD, Myers EW, Li PW, Mural RJ, Sutton GG, et al. (2001). The sequence of the human genome. Science 291(5507):1304-51.

Weyant RJ, Burt BA (1993). An assessment of survival rates and within-patient clustering of failures for endosseous oral implants. J Dent Res 72(1):2-8.

Wierzchos J, Falcioni T, Kiciak A, Wolinski J, Koczorowski R, Chomicki P, et al. (2008). Advances in the ultrastructural study of the implant-bone interface by

backscattered electron imaging. Micron 39(8):1363-70.
Williams DM (2011). Global oral health inequalities: the research agenda. Adv Dent Res 23(2):198-200.
Wilson TG, Jr., Nunn M (1999). The relationship between the interleukin-1 periodontal genotype and implant loss. Initial data. J Periodontol 70(7):724-9.
Winet H, Albrektsson T (1988). Wound healing in the bone chamber 1. Neoosteogenesis during transition from the repair to the regenerative phase in the rabbit tibial cortex. J Orthop Res 6(4):531-9.
Yamada Y, Ando F, Niino N, Shimokata H (2002). Association of a polymorphism of the matrix metalloproteinase-1 gene with bone mineral density. Matrix Biol 21(5):389-92.

5

Implant Complications

Mª Angeles Sánchez Garcés, Jaume Escoda-Francolí
and Cosme Gay-Escoda
*University of Barcelona, Faculty of Dentistry,
Spain*

1. Introduction

Implant treatment is regarded as a safe technique with high rates of success (Adell et al., 1981; Adell et al., 1990; Buser et al., 1997; Buser et al., 2000; Wennström et al., 2005). Nevertheless, it has, as every surgical procedure, several complications that can occur and that must be known in order to prevent or solve them. Implantology is an ever growing field that is reaching the practice of general dentists due to the simplification of technical procedures. Specialists in oral surgery now perform more demanding procedures, along with general dentists, they must pay special attention during the learning curve in order to avoid risks.

The osseointegration process is considered to be safe and durable by both patients and dentists, for this reason, implants are considered as the first option to treat almost all cases of complete or partial edentulism. Regarded as a problem free procedure, it´s demand is increasing. Despite the severe complications index is low, risk evaluation must be conducted systematically during the preoperatory stage based on clinical history, thorough exploration and if necessary consulting other specialists, dentists or physicians. Only by using a good work protocol, we can detect the local and systemic risk factors that could determine the success of the treatment and allow us to implement preventive measures if needed.

Parameters concerning systemic risks and their categories were well established in the 2nd ITI Consensus's Conference (Buser et al., 2000) there are also excellent systematic reviews (Bornstein et al., 2009). If our interest is to know about local factors that can negatively interfere in the success of the treatment or even cause serious local or general complications, we can consult several reviews or case reports (Cochran, et al., 2009).

It is mandatory to classify all those clinical complications that can arise in this chapter, so we should differentiate between two concepts: accidents and complications (Annibali et al, 2009).

- Accidents always happen during surgical procedures.
- Complications appear lately, once surgery is already performed. There are two kinds of complications, depending on the time they emerge: early and late.
- Failures occur when the professional and/or the patient do not obtain the desirable results.
- Iatrogenic acts are regarded as accidents, complications or failures caused by a deficient praxis of the professional.

The majority of problems that can arise in an implantology treatment are accidents, complications or iatrogenic errors, and are a consequence of an inadequate indication, poor quality or quantity of bone, an erroneous surgical technique, infections, lack of oral hygiene, smoking habit, systemic diseases that were poorly controlled, et cetera. Failures of implants normally occur once they are correctly osseointegrated, have developed an acceptable masticatory function and are the consequence of lost of bone support derived from a periimplantitis produced by the presence of bacterial plaque and/or overload.

Early complications can be included in the following group: infection, edema, ecchymosis and hematoma, emphysema, bleeding, dehiscence of the area and sensitive alterations; and in the group of late complications we can distinguish: mucoperiosteal flap perforations, maxillary sinusitis, mandibular fractures, loss of osseointegration, bone defects, periimplant lesions and infections (Annibali et al., 2009). Nevertheless, some of them, like bleeding, could appear at any moment during the treatment. We will not comment prosthetic complications or periimplantitis because they will be explained in other chapters.

Other authors classify complications as general or local, depending on their etiology. We prefer to describe these topics as they arise in the course of the treatment.

2. Intraoperative accidents

As we said previously, we define intraoperative accidents as those events that can occur during surgery. Their severity ranges from minimum to maximum values.

Among accidents we can include: Badly placed implants, bleeding episodes, lesions of soft tissues, and on an adjacent tooth, lack of primary stability, dehiscences and osseous fenestrations, implant displacement to maxillary sinus, mandibular fracture, broken instruments, aspiration or swallowing of instruments:

2.1 Malposition or angulation of an implant

It is advisable to assess the characteristics of the edentulous zone subject to rehabilitation using clinical and radiological CT, or cone beam CT imaging (Dreiseidler et al., 2009) at the time of devising an implantology treatment. Sometimes, this is not possible and the option then is to use short or tilted implants that can increase the availiable bone length by 50% when tilted aproximately 30° or" by avoiding anatomical structures (menton nerve, maxillary sinus).

A wrong planning that involves a malposition or an overangulation, would represent an obstacle for carrying out the prosthetic restoration, while it also would deteriorate long-term implant viability throughout the implant treatment.

Angulation, in the case of a single implant, increases tension forces between the implant and the bone. However, angulation of implants located at very distal positions reduce forces supported by the periimplant bone (Bellini et al., 2009).

In the event that, as a result of a negligence or bone deficit, an implant may have been placed with an angulation that makes it dysfunctional, it is suggested the use of a repositioning system that has yielded excellent results and which is based on the osteogenic distraction of a bone fragment containing the integrated implant (Gotta et al., 2008; Mendonca et al.,. 2008; Oduncuoglu et al., 2011). All of which improves esthetic effects, as well as the biomechanical behavior of the implant by correcting crown-root proportion, contour of soft tissues and the relation with neighboring teeth. The authors reported that the distraction rate is the usual value (1 mm per day) and the suggested consolidation period is 8 weeks, and confirm implant stability in time (Oduncuoglu et al., 2011).

2.2 Bleeding

Bleeding excessively is a common accident that can happen in some surgeries as a consequence of local-anatomical or systemic causes. Sometimes, patients are more prone to bleeding, since they are under a platelet antiaggregant treatment on a daily basis or have coagulation disorders (Garfunkel et al., 1999). This clinical situation is defined in the Group 2 of medical-systemic risk, where other disorders are also classified: irradiated patients (radiotherapy), those with Diabetes Mellitus (specially type I), patients with coagulation disorders (anticoagulated patients or those with haemostatic disorders) and severe smokers (Buser et al., 2000). Group I includes high risk patients: patients with serious systemic diseases (rheumatoid arthritis, osteomalacia, imperfect osteogenesis), immunodepressed (HIV, immunosupresory treatments), drug addicts (alcohol, etc.), unreliable patients (mental or psychological disorders).

Patients treated with anticoagulant medication usually have history of vascular or cardiac pathology (fibrillation, myocardial ischemia, valvular diseases or prosthesis, or thromboembolisms) (Lang et al., 2000). Probably, these patients would be included in the P1 or P2 risk classification groups of the ASA (American Society of Anesthesiology); P3 and P4 groups cannot undergo any surgical intervention until they are under treatment and included in a lower group. In general, the elderly are the majority of patients who need implantology solutions, which means that the probability of comorbidity is higher and therefore it is mandatory to know their medical history.

Generally, therapeutic options in these patients comprise two approaches: decrease or eliminate the anticoagulant therapy once patient and physician have assessed risks and benefits.

However, invasive treatments can be performed, as in the case of implantology procedures, without the interruption of medication and as long as values concerning International Normalized Ratio (INR) are > 4, and adequate hemostatic measures are followed and, at the same time, efforts are made to use atraumatic surgery techniques; in this situation, the risk of bleeding should be similar to that seen in healthy patients who are not under surgical outpatient treatment (Bacci et al., 2010). Anyway, it is advisable that any discontinuation of the anticoagulant therapy before any aggressive surgery (bone graft, extensive flaps, and maxillary sinus elevation) is discussed with the patient's physician, whereas patients should always be informed on the risk of procedures. It is recommendable to temporarily discontinue the anticoagulant treatment for 1-2 weeks, with previous physician's knowledge, when it is based on platelet antiaggregants (acetylsalicylic, acid, clopidogrel, ticlopidin, etc.) (Brennan et al., 2007; Sanz et al., 2009).

Data from recent studies also suggest that the risk of postoperative bleeding in this type of patients is low or almost negligible, while any bleeding complication can be handled with local intraoperative or postoperative measures suggested for dental extractions or dental implantations, where this is the standard procedure to assure local hemostasis (suture, compression, the use of hemostatic microfibrilar collagen gauzes, oxidized cellulose, re-absorbable fibrin, or mouth rinsing with 4,8% of tranexamic acid) (Bornstein et al., 2009; Napenas et al., 2009). In more severe cases of bleeding, it is proposed to use a nasal spray of desmopressin acetate (Nahlieli et al., 2011).

The same procedure could be useful in those cases where bleeding is caused by a mild variety of Von Willebrand disease (Garfunkel et al., 1999). The rest of coagulation pathologies resulting from a lack of coagulation factors should be managed in conjunction with the Hematology Department to settle the adequate preoperative therapeutic measures.

Patients should be advised, once intraoperative bleeding has been put under control and surgery procedures have concluded, to follow some postoperative instructions at home, which include the application of ice, compression, and the intake of a soft and cold diet; they also should be provided with a contact telephone in case of any emergency.

Other infrequent causes of bleeding are as follows: lesions in any sublingual, lingual, peri-mandibular, or submaxillary artery when performing surgeries in the lower and anterior area of totally edentulous patients who have a deficit in the quality and quantity of bone. Sometimes bleeding is less acute and can be perceived as a sublingual hematoma detected after few hours of performing the surgery (Mardinger et al., 2007). In other cases it involves an emergency that threatens patient's life and which requires a bimanual compression and subsequent referral of the patient to an hospital. A total of 18 clinical cases have been reported in the literature with this problem. Dubois et al. (Dubois et al, 2010) reported two cases that required a tracheotomy to solve an obstruction of the upper respiratory system due to a perforation of the lingual cortical that broke several sublingual vessels. Therefore, it is essential to do an exhaustive preoperative radiological exam that should include regular computerized tomography to appreciate the particular anatomy of each mandible, especially when placing implants in the premolar and canine area to avoid concavities and follow the major axis to the maximum (Dubois et al., 2010; Frenken et al., 2010). The onset of this complication is easily determined by a remarkable lingual protrusion caused by the swelling of the area below the tongue. In the event of a wound, it should be compressed by a ligature of the vessel involved as soon as it has been identified.

There is also a case report that describes an uncontrolled bleeding following a sinus lift procedure that caused a lesion on the artery that anastomoses the posterior superior alveolar artery with the infra-orbital one. Another case on a sinus lift procedure described an uncontrolled bleeding resulting from a lesion involving an artery that joined by anastomosis the posterior superior alveolar artery and the infra-orbital artery. Both arteries are branches of the maxillary artery that finds its way through an intraosseous passage located at a distance of 16.4 mm from the bone crest (Elian et al., 2005). The process of opening the lateral wall of the maxillary sinus, to connect the upper and lower osteotomies with vertical right and left osteotomies, can produce a lesion on this vessel that could lead to an intense and pulsating bleeding in a remote and difficult place to access (Testori et al., 2010). Lee (Lee, 2010) reported a case of a bleeding of an 8,1 mm artery above the alveolar crest that was finally controlled (after multiple attempts of compression and using bone wax) with the administration of local anesthesia and vasoconstrictor agents, as well as the application of gauzes soaked in bovine thrombin to help in the last coagulation process of transforming fibrinogen into fibrin. Once again, it is strongly recommended to carry out an exhaustive tomography study of this area before performing this surgical technique.

2.3 Soft tissue lesions

A series of lesions can occur in soft tissues, such as burn lesions on the labial mucosa resulting from overheating of the hand piece head, flap tear due to an excessive traction or as a consequence of an incorrect use of instruments or any abrupt movement by the patient or the surgeon, among other causes (Ozcelik et al., 2005). These lesion can be mostly avoided through a careful management of tissues or by sedating the patient and thus prevent the occurrence of stress situations for both surgeon and patient.

2.4 Lesions of adjacent teeth

The malposition of an implant may lead to the lesion of an adjacent tooth, where this involves a lesion on the radicular surface or the root apex and a subsequent post-operative pulpitis, or periodontitis, that must be treated, in the majority of cases, by endodontic means, while sometimes it involves the non-integration of the implant because of the inflammation. It is of the utmost interest to study the axis of those teeth delimiting the edentulous space to be rehabilitated with implants to decide, before surgery, implant axis and thus choose the most convenient one, or reduce its length to curb its convergence and thus prevent this type of dental iatrogenic lesions. On some other occasions, the inflammatory-infectious origin in the apical zone is a tooth adjacent to the implant and this is especially due to the proximity of the tooth to the implant and to the time elapsed since the endodontic procedure on the tooth was performed, so the risk of a retrograde periimplantitis increases when the distance between tooth and implant apexes is shorter and when the lapse of time between the endodontic procedure and the implantation is also shorter (Quirynen et al., 2005; Tozum et al., 2006; Zhou et al., 2009).

2.5 Lack of primary stability

Primary stability is determined by bone density and cortical bone thickness, a fact that explains why it is easier to obtain a better stability in mandibular implants than in maxillary ones (Seong et al., 2009) as it entails preparing the implant bed (incorrect tapping, too-wide ostectomy) or in those cases in which the implant is immediately placed after an exodontic procedure (Becker et al., 2011; Cooper, 2010) and becomes manifest by insertion torque values, so a low insertion torque value (<10Ncm) will determine a higher risk of osseointegration failure (type bone IV), whereas a too-high torque value (>45Ncm) could lead to a bone compression which would result in a bone necrosis (type bone I), and in an osseointegration failure (Neugebauer et al., 2009).

Cooper (Cooper, 2010) described, in a study on 1084 implants, that there was a 6.43-fold lower risk of primary implant stability failure in the anterior mandible than in other locations. The maxilla had a 2.7-fold higher risk of primary stability failure versus the mandible. Females had a 1.54 higher risk of primary implant stability failure versus men; implants less than 15 mm in length had a 1.49-fold higher risk of primary implant stability failure versus longer implants.

Rough surfaces, a cone design of implants, and the use of osteotomes in the management of the implant bed can increase primary stability on low-quality bones (Javed et al., 2011; Padmanabhan & Gupta, 2010). When it is not possible to implement the aforementioned solutions, it would then be advisable to replace the unstable implant for a rescue implant, with a wider diameter and/or a longer length, or wait, as a final resort, 6-8 weeks before a surgical re-intervention.

2.6 Dehiscences and fenestrations

Osseous dehiscences and fenestrations in the vestibular cortical bone during the placement of implants constitute a risk factor for the healing process of periimplant tissues (fig. 1). In these cases, bone regeneration in parallel with implant placement is therefore mandatory and can be achieved using different materials, such as autologous, allogenic or xenolog bone, or phosphocalcium materials, such as hydroxypatite or tricalcium phosphate, in conjunction with non-reabsorbable or reabsorbable membranes (Becker et al., 2009; Jung et al., 2009; Oh et al., 2003; Rosen & Reynols, 2001; Mayfield et al., 1997), in addition to associated growing factors, or in combination with different materials (Hassan, 2009.)

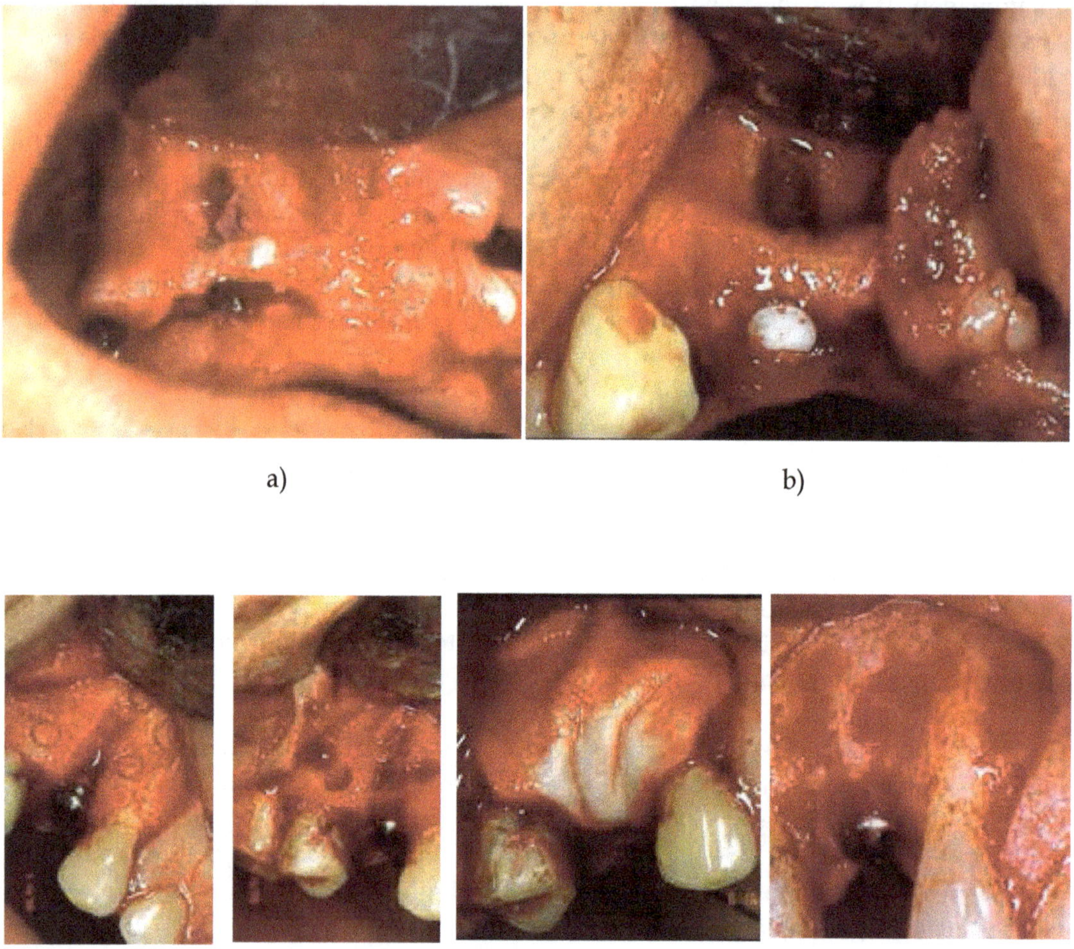

a) b)

c) d) e) f)

Fig. 1. (a, b) Osseous fenestration. (c) Osseous dehiscence. (d) Autologous bone chips. (e) Collagen membrane. (f) Clinical result at 5 months.

Results are subject to the magnitude and morphology of the defect to be regenerated, the stability of both the material and the membrane, the maintenance of the space, the reabsorption time of the membrane, on the assumption that it is reabsorbable since its efficiency, or that concerning the fenestration of non-reabsorbable membranes (it could trigger the onset of an infection). All these factors determine the final results (fig. 2).

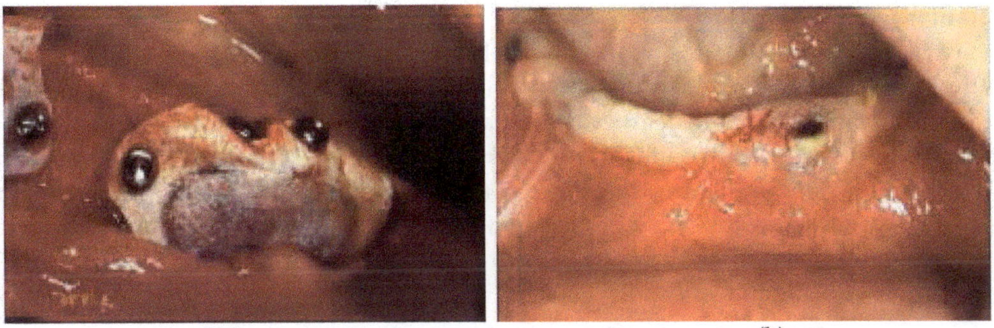

(a) (b)

Fig. 2. (a) PTFE membrane covering a bone defect. (b) Membrane fenestration at 15 days control.

These accidents happen when implants are placed in a prosthesis-guided axis-position, but even though guided bone regeneration principles may have been followed, the main problem lays in a good wound-closure that may allow a primary scarring. It is necessary for the design, and the management and release of the flap to allow a wider extension, and thus achieve a better cover and tension-free surgical site (Hur et al., 2010). Smoker and diabetic patients have an added risk factor since scarring is more difficult and this can significantly jeopardize results, since the success of bone regeneration in non-smokers may reach 95% compared to 65% in those who smoke; furthermore, inflammation and exposure of membranes is greater (Garg, 2010; Abt, 2009; Cochran et al., 2009; Lindfors et al., 2010) (Fig. 3).

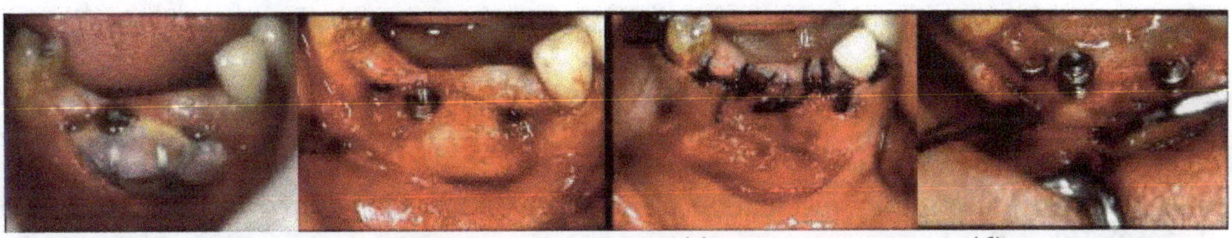

a) (b) (c) (d)

Fig. 3. (a) Wound dehiscence in a GBR with PTFEe Ti reinforced at 5 weeks of maintenance. (b) Image after the membrane was retrieved. (c) Bipedicular flap covering the new tissue. (d) Clinical result after 5 months.

Osseous dehiscences and bone fenestrations can pass unnoticed in those cases when an implant is immediately placed following an exodontic procedure or a transmucosal flapless surgery (Steigmann, 2008); so, as to values concerning probing depth and insertion level, results are less favorable when compared with implants placed in integral alveolar crests (Siciliano et al., 2009). This risk should be prevented by a correct exploration of the alveolus before inserting the implant (Nahlieli et al., 2011).

It is not recommendable to carry out guided bone regeneration (GBR) during the intra-operative period when the exposed surface of the implant is, in the event of dehiscence, equal or greater than 2/3 of its length.

Consequences could be more severe in the event of perforating the lingual cortical layer of the inferior jawbone in the inter-mental region, as abovementioned, so it is necessary to adequately arrange the implant axis in this situation and in all possible situations. This situation, though, could be prevented by requesting CT imaging studies (Parnia et al., 2010).

2.7 Implant displacement

The invasion of the maxillary sinus by an implant can occur during or after the surgery as a result of an insufficient primary stability. It has been reported a case of an implant which had been implanted 9 months earlier during a maxillary sinus lift surgery, and which was found inside the sinus only a few days after having placed the fixture (Chappuis et al., 2009). Therefore, any implant could undergo a displacement at any time after having been fixed with a cover screw (osseointegration period), even avoiding regenerative techniques in a spontaneous and asymptomatic way, or even afterwards, at the time of connecting the healing abutment (Ridaura-Ruiz et al., 2009) (Fig. 4).

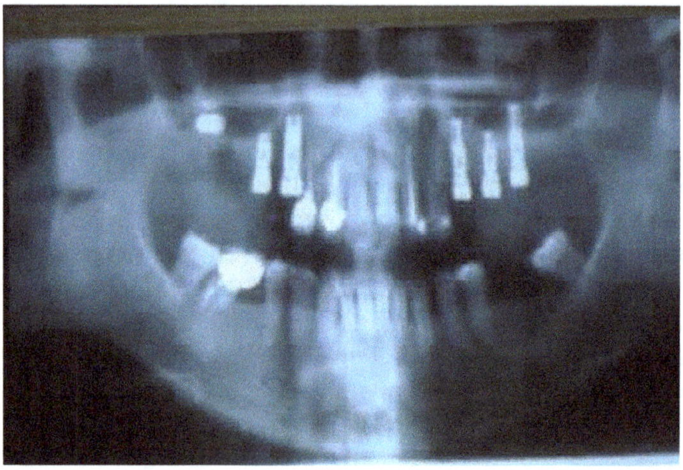

Fig. 4. Implant displaced within the course of a second stage surgery.

In general, implant displacements occur sometimes after an implant placement because there is an absence or loss of osseointegration and, therefore, of stability (low osseous density around it). Nevertheless, some authors report the displacement of implants into the maxillary sinus during their installation (Chappuis et al., 2009; Felisati et al., 2007; Haben et al., 2003). When this happens, the implant remains, in almost all the cases, lodged inside the sinus (Chappuis et al, 2009; Borgonovo et al, 2010), and can be removed a few days later by opening the lateral wall of the maxillary sinus (Haben et al., 2003) (Fig. 5), or by endoscopic via through a nasal window; a process that allows a considerable good access to the zone and a lower postoperative morbidity than when it is performed intraorally (Haben et al., 2003; Felisati et al., 2007; Galindo et al., 2005; Ramotar et al., 2010).

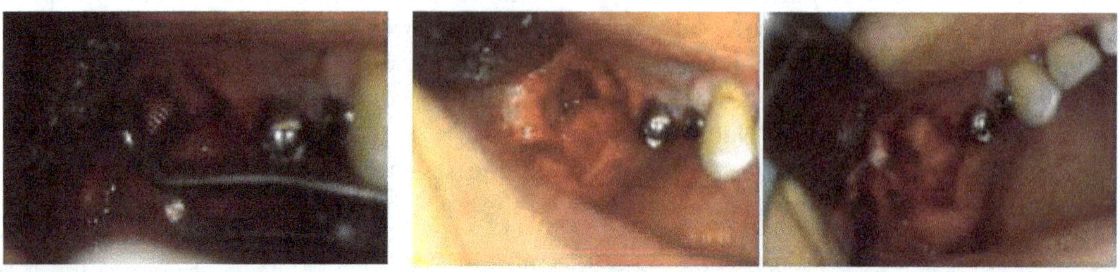

a) (b) (c)

Fig. 5. (a) Implant retrieval through a lateral window. (b) Oro-antral communication. (c) Membrane covering the window.

In these intra- or postoperative cases, authors recommend the immediate removal of the implant lodged in the maxillary sinus (Ramotar et al., 2010; Galindo et al., 2005; Felisati et al., 2007; Haben et al., 2003) through an intraoral or trans-nasal via that will prevent further associated complications; although it is in general asymptomatic condition, most patients suffer from a marked sinusitis. Another complication, in addition to the acute or chronic sinusitis, is the implant intrusion that occurs when it is not removed during its migration Felisati et al. and Haben et al. (Felisati et al., 2007; Haben et al., 2003) reported two cases of intrusions in which they found that two fixations had displaced from the maxillary sinus into the sphenoidal and ethmoidal sinuses, respectively, when they tried to remove them; the solution, though, should be to use an endoscopic nasal via. There is also a particular case describing a migration that ended in the orbital floor (Griffa et al., 2010) in its way from the maxillary sinus, and after an attempt to install a fixture in the alveolar bone. The article describes how the authors tried to aspirate the implant, which had penetrated deep into the zone and perforated the thin cortical bone of the orbital floor to end up lodged between the bone and the inferior rectus orbital muscle causing pain and diplopia. It was finally removed with general anesthesia and nasal endoscopy (Fig. 6).

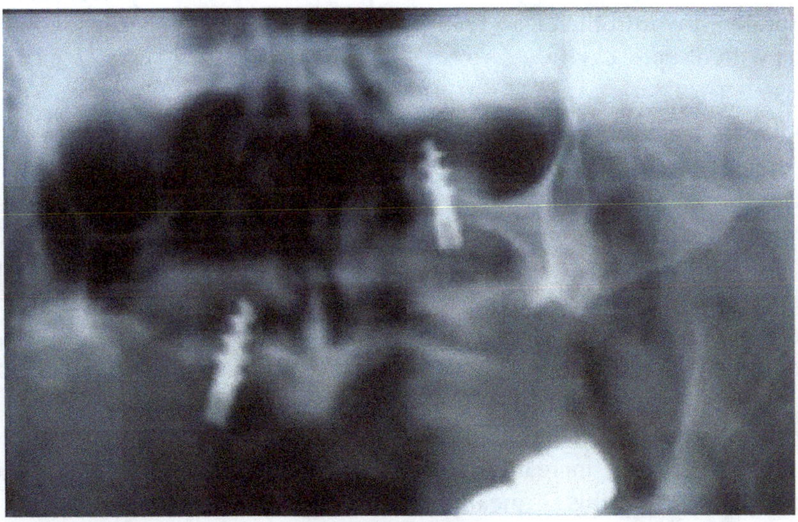

Fig. 6. Image of an implant migrated to the orbital floor.

To conclude, the positioning of an implant into the sinus is an infrequent event that does rarely occur during the placement of dental fixtures, or in the second phase. It is usually detected in the postoperative period and is in general ascribed to a lack of primary stability of the implant (a poor bone quality) (fig. 7). This complication could be prevented with an accurate surgical technique that would include using osteotomes to prepare the implant beds or a drill with a smaller diameter to that of the fixture, or using implants with a conical compressive form. If this complication finally occurs, it must be solved immediately and carefully in order to avoid any migration of this foreign body to a more harmful anatomical space.

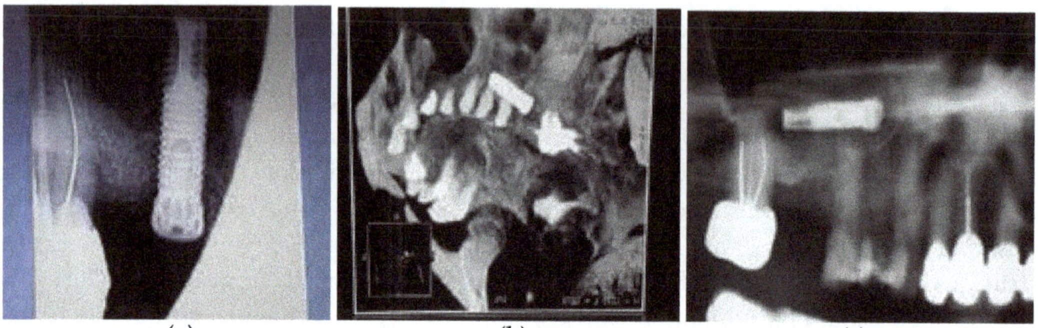

(a) (b) (c)

Fig. 7. (a) Implant installed (Summer's technique). (b) Control CT Scan after displacement and before second stage surgery. (c) Change of position.

Finally, it is worth mentioning a case report describing the migration of a zygomatic implant to the cranial fossa. This is a major complication that can end up with a cerebral lesion or an infection that must be prevented with a preoperative and postoperative three-dimensional radiographic study (Reychler & Olszewski, 2010).

There are no publications about cases where the cortical nasal floor ended up perforated and the implant has subsequent migrated to this cavity. The fact of anchoring the fixture bicortically does not constitute any risk as long as the mucosa is preserved, whereas if it became perforated it would then lead to an infection complication because it would enable a direct contact with a septic cavity.

2.8 Mandibular fracture

Mandibular fracture, during implant placement, is associated with atrophic mandibles. The central area of the mandible has a greater risk for this complication because it has a poor vascular irrigation, which sometimes makes very difficult for the bone and periosteum to provide enough blood for the healing process derived from an implant placement (Chrcanovic & Custodio, 2009). The bone in this area is usually sclerotic and undergoes severe resorption as a consequence of a large period of edentulism and also as a result of the pressure exerted by the prosthesis, which does accelerate the process. Technically, it is difficult to perform implant perforations in this zone without running the risk of overheating the surrounding bone; moreover, sometimes surgeons resort to bi-corticalized implants in this area, which increases the risk of a mandibular fracture, so patients should be informed before starting this surgical procedure (fig. 8).

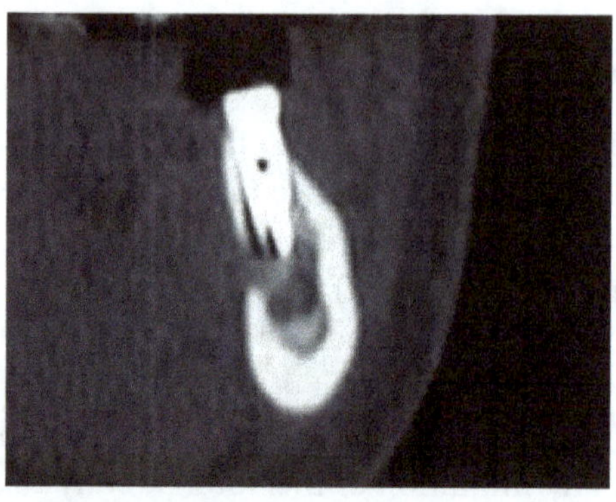

Fig. 8. Perforation of the lingual cortical during drilling.

It is an infrequent complication that could start during surgery and subsequently evolve to a serious complication if, as Oh et al. report (Oh et al., 2010), the implant causes an infection when it becomes displaced from the fracture line to a sub-mandibular space.
The main treatment consists in the reduction and stabilization of the fracture with titanium miniplates (Oh et al., 2010; Tiwana et al., 2009), or resorbable miniplates. Nevertheless, other authors report less atraumatic techniques such as splinting implants with a Dolder bar to reduce and immobilize the fracture (Romanos, 2009).
Chrcanovic and Custodio (Chrcanovic & Custodio, 2009) suggest, in order to prevent this complication in the management of thin mandibular alveolar crests, to increase width by performing bone grafts beforehand and through an accurate tomography imaging study to calculate these parameters with precision.
A case of a fracture and displacement of part of the lingual mandible cortical was reported, as a result of withdrawing a mono-cortical bone graft from the chin. The surgical procurement of a mono-cortical bone graft from the chin resulted in the fracture and displacement of part of the lingual mandibular cortical bone (Cordaro et al., 2004); it was decided not to perform any re-intervention due the lack of patient symptomatology.

2.9 Neurosensory impairment

Nerve lesions are both an intraoperative accident and a postoperative complication that can affect the infra-orbitary nerve, the inferior alveolar nerve, or its menton branch and the lingual nerve. Neurosensory impairment may occur at any time during implant surgery, including anesthesia administration, incision, raising a flap, as well separating it too tightly, during osteotomy preparation, bone augmentation, implant placement, suturing or any soft tissue swelling after surgery (Misch & Resnik, 2010) (Fig. 9). These complications have a low incidence (reported between 0%-44%) (Misch & Resnik, 2010). Symptomatology is of a large variety and depends on the severity of the axonal damage.

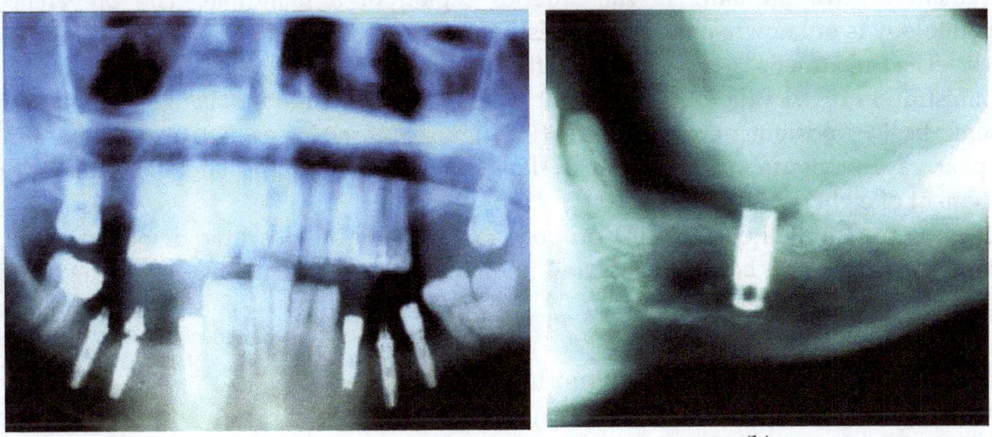

a) (b)

Fig. 9. (a, b). Several implants in contact to the Inferior Alveolar nerve in patients with postoperative paresthesia.

The complication could manifest as a paresthesia when the lesion is due to a nerve compression, or a minor stiffening of nerve fibers, without sectioning any of them (neuropraxia). Dysesthesia may occur in cases of nerve compression, traction, partial crush or stretching (axonotmesis) of nerve fibers with different intensities. Hypoesthesia or hyperesthesia may be caused by extreme stretching, complete crush and direct trauma on nerve fibers (neurotmesis); anesthesia and pain appear as consequence of a complete nerve section.

A very useful review about lesions and treatment algorithms may be found in a report published by Misch and Resnik (Misch & Resnik, 2010). Treatments depend on the type of injury. The implant should be removed as soon as possible to avoid compression when radiological imaging reveals there is too much proximity between the implant and a nerve. Treatment with corticosteroids and non-steroidal anti-inflammatory drugs are indicated to control inflammatory reactions that provoke nervous compression. It seems that the topical application of dexamethasone (4 mg/ml) for 1 or 2 minutes enhances recovery, and when it is administered orally and in high doses within one week of injury, it has have shown to inhibit axon sprouting centrally and ectopic discharges from injured axons, and prevention of neuroma formation (Misch & Resnik, 2010).

An intraoperative nerve section requires microsurgery techniques to reestablish nerve continuity. Nerves can be partially or completely damaged, and this aspect determines the prognostic of recovering the sensibility completely. Clinically, the evaluation of the neurosensorial loss should be checked at different moments to determine with precision the evolution of the lesion and, if necessary, refer the patient to a neurosurgery specialist (Misch & Resnik, 2010; Greenstein et al., 2008). Hegedus et al. (Hegedus et al., 2006) propose an evaluation of the subjective symptoms and carry out an exhaustive neurosensory exploration of the patient's affected area to document all the written data referring this complication and thus evaluate patient's evolution. It is recommendable to resort to microsurgery if, after four months, patient's situation has not improved, pain persists and there is a remarkable loss of sensitivity.

Another nervous lesion could manifest in the form of an idiopathic facial pain, as the case reported by Queral-Godoy et al. (Queral-Godoy et al., 2006), on a lesion subsequent to the placement of two implants in the anterior region of a mandible. The prevalence in implantology is unknown, although it is estimated to be between 3-6% of all the endodontic cases. The treatment suggested by these authors should basically comprise the administration of tricyclic antidepressant drugs, amitriptyline and benzodiazepines on a chronic basis. Rodriguez-Lozano et al. (Rodriguez-Lozano et al., 2010) describe another peculiar case of neuropathic pain that showed up eight months later after the surgical placement of eight dental fixtures.

Nahlieli et al (Nahlieli et al., 2011) propose to use a mini-endoscopic device to check the bottom of the surgical bed to detect any possible osseous defect; this technique could be interesting to prevent nervous lesions.

2.10 Aspiration and swallowing of instruments

When an accident involves the aspiration (Pingarron et al., 2010) or swallowing (Welcker et al., 2005; Worthington,. 1996) of an instrument (burs, screwdrivers, covering screws or healing abutments), it can become a vital emergency if the instrument has entered the airways. If the object has not been discharged from the respiratory track, it should then be necessary to perform a bronchoscopy. A special case describes the need to even perform a tracheotomy in a similar situation; the patient subsequently suffered a pneumothorax and a pleural effusion. Authors recommend general anesthesia in those cases in which there is the suspicion of any difficulty in the course of the procedure.

For daily surgeries, it is strongly recommended to tie all tiny and slippery instruments regularly used during the procedure with silk ligatures so as to quickly recover them if they fall from the operator's hands, or else use a rubber dam (Bergermann et al., 1992).
In the event an object entered the digestive system, it would require carrying out a series of post-operative controls with the help of radiological imaging. A rich diet in fiber will also help solve this problem sooner. A gastroscopy or colonoscopy could also be mandatory in those cases in which the object remains stationery in the intestinal tract, while a proper medical follow-up will help see any progress of the object, or objects, through the digestive tract (Fig. 10). This type of accidents can occur in any of the sequences of the implant treatment.

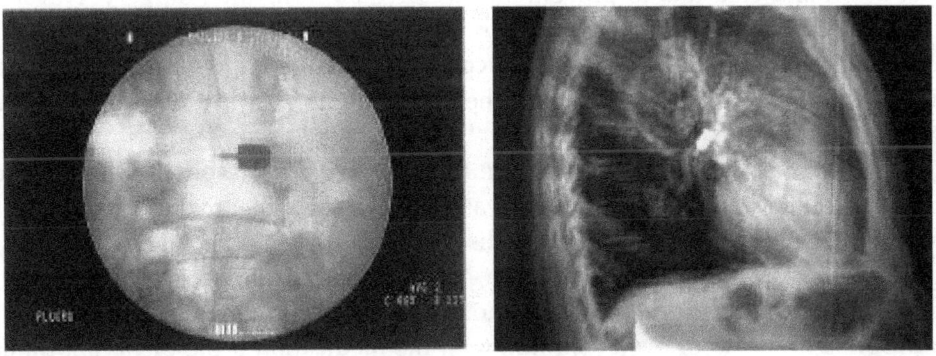

a) (b)

Fig. 10. (a) Images of a screw driver in the digestive tract. (b) Screw driver into pulmonary tissue.

3. Early and late complications

Early complications include: implant fracture, infection, edema, ecchymosis and hematoma, emphysema, bleeding, soft tissue dehiscence of the area and sensitive alterations. As to late complications we can distinguish: mucoperiosteal flap perforations, maxillary sinusitis, mandibular fractures, loss of osseointegration, periimplantitis (Annibali et al., 2009). Most of the complications described in this chapter, though, may occur early, or lately, or even be the consequence of a surgical accident or an iatrogenic act.

3.1 Edema

Swelling can appear after a surgical intervention, although it is more noticeable 24 hours after performing it. It can lead to trismus, lack of hygiene in the wound and discomfort to the patient. It normally decreases with time, and can easily vanish after a few days. Wide flaps, bone regenerating techniques, and surgery time are factors that trigger the occurrence of edemas and patient's susceptibility. The occurrence of edemas, and the need of analgesic and anti-inflammatory drugs is, in a statistically significant way, lower in guided flapless surgery, as can be seen in under-control studies (Arisan et al., 2010; Cannizzaro et ala., 2008), even in immediate implants after exodontic procedures (Cannizzaro et al., 2007) and immediately loaded implants (Cannizzaro et al., 2007; Cannizzaro et al., 2008; Merli et al., 2008; Arisan et al., 2010); however, a careful management of tissues, using non-excessive tension and bone-supported retrievers can minimize this effect along with the use of a cold pack, and non-steroid anti-inflammatories drugs; although in the event of a complex postop, the administration of corticosteroids during a short period of time can be very helpful. Before the suspicion that the inflammation could compress any nervous structure, corticosteroids are crucial to minimize the risk of lesions (Misch & Resnik, 2010).

3.2 Bleeding, ecchymosis and hematoma

Low-intensity bleeding is a frequent complication that must be solved as soon as possible, and it generally occurs on the basis of the surgical extension of the surgical procedure and the general condition of the patient. We recommend suturing all surgical wounds and compressing the zone with gauzes, as well as apply a cold pack, have physical rest, and the intake of a soft and cold diet to prevent an excessive bleeding after surgery. Nevertheless, the best method to avoid this problem is to write up a complete medical report from data provided by the patient's physician to collect any information on blood disorders. Sometimes we have to request a complete hemogram with coagulation tests to make clear the situation of a specific patient.

There are three main anticoagulants: coumarin, heparin and aspirin. Usually, they are prescribed to treat a number of cardiac or vascular disorders that include atrial fibrillation, ischemic cardiac disease, cardiac valvular disease, prosthetic cardiac valves, post-MI, deep venous thrombosis, pulmonary embolism, cerebrovascular accident, and many other disorders. Therefore, antiaggregant medication could be discontinued if the physician thinks it is appropriate to do so or even continue with the medication if the physician thinks that bleeding could be handled with local hemostatic measures, as in the case when the patient is taking aspirins.

Hematomas and ecchymosis are the result of a surgery procedure and are usually proportional to the magnitude of the intervention. Blood collected under the mucosa and skin are known as bruises and generally cause a feeling of esthetical discomfort to patients, but in some days reabsorption occurs and solves the disgusting aspect of the zone and surroundings (because coagulated blood frequently moves through the anatomy in a descendent trajectory)(fig. 11).

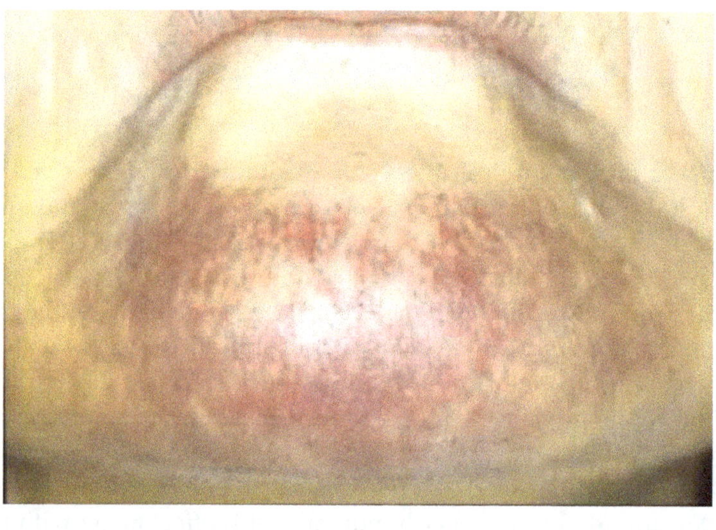

Fig. 11. Ecchymosis are the result of a intermental surgery procedure.

3.3 Emphysema

Tissue emphysema is one of these early complications caused by inadvertent insufflation propulsion of air into tissues under skin or mucous membranes, air from a high-speed handpiece, an air/water syringe, an air polishing unit or an air abrasive device can be projected into a sulcus, surgical wound, or a laceration in the mouth (Liebenberg & Crawford, 1997); it is a rare complication, though it can lead to severe consequences (McKenzie & Rosenberg, 2009). The use of abrasive air in implantology, or a laser device as a way to remove residues from an implant surface, has been suggested in the treatment of periimplantitis to facilitate decontamination. The chance for the occurrence of emphysema process during this cleansing maneuver is higher than that of the surgical process since the device uses mechanical motors. This complication occurs when pressurized-air devises are used to remove periodontal and peri-implantation calculi in the maintenance period, as Bergendal et al. (Bergendal et al., 1990) report in a case concerning an acute subcutaneous emphysema.

The air can follow facial planes and create a unilateral enlargement of the fascial and/or sub-mandibular regions. The region with a swelling does normally produce a crackling sensation (crepitation on palpation) as the gas is pushed through the tissue. The crackling sound is pathognomonic of tissue emphysemas, even when discomfort is not reported.

These complications could be avoided by using a sterile water jet handpiece with retrograde air insufflation when, besides an associated implantology surgical process, it is necessary to dry a surface (periodontal treatment, laser, shutting, periapical surgery on an adjacent tooth). The use of air abrasives directed on the sulcus should be avoided as well as its use on inflamed tissues with friable margins, so manual curettage is the best option.

Treatment usually consists on prescribing antibiotics and a mild analgesic therapy, close observation, saline rinses, light massage, apply heat packs and provide mental comfort to patients. The problem does normally solve in 3-10 days.

3.4 Mucosal dehiscence

This is a soft tissue complication that can develop infections in the surgical area and implant and/or graft failures that can lead to unfortunate esthetic results. As a rule, surgical wound dehiscences are associated with patients that have scarring problems due to a poor-quality mucosa (thin biotype, traumatized or cicatricial type), heavy smokers, patients treated with corticosteroids, diabetics, or irradiated patients (Lee & Thiele, 2010) (fig. 12). Another factor leading to surgical wound dehiscence is flap closure under tension, for it has been established that a higher tension causes a more frequent onset of these complications (Lee & Thiele, 2010).

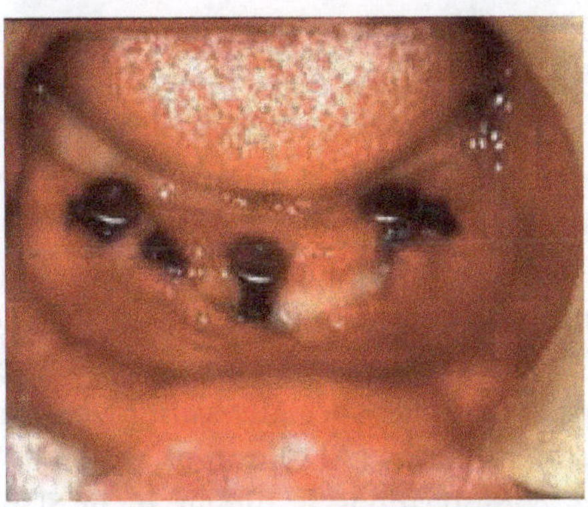

Fig. 12. Wound dehiscence at one week post surgery in a diabetic patient with oral candidiasis.

Many different solutions have been suggested to prevent dehiscence, in addition to flap management, to guarantee the success of bone regeneration (Park & Wang, 2007)(fig. 13). A study by Torres et al. established the efficacy of using platelet-rich plasma (PRP) on titanium meshes to prevent the occurrence dehiscences in all the cases described (Torres et al., 2010).

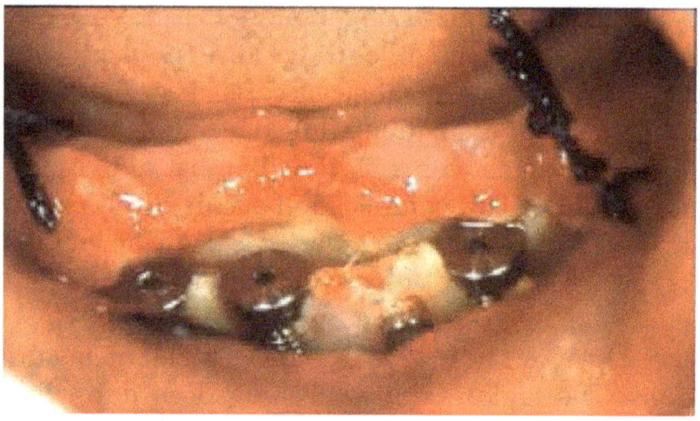

Fig. 13. Wound dehiscence in a case of bone regeneration with collagen membrane (one week control).

The use of free connective tissue grafts may be highly useful for both guaranteeing the closure of the wound and the enlargement of the mucosa thickness around implants, all of which allows better esthetical results in the long run as well as the maintenance of periimplant health (Speroni et al., 2010; Stimmelmayr et al., 2010). El Chaar describes the good results observed in the use of palatal pedicle connective tissue grafts to facilitate the primary closure of a post-exodontic alveolus (El Chaar, 2010), or an acellular dermal matrix interposed between the lap and the subjacent bone (Taylor et al., 2010; Park, 2006).
The use of dense politetraphluoroethilene (d-PTFE) membranes has been suggested to cover the regeneration zones; the benefit of this material resides in that it does not need to be completely covered by the flap since its internal surface does not become contaminated, which is an advantage over other type of membranes (Barber et al., 2007).
A mucosal dehiscence associated with a sinus lift technique represents an aggravating factor that can lead to an infection of the graft material, an acute sinusitis, or an oroantral fistula (Watzak et al., 2005). The management of these abnormal tracts is, depending on the size, laborious and requires well-designed flaps. The use of mono-cortical grafts of intraoral origin (Watzak et al., 2005) or PRP associated with a mucogingival plastia has also been suggested (DePoi et al., 2007).

3.5 Implant fracture

Fracture of prosthetic retaining screws is more common than implant fracture and it is normally due to a metal fatigue following an overload of materials (Al Jabbari et al, 2008). An implant fracture seems to be an infrequent complication (among 0,2 y 1,5% of cases) (Eckert et al., 2000) that could be ascribed to different reasons: defects in the implant design or materials used in their construction, a non-passive union between the implant and the prosthesis or by mechanical overload, specially cantilevers in fixed prostheses, occlusal overload or/ and parafunctional habits (Al Quran et al., 2009; Mendonca et al., 2009) (fig. 14). The incidence of these complications is higher in implants supporting fixed partial prosthesis than in complete edentulous patients.

This complication is frequently managed by the removal of the implant and its replacement by another one (Cardoso Lde et al., 2010; Gargallo-Albiol et al., 2008) (fig. 15); nevertheless, some cases describe the use of the remnant part of the dental fixture to rebuild a new prosthesis when is possible (Mendonca et al., 2009).

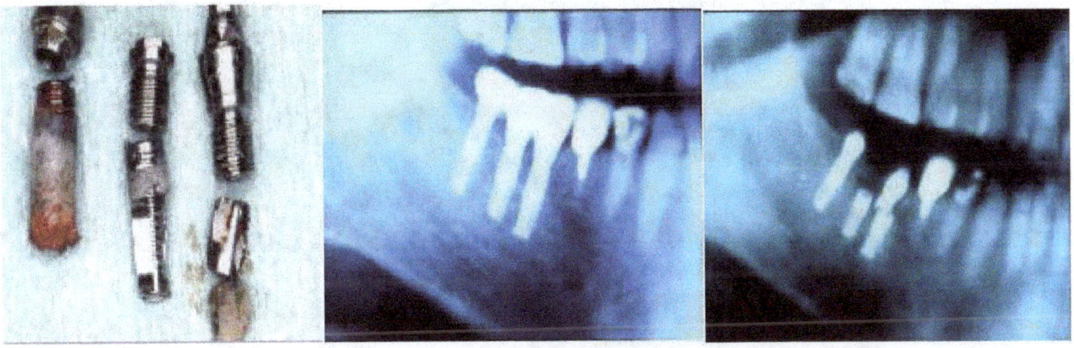

(a) (b) (c)

Fig. 14. (a) Implants retrieved in molar region in a patient with parafunctional habit. (b) Implant rehabilitation). (c) Implants fractured.

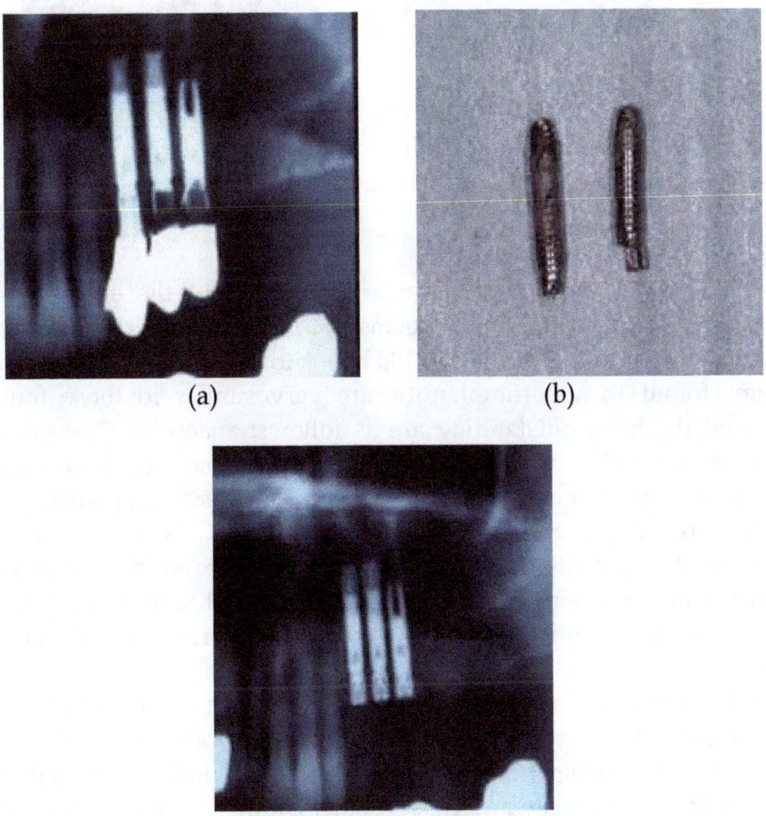

(a) (b)

(c)

Fig. 15. (a) Implant fractured in maxillary posterior region. (b) Implants retrieved. (c) Substitution for a wider diameter in the same surgery.

More than 80% of factures are located in the molar and premolar regions, and most of them occur 3-4 years after being loaded (Kohal et al., 2010; Gargallo-Albiol et al., 2008) (fig. 16).

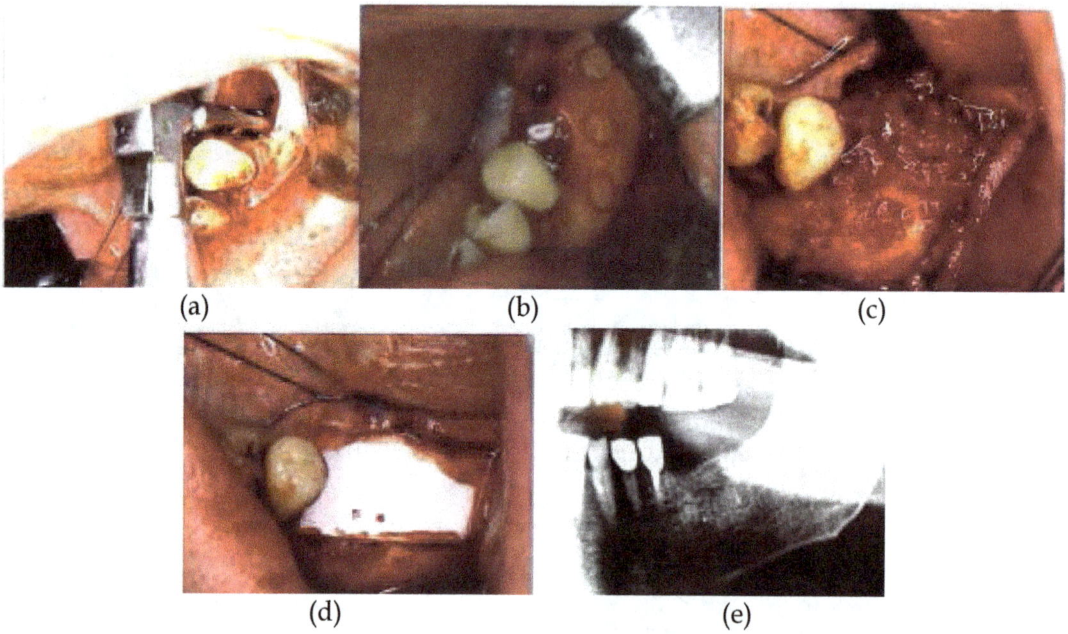

Fig. 16. Sequence of treatment of an implant fractured. (a) Retrieval with a trephine. (b) Bone harvesting for osseous regeneration. (c) Filling of the osseous defect. (d) Collagen membrane. (e) Image of the control 6 months later.

3.6 Infection

Infection of the implant is a common cause of failure but the efficacy of prophylactic antibiotics for dental implant placement seems not influence in risk of implant failure and other complications (Esposito et al., 2010a; 180 Esposito et al., 2010b; Anitua et al., 2009).

Microorganisms found in a periimplantitis are very similar to those found in chronic periodontitis, and the most outstanding are as follows: anaerobic Gram negative bacillus (Porphyromonas gingivalis and Prevotella intermedia), anaerobic Gram negative coccus (Veillonella spp) and the spiroquettes, such as Treponema denticola (Sanchez-Garces & Gay-Escoda, 2004). Nowadays, antibiotics are not accepted as the main treatment for periimplantitis, as it is considered a disease with a bad prognosis and predictability that formerly required implant removal (Pye et al., 2009) (fig. 17). This condition requires, on account of its importance and frequency, it own a chapter, so it will not be extensively developed here.

A recent complication detected in the last years is the use of oral bisphosphonates. This medication is broadly used to treat osteoporosis, bones diseases, such as Paget's disease, and osseous metastasis in malign neoplasias. The most common presentations of oral bisphosphonates are Alendronate and Risedronate. On the one hand, they are mainly used for treating osteoporosis and, whereas they curiously are helpful for the long-term stability of the implant, they generate a higher amount of quality bone around the implant surface. This has already been shown in several clinical trials, although a larger amount of patients is needed to assure these results (Aspenberg, 2009). In other hand Zahid et al. observed in retrospective radiographic study those patients who take BP are at greater risk of implant failure or thread exposure (Zahid et al., 2010).

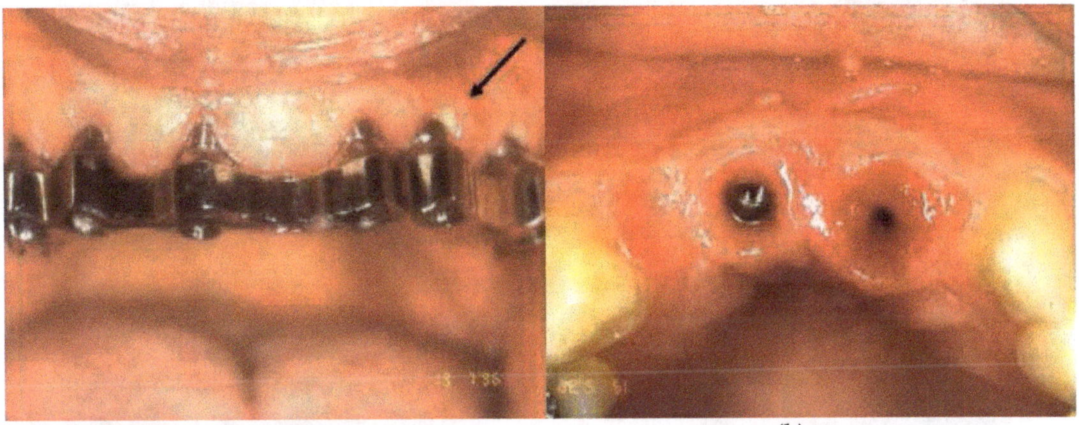

a) (b)

Fig. 17. (a) Image of periimplantitis and suppuration (arrow). (b) Image of mucositis.

On the other hand, this benefit soon disappears because these drugs can cause osteochemonecrosis of the jaws during the postoperative healing period once the implant has been placed. It has been shown that the length of the medication period is related to the onset and severity of this complication, although more investigation is needed to understand the exact mechanism, while a worldwide consensus is also necessary to prevent the risk posed by osteochemonecrosis after a surgical implant placement. The use of a biochemical marker of bone metabolism as CTX could help to predict the risk in some cases (Lee & Suzuki, 2009). An article on seven osteochemonecrosis cases treated with low and medium doses of bisphosphonates (oral and venous administration) concluded that it is necessary a strict treatment protocol to obtain good results. The treatment suggested consists in a deep surgical debridement of all the necrotic tissues before performing a regularization procedure on the edge of the bone crest, as well as a primary closure of the wound, avoiding dead spaces (fig. 18). An intravenous antimicrobial therapy should be established for a week to be followed by the oral intake of the drug for another three weeks (Alons et al., 2009). There are at present ten cases in the literature on the use of oral bisphosphonates that caused osteonecrosis. Symptomatology is not well defined at the early stages of this condition, so gammagraphy, using Technetium-99 methylene diphosphonate, ((99)Tc(m)-MDP) could be helpful to diagnose it. In those patients treated with bisphosphonates, controls must be frequent and rigorous and periimplantary hygiene must be carefully performed.

Osteomyelitis (OM) is another scarcely frequent osseous complication of the maxillae. OM is currently related to maxillary bone infections mainly caused by: odontogenic primary infections, after surgical oral procedures (removal of tooth and implant placement); when they are secondary to osteoradionecrosis, or any other osteochemonecrosis processes, or in a postoperative/posttraumatic process.

A retrospective study on 46 patients with OM of the mandible assessed the type of antimicrobial treatments used and the level of resistance against them. Streptococcus viridans

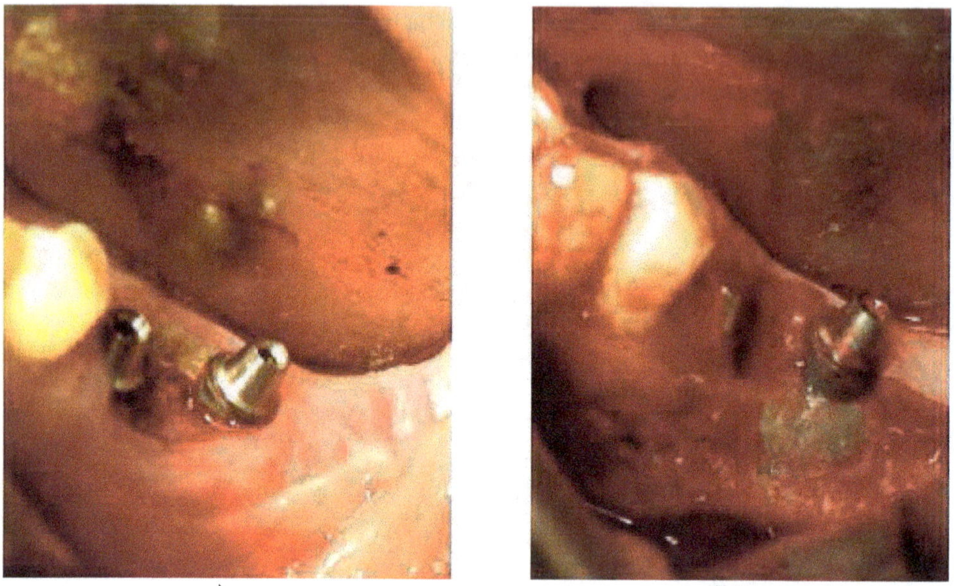

a) (b)

Fig. 18. (a) Osteonecrosis in a patient treated with biphosphonates i.v. clinical image. (b) Surgical debridement.

was the most frequent pathogen, 81% were sensible to penicillin and 96% to fluoroquinolone; however, only 11.5% were sensitive to clindamycin. Therefore, it was suggested that the drug of choice against maxillae OM should be antimicrobials of the beta-lactam family. As to patients allergic to penicillin, the best option is the combination of fluoroquinolones and rifampicin, or clindamycin, for a better anaerobic coverage (Pigrau et al., 2009).

4. Conclusions

The vast majority of complications in implant surgery can be prevented by correctly selecting patients and treating difficult cases in the most adequate way, while knowing the risks, trying to avoid them with the necessary information and having carefully devised a specific plan for every patient.

5. References

Abt, E. (2009). Smoking increases dental implant failures and complications, *Evidence-based dentistry* Vol. 10 (No. 3): 79-80.

Adell, R., Lekholm, U., Rockler, B. & Brånemark, P.I. (1981). A 15-year study of osseointegrated implants in the treatment of the edentulous jaw, *International journal of oral surgery* Vol. 10 (No. 6); 387-416.

Adell, R., Eriksson, B., Lekholm, U., Branemark, P.I. & Jemt, T. (1990). Long-term follow-up study of osseointegrated implants in the treatment of totally edentulous jaws, *The International journal of oral & maxillofacial implants* Vol. 5 (No. 4); 347-359.

Al Jabbari, Y.S., Fournelle, R., Ziebert, G., Toth, J. & Iacopino, A.M. (2008). Mechanical behavior and failure analysis of prosthetic retaining screws after long-term use in vivo. Part 4: Failure analysis of 10 fractured retaining screws retrieved from three patients, *Journal of prosthodontics : official journal of the American College of Prosthodontists* Vol. 17 (No. 3); 201-210.

Al Quran, F.A., Rashan, B.A. & Al-Dwairi, Z.N.(2009). Management of dental implant fractures. A case history", *The Journal of oral implantology* Vol. 35 (No. 4); 210-214.

Alons, K., Kuijpers, S.C., de Jong, E. & van Merkesteyn, J.P. (2009). Treating low- and medium-potency bisphosphonate-related osteonecrosis of the jaws with a protocol for the treatment of chronic suppurative osteomyelitis: report of 7 cases, *Oral surgery, oral medicine, oral pathology, oral radiology, and endodontic,* Vol. 107 (No. 2); e1-7.

Anitua, E., Aguirre, J.J., Gorosabel, A., Barrio, P., Errazquin, J.M., Roman, P., Pla, R., Carrete, J., de Petro, J. & Orive, G. (2009). A multicentre placebo-controlled randomised clinical trial of antibiotic prophylaxis for placement of single dental implants, *European journal of oral implantology* Vol. 2 (No. 4); 283-292.

Annibali, S., La Monaca, G., Tantardini, M. & Cristalli, M.P. (2009). The Role of the Template in Prosthetically Guided Implantology, *Journal of Prosthodontics* Vol. 18 (No. 2); 177-183.

Arisan, V., Karabuda, C.Z. & Ozdemir, T. (2010). Implant surgery using bone- and mucosa-supported stereolithographic guides in totally edentulous jaws: surgical and post-operative outcomes of computer-aided vs. standard techniques, *Clinical oral implants research* Vol. 21 (No. 9);980-988.

Aspenberg, P.(2009). Bisphosphonates and implants: an overview, *Acta orthopaedica* Vol. 80 (No. 1);119-123.

Barber, H.D., Lignelli, J., Smith, B.M. & Bartee, B.K. (2007). Using a dense PTFE membrane without primary closure to achieve bone and tissue regeneration, *Journal of oral and maxillofacial surgery : official journal of the American Association of Oral and Maxillofacial Surgeons* Vol. 65 (No. 4);748-752.

Becker, J., Al-Nawas, B., Klein, M.O., Schliephake, H., Terheyden, H. & Schwarz, F. (2009). Use of a new cross-linked collagen membrane for the treatment of dehiscence-type defects at titanium implants: a prospective, randomized-controlled double-blinded clinical multicenter study", *Clinical oral implants research* Vol. 20 (No. 7);742-749.

Becker, C.M., Wilson, T.G.,Jr & Jensen, O.T. (2011). Minimum criteria for immediate provisionalization of single-tooth dental implants in extraction sites: a 1-year retrospective study of 100 consecutive cases, *Journal of oral and maxillofacial surgery : official journal of the American Association of Oral and Maxillofacial Surgeons,* Vol. 69 (No. 2);491-497.

Bellini, C.M., Romeo, D., Galbusera, F., Taschieri, S., Raimondi, M.T., Zampelis, A. & Francetti, L. (2009). Comparison of tilted versus nontilted implant-supported prosthetic designs for the restoration of the edentuous mandible: a biomechanical study, *The International journal of oral & maxillofacial implants,* Vol. 24 (No. 3);511-517.

Bergendal, T., Forsgren, L., Kvint, S. & Lowstedt, E. (1990). The effect of an airbrasive instrument on soft and hard tissues around osseointegrated implants. A case report, *Swedish dental journal,* Vol. 14 (No. 5);219-223.

Bergermann, M., Donald, P.J. & aWengen, D.F. (1992). Screwdriver aspiration. A complication of dental implant placement, *International journal of oral and maxillofacial surgery* Vol. 21 (No. 6); 339-341.

Borgonovo, A., Fabbri, A., Boninsegna, R., Dolci, M. & Censi, R. (2010). Displacement of a dental implant into the maxillary sinus: case series, *Minerva stomatologica,* Vol. 59 (No. 1-2);45-54.

Bornstein, M.M., Cionca, N. & Mombelli, A. (2009). Systemic conditions and treatments as risks for implant therapy, *The International journal of oral & maxillofacial implants* Vol. 24 (Suppl);12-27.

Brennan, M.T., Wynn, R.L. & Miller, C.S.(2007). Aspirin and bleeding in dentistry: an update and recommendations", *Oral surgery, oral medicine, oral pathology, oral radiology, and endodontics,* Vol. 104 (No. 3);316-323.

Buser, D.; Mericske-stern, R., Pierre Bernard, J.P., Behneke, A., Behneke, N., Hirt, H.P., Belser, U.C. & Lang, N.P. (1997). Long-term evaluation of non-submerged ITI implants. Part 1: 8-year life table analysis of a prospective multi-center study with 2359 implants, *Clinical oral implants research,* Vol. 8 (No. 3);161-172.

Buser, D.; Von Arx, T., Ten Bruggenkate, C. & Weingart, D.(2000). Basic surgical principles with ITI implants Note, *Clinical oral implants research,* Vol. 11, 59-68.

Cannizzaro, G., Leone, M. & Esposito, M. (2007). Immediate functional loading of implants placed with flapless surgery in the edentulous maxilla: 1-year follow-up of a single cohort study, *The International journal of oral & maxillofacial implants,* Vol. 22 (No. 1);87-95.

Cannizzaro, G., Leone, M., Consolo, U., Ferri, V. & Esposito, M.(2008). Immediate functional loading of implants placed with flapless surgery versus conventional implants in partially edentulous patients: a 3-year randomized controlled clinical trial, *The International journal of oral & maxillofacial implant* Vol. 23 (No. 5);867-875.

Cardoso Lde, C., Luvizuto, E.R., Trevisan, C.L., Garcia, I.R.,Jr, Panzarini, S.R. & Poi, W.R. (2010). Resolution of a titanium implant fracture after a recurrent trauma, *Dental traumatology : official publication of International Association for Dental Traumatology* Vol. 26 (No. 6);512-515.

Chappuis, V., Suter, V.G. & Bornstein, M.M. (2009). Displacement of a dental implant into the maxillary sinus: report of an unusual complication when performing staged sinus floor elevation procedures, *The International journal of periodontics & restorative dentistry* Vol. 29 (No. 1);81-87.

Chrcanovic, B.R. & Custodio, A.L. (2009). Mandibular fractures associated with endosteal implants, *Oral and maxillofacial surgery* Vol. 13 (No. 4);231-238.

Cochran, D.L., Schou, S., Heitz-Mayfield, L.J., Bornstein, M.M., Salvi, G.E. & Martin, W.C. (2009). Consensus statements and recommended clinical procedures regarding risk factors in implant therapy, *The International journal of oral & maxillofacial implants* Vol. 24 (Suppl);86-89.

Cooper, L.F. (2010). Factors influencing primary dental implant stability remain unclear, *The journal of evidence-based dental practice* Vol. 10 (No. 1);44-45.

Cordaro, L., Rossini, C. & Mijiritsky, E. (2004). Fracture and displacement of lingual cortical plate of mandibular symphysis following bone harvesting: case report, *Implant dentistry* Vol. 13 (No. 3);202-206.

DePoi, R., John, V., Paez de Mendoza, C.Y. & Gossweiler, M.K. (2007). Development of an oro-antral fistula following sinus elevation surgery: a case report on management using platelet-rich plasma, *Journal (Indiana Dental Association)* Vol. 86 (No. 4);10-16.

Dreiseidler, T., Mischkowski, R.A., Neugebauer, J., Ritter, L. & Zoller, J.E. (2009). Comparison of cone-beam imaging with orthopantomography and computerized tomography for assessment in presurgical implant dentistry, *The International journal of oral & maxillofacial implants* Vol. 24 (No. 2);216-225.

Dubois, L., de Lange, J., Baas, E. & Van Ingen, J. (2010). Excessive bleeding in the floor of the mouth after endosseus implant placement: a report of two cases", *International journal of oral and maxillofacial surgery* Vol. 39 (No. 4);412-415.

Eckert, S.E., Meraw, S.J., Cal, E. & Ow, R.K. (2000). Analysis of incidence and associated factors with fractured implants: a retrospective study", *The International journal of oral & maxillofacial implants* Vol. 15 (No. 5);662-667.

El Chaar, E.S.(2010). Soft tissue closure of grafted extraction sockets in the posterior maxilla: the rotated pedicle palatal connective tissue flap technique, *Implant dentistry* Vol. 19 (No. 5);370-377.

Elian, N., Wallace, S., Cho, S.C., Jalbout, Z.N. & Froum, S. (2005). Distribution of the maxillary artery as it relates to sinus floor augmentation, *The International journal of oral & maxillofacial implant* Vol. 20 (No. 5);784-787.

Esposito, M., Cannizzaro, G., Bozzoli, P., Checchi, L., Ferri, V., Landriani, S., Leone, M., Todisco, M., Torchio, C., Testori, T., Galli, F. & Felice, P. (2010a). Effectiveness of prophylactic antibiotics at placement of dental implants: a pragmatic multicentre placebo-controlled randomised clinical trial, *European journal of oral implantology* Vol. 3 (No. 2);135-143.

Esposito, M., Grusovin, M.G., Loli, V., Coulthard, P. & Worthington, H.V. (2010b). Does antibiotic prophylaxis at implant placement decrease early implant failures? A Cochrane systematic review, *European journal of oral implantology* Vol. 3 (No. 2);101-110.

Felisati, G., Lozza, P., Chiapasco, M. & Borloni, R. (2007). Endoscopic removal of an unusual foreign body in the sphenoid sinus: an oral implant, *Clinical oral implants research* Vol. 18 (No. 6);776-780.

Frenken, J.W., Zijderveld, S.A., van den Bergh, J.P., Huisman, F.W. & Cune, M.S. (2010). Haematoma of the floor of the mouth following implant surgery, *Nederlands tijdschrift voor tandheelkunde* Vol. 117 (No. 1);17-21.

Galindo, P., Sanchez-Fernandez, E., Avila, G., Cutando, A. & Fernandez, J.E. (2005). Migration of implants into the maxillary sinus: two clinical cases, *The International journal of oral & maxillofacial implants* Vol. 20 (No. 2);291-295.

Garfunkel, A.A., Galili, D., Findler, M., Lubliner, J. & Eldor, A.(1999). Bleeding tendency: a practical approach in dentistry, *Compendium of continuing education in dentistry (Jamesburg, N.J.: 1995)* Vol. 20 (No. 9);836-8, 840-2, 844 passim.

Garg, A. (2010). Pathophysiology of tobacco use and wound healing", *Dental implantology update* Vol. 21 (No. 1);1-4.

Gargallo Albiol, J., Satorres-Nieto, M., Puyuelo Capablo, J.L., Sanchez Garces, M.A., Pi Urgell, J. & Gay Escoda, C. (2008). Endosseous dental implant fractures: an analysis of 21 cases, *Medicina oral, patologia oral y cirugia bucal* Vol. 13 (No. 2);E124-8.

Gotta, S., Sarnachiaro, G.O. & Tarnow, D.P. (2008). Distraction osteogenesis and orthodontic therapy in the treatment of malpositioned osseointegrated implants: a case report, *Practical procedures & aesthetic dentistry : PPAD* Vol. 20 (No. 7);401-405.

Greenstein, G., Cavallaro, J., Romanos, G. & Tarnow, D. (2008). Clinical recommendations for avoiding and managing surgical complications associated with implant dentistry: a review, *Journal of periodontology* Vol. 79 (No. 8);1317-1329.

Griffa, A., Viterbo, S. & Boffano, P. (2010). Endoscopic-assisted removal of an intraorbital dislocated dental implant, *Clinical oral implants research* Vol. 21 (No. 7);778-780.

Haben, C.M., Balys, R. & Frenkiel, S. (2003). Dental implant migration into the ethmoid sinus, *The Journal of otolaryngology* Vol. 32 (No. 5);342-344.

Hassan, K.S. (2009). Autogenous bone graft combined with polylactic polyglycolic acid polymer for treatment of dehiscence around immediate dental implants, *Oral surgery, oral medicine, oral pathology, oral radiology, and endodontics* Vol. 108 (No. 5);e19-25.

Hegedus, F. & Diecidue, R.J. (2006). Trigeminal nerve injuries after mandibular implant placement--practical knowledge for clinicians, *The International journal of oral & maxillofacial implants* Vol. 21 (No. 1);111-116.

Hur, Y., Tsukiyama, T., Yoon, T.H. & Griffin, T. (2010). Double flap incision design for guided bone regeneration: a novel technique and clinical considerations, *Journal of periodontology* Vol. 81 (No. 6);945-952.

Javed, F., Almas, K., Crespi, R. & Romanos, G.E. (2011). Implant surface morphology and primary stability: is there a connection?, *Implant dentistry* Vol. 20 (No. 1);40-46.

Jung, R.E., Halg, G.A., Thoma, D.S. & Hammerle, C.H. (2009). A randomized, controlled clinical trial to evaluate a new membrane for guided bone regeneration around dental implants, *Clinical oral implants research* Vol. 20 (No. 2);162-168.

Kohal, R.J., Wolkewitz, M. & Mueller, C. (2010). Alumina-reinforced zirconia implants: survival rate and fracture strength in a masticatory simulation trial, *Clinical oral implants research* Vol. 21 (No. 12);1345-1352.

Lang, N.P., Wilson, T.G. & Corbet, E.F. (2000). Biological complications with dental implants: their prevention, diagnosis and treatment Note, *Clinical oral implants research* Vol. 11;146-155.

Lee, C.Y. & Suzuki, J.B. (2009). CTX biochemical marker of bone metabolism. Is it a reliable predictor of bisphosphonate-associated osteonecrosis of the jaws after surgery? Part I: biological concepts with a review of the literature, *Implant dentistry* Vol. 18 (No. 6);492-500.

Lee, C.Y. (2010). Brisk, prolonged pulsatile hemorrhage during the sinus graft procedure: a case report with discussion on intra-operative hemostatic management, *Implant dentistry* Vol. 19 (No. 3);189-195.

Lee, S. & Thiele, C. (2010). Factors associated with free flap complications after head and neck reconstruction and the molecular basis of fibrotic tissue rearrangement in preirradiated soft tissue, *Journal of oral and maxillofacial surgery : official journal of the American Association of Oral and Maxillofacial Surgeons* Vol. 68 (No. 9);2169-2178.

Liebenberg, W.H. & Crawford, B.J. (1997). Subcutaneous, orbital, and mediastinal emphysema secondary to the use of an air-abrasive device, *Quintessence international (Berlin, Germany : 1985)* Vol. 28 (No. 1);31-38.

Lindfors, L.T., Tervonen, E.A., Sandor, G.K. & Ylikontiola, L.P. (2010). Guided bone regeneration using a titanium-reinforced ePTFE membrane and particulate autogenous bone: the effect of smoking and membrane exposure, *Oral surgery, oral medicine, oral pathology, oral radiology, and endodontic* Vol. 109 (No. 6);825-830.

Mardinger, O., Manor, Y., Mijiritsky, E. & Hirshberg, A. (2007). Lingual perimandibular vessels associated with life-threatening bleeding: an anatomic study, *The International journal of oral & maxillofacial implants* Vol. 22 (No. 1);127-131.

Martin, W., Lewis, E. & Nicol, A. (2009). Local risk factors for implant therapy, *The International journal of oral & maxillofacial implants* Vol. 24 (Suppl);28-38.

Mayfield, L., Nobreus, N., Attstrom, R. & Linde, A. (1997). Guided bone regeneration in dental implant treatment using a bioabsorbable membrane, *Clinical oral implants research* Vol. 8 (No. 1);10-17.

McKenzie, W.S. & Rosenberg, M. (2009). Iatrogenic subcutaneous emphysema of dental and surgical origin: a literature review, *Journal of oral and maxillofacial surgery : official journal of the American Association of Oral and Maxillofacial Surgeons* Vol. 67 (No. 6);1265-1268.

Mendonca, G., Mendonca, D.B., Fernandes Neto, A.J. & Neves, F.D.(2008). Use of distraction osteogenesis for repositioning of an osseointegrated implant: a case report, *The International journal of oral & maxillofacial implants* Vol. 23 (No. 3);551-555.

Mendonca, G., Mendonca, D.B., Fernandes-Neto, A.J. & Neves, F.D.(2009). Management of fractured dental implants: a case report, *Implant dentistry* Vol. 18 (No. 1);10-16.

Merli, M., Bernardelli, F. & Esposito, M. (2008). Computer-guided flapless placement of immediately loaded dental implants in the edentulous maxilla: a pilot prospective case series, *European journal of oral implantology* Vol. 1 (No. 1);61-69.

Misch, C.E. & Resnik, R. (2010). Mandibular nerve neurosensory impairment after dental implant surgery: management and protocol, *Implant dentistry* Vol. 19 (No. 5);378-386.

Nahlieli, O., Moshonov, J., Zagury, A., Michaeli, E. & Casap, N. (2011). Endoscopic approach to dental implantology, *Journal of oral and maxillofacial surgery : official journal of the American Association of Oral and Maxillofacial Surgeons* Vol. 69 (No. 1);186-191.

Napenas, J.J., Hong, C.H., Brennan, M.T., Furney, S.L., Fox, P.C. & Lockhart, P.B. (2009). The frequency of bleeding complications after invasive dental treatment in patients receiving single and dual antiplatelet therapy, *Journal of the American Dental Association (1939)* Vol. 140 (No. 6);690-695.

Neugebauer, J., Scheer, M., Mischkowski, R.A., An, S.H., Karapetian, V.E., Toutenburg, H. & Zoeller, J.E. (2009). Comparison of torque measurements and clinical handling of various surgical motors, *The International journal of oral & maxillofacial implants* Vol. 24 (No. 3);469-476.

Oduncuoglu, B.F., Alaaddinoglu, E.E., Oguz, Y., Uckan, S. & Erkut, S. (2011). Repositioning a Prosthetically Unfavorable Implant by Vertical Distraction Osteogenesis, *Journal of oral and maxillofacial surgery : official journal of the American Association of Oral and Maxillofacial Surgeons,* April 4 (Epub ahead of print).

Oh, T.J., Meraw, S.J., Lee, E.J., Giannobile, W.V. & Wang, H.L. (2003). Comparative analysis of collagen membranes for the treatment of implant dehiscence defects, *Clinical oral implants research* Vol. 14 (No. 1);80-90.

Oh, W.S., Roumanas, E.D. & Beumer, J.,3rd (2010). Mandibular fracture in conjunction with bicortical penetration, using wide-diameter endosseous dental implants, *Journal of prosthodontics : official journal of the American College of Prosthodontists* Vol. 19 (No. 8);625-629.

Ozcelik, O., Haytac, M.C. & Akkaya, M.(2005). Iatrogenic trauma to oral tissues, *Journal of periodontology* Vol. 76 (No. 10);1793-1797.

Padmanabhan, T.V. & Gupta, R.K. (2010). Comparison of crestal bone loss and implant stability among the implants placed with conventional procedure and using osteotome technique: a clinical study, *The Journal of oral implantology* Vol. 36 (No. 6);475-483.

Park, J.B. (2006). Increasing the width of keratinized mucosa around endosseous implant using acellular dermal matrix allograft, *Implant dentistry* Vol. 15 (No. 3);275-281.

Park, S.H. & Wang, H.L. (2007). Clinical significance of incision location on guided bone regeneration: human study, *Journal of periodontology* Vol. 78 (No. 1);47-51.

Parnia, F., Fard, E.M., Mahboub, F., Hafezeqoran, A. & Gavgani, F.E. (2010). Tomographic volume evaluation of submandibular fossa in patients requiring dental implants, *Oral surgery, oral medicine, oral pathology, oral radiology, and endodontics* Vol. 109 (No. 1);e32-6.

Pigrau, C., Almirante, B., Rodriguez, D., Larrosa, N., Bescos, S., Raspall, G. & Pahissa, A. (2009). Osteomyelitis of the jaw: resistance to clindamycin in patients with prior antibiotics exposure, *European journal of clinical microbiology & infectious diseases : official publication of the European Society of Clinical Microbiology* Vol. 28 (No. 4);317-323.

Pingarron Martin, L., Moran Soto, M.J., Sanchez Burgos, R. & Burgueno Garcia, M. (2010). Bronchial impaction of an implant screwdriver after accidental aspiration: report of a case and revision of the literature, *Oral and maxillofacial surgery* Vol. 14 (No. 1);43-47.

Pye, A.D., Lockhart, D.E., Dawson, M.P., Murray, C.A. & Smith, A.J.(2009). A review of dental implants and infection, *The Journal of hospital infection* Vol. 72 (No. 2);104-110.

Queral-Godoy, E., Vazquez-Delgado, E., Okeson, J.P. & Gay-Escoda, C. (2006). Persistent idiopathic facial pain following dental implant placement: a case report, *The International journal of oral & maxillofacial implants* Vol. 21 (No. 1);136-140.

Quirynen, M., Vogels, R., Alsaadi, G., Naert, I., Jacobs, R. & van Steenberghe, D.(2005). Predisposing conditions for retrograde peri-implantitis, and treatment suggestions, *Clinical oral implants research* Vol. 16 (No. 5);599-608.

Ramotar, H., Jaberoo, M.C., Koo Ng, N.K., Pulido, M.A. & Saleh, H.A.(2010). Image-guided, endoscopic removal of migrated titanium dental implants from maxillary sinus: two cases, *The Journal of laryngology and otology* Vol. 124 (No. 4);433-436.

Reychler, H. & Olszewski, R.(2010). Intracerebral penetration of a zygomatic dental implant and consequent therapeutic dilemmas: case report, *The International journal of oral & maxillofacial implants* Vol. 25 (No. 2);416-418.

Ridaura-Ruiz, L., Figueiredo, R., Guinot-Moya, R., Pinera-Penalva, M., Sanchez-Garces, M.A., Valmaseda-Castellon, E. & Gay-Escoda, C.(2009). Accidental displacement of dental implants into the maxillary sinus: a report of nine cases, *Clinical implant dentistry and related research* Vol. 11 (Suppl 1);e38-45.

Rodriguez-Lozano, F.J., Sanchez-Perez, A., Moya-Villaescusa, M.J., Rodriguez-Lozano, A. & Saez-Yuguero, M.R.(2010). Neuropathic orofacial pain after dental implant placement: review of the literature and case report, *Oral surgery, oral medicine, oral pathology, oral radiology, and endodontics* Vol. 109 (No. 4);e8-12.

Romanos, G.E. (2009). Nonsurgical prosthetic management of mandibular fracture associated with dental implant therapy: a case report, *The International journal of oral & maxillofacial implants* Vol. 24 (No. 1);143-146.

Rosen, P.S. & Reynolds, M.A. (2001). Guided bone regeneration for dehiscence and fenestration defects on implants using an absorbable polymer barrier, *Journal of periodontology* Vol. 72 (No. 2);250-256.

Sanchez-Garces, M.A. & Gay-Escoda, C. (2004). Periimplantiti", *Medicina oral, patologia oral y cirugia bucal* Vol. 9 (Suppl);69-74; 63-9.

Sanz, M., Naert, I. & Working Group 2 (2009). Biomechanics/risk management (Working Group 2), *Clinical oral implants research* Vol. 20 (Suppl 4);107-111.

Seong, W.J., Kim, U.K., Swift, J.Q., Hodges, J.S. & Ko, C.C. (2009). Correlations between physical properties of jawbone and dental implant initial stability, *The Journal of prosthetic dentistry* Vol. 101 (No. 5);306-318.

Siciliano, V.I., Salvi, G.E., Matarasso, S., Cafiero, C., Blasi, A. & Lang, N.P.(2009). Soft tissues healing at immediate transmucosal implants placed into molar extraction sites with buccal self-contained dehiscences. A 12-month controlled clinical trial, *Clinical oral implants research* Vol. 20 (No. 5);482-488.

Speroni, S., Cicciu, M., Maridati, P., Grossi, G.B. & Maiorana, C. (2010). Clinical investigation of mucosal thickness stability after soft tissue grafting around implants: a 3-year retrospective study, *Indian journal of dental research : official publication of Indian Society for Dental Research* Vol. 21 (No. 4);474-479.

Steigmann, M.(2008). Aesthetic flap design for correction of buccal fenestration defects, *Practical procedures & aesthetic dentistry : PPAD* Vol. 20 (No. 8);487-93; quiz 494.

Stimmelmayr, M., Allen, E.P., Reichert, T.E. & Iglhaut, G.(2010). Use of a combination epithelized-subepithelial connective tissue graft for closure and soft tissue augmentation of an extraction site following ridge preservation or implant placement: description of a technique, *The International journal of periodontics & restorative dentistry* Vol. 30 (No. 4);375-381.

Taylor, J.B., Gerlach, R.C., Herold, R.W., Bisch, F.C. & Dixon, D.R. (2010). A modified tensionless gingival grafting technique using acellular dermal matrix, *The International journal of periodontics & restorative dentistry* Vol. 30 (No. 5);513-521.

Testori, T., Rosano, G., Taschieri, S. & Del Fabbro, M. (2010). Ligation of an unusually large vessel during maxillary sinus floor augmentation. A case report, *European journal of oral implantology* Vol. 3 (No. 3);255-258.

Tiwana, P.S., Abraham, M.S., Kushner, G.M. & Alpert, B. (2009). Management of atrophic edentulous mandibular fractures: the case for primary reconstruction with immediate bone grafting, *Journal of oral and maxillofacial surgery : official journal of the American Association of Oral and Maxillofacial Surgeons* Vol. 67 (No. 4);882-887.

Torres, J., Tamimi, F., Alkhraisat, M.H., Manchon, A., Linares, R., Prados-Frutos, J.C., Hernandez, G. & Lopez Cabarcos, E.(2010). Platelet-rich plasma may prevent titanium-mesh exposure in alveolar ridge augmentation with anorganic bovine bone, *Journal of clinical periodontology* Vol. 37 (No. 10);943-951.

Tozum, T.F., Sencimen, M., Ortakoglu, K., Ozdemir, A., Aydin, O.C. & Keles, M. (2006). Diagnosis and treatment of a large periapical implant lesion associated with adjacent natural tooth: a case report, *Oral surgery, oral medicine, oral pathology, oral radiology, and endodontics* Vol. 101 (No. 6);e132-8.

Watzak, G., Tepper, G., Zechner, W., Monov, G., Busenlechner, D. & Watzek, G. (2005). Bony press-fit closure of oro-antral fistulas: a technique for pre-sinus lift repair and secondary closure, *Journal of oral and maxillofacial surgery : official journal of the American Association of Oral and Maxillofacial Surgeons* Vol. 63 (No. 9);1288-1294.

Welcker, K., Nakashima, M. & Branscheid, D. (2005). Aspiration of dental implant -- reasons, management and prevention], *Pneumologie (Stuttgart, Germany* Vol. 59 (No. 3);174-177.

Wennström, J.L., Ekestubbe, A., Gröndahl, K., Karlsson, S. & Lindhe, J. (2005). Implant-supported single-tooth restorations: a 5-year prospective study, *Journal of clinical periodontology* Vol. 32 (No. 6);567-574.

Worthington, P. (1996). Ingested foreign body associated with oral implant treatment: report of a case, *The International journal of oral & maxillofacial implants* Vol. 11 (No. 5)679-681.

Zahid, T., Wang, B.Y. & Cohen, R. (2010). Influence of Bisphosphonates on Alveolar Bone Loss around Osseointegrated Implants, *The Journal of oral implantology,* Jun 16 (Epub ahead of print).

Zhou, W., Han, C., Li, D., Li, Y., Song, Y. & Zhao, Y. (2009). Endodontic treatment of teeth induces retrograde peri-implantitis, *Clinical oral implants research* Vol. 20 (No. 12);1326-1332.

6

Bone Substitutes

Jesus Torres[1], Faleh Tamimi[2], Mohammad Alkhraisat[3],
Juan Carlos Prados-Frutos[1] and Enrique Lopez-Cabarcos[3]
[1]*Universidad Rey Juan Carlos,*
[3]*Universidad Complutense,*
[2]*McGill University,*
[1,3]*Spain*
[2]*Canada*

1. Introduction

In daily clinical practise we frequently encounter situations in which the bone volume is insufficient for an ideal dental implant placement. Bone regeneration can provide the structural support necessary in these cases. Procedures such as sinus lifting and alveolar ridge augmentation have reached high levels of predictability and already are of major importance in implant practise. Interest for bone substitutes for alveolar ridge augmentation or preservation appears in the early 1980's alongside the development of endoosseous dental implants. Although first studies regarding bone substitutes dates from 1920 by Albee (Albee, 1920), until 1980´s there are very few studies in reference this issue. From 1980´s until nowadays an exponential number of studies about bone substitutes have been made.
The reason for this increasing interest in bone substitutes stems from the fact that about 10-20% of the patients that need treatments with dental implants, require bone regeneration procedures before implant placement. Moreover, more than 60% of the population in industrialized countries need dental prosthetic replacements (Peterson, 2006), ideally with implants. This is the reason why the market of dental implants is experiencing an increase of approximately 15% every year.
Bone regeneration procedures are becoming an almost daily practice in dentistry all around the world as a result of the wide acceptance of dental implants as the "ideal" option for oral rehabilitation. Bone regeneration procedures are critical for the success of dental implant treatments in cases where there is a deficiency in bone width and/or height. The cornerstone in these treatments is the use of bone substitutes to create a bone mantle that covers the screw to enhance implant stability and treatment outcome. In this chapter, we will discuss the different types of bone substitutes and recent developments achieved to enhance the outcomes of bone regeneration procedures with the newest available biomaterials.
The term "bone graft" was defined by Muschler (Bauer, 2000) as: "any implanted material that alone or in combination with other materials promotes a bone healing response by providing oteogenic, osteoinductive or osteoconductive properties". An osteogenic material can be defined as one that has inherent capacity to form bone, which implies to contain living cells that are capable of differentiation into bone cells. An osteoinductive material

provides biologic signals capable to induce local cells to enter a pathway of differentiation leading to mature osteoblasts. An osteoconductive biomaterial provides a three-dimensional interconnected scaffold where local bone tissue may regenerate new living bone. However, osteoconductive biomaterials are unable to form bone or to induce its formation.
Another property that is interesting to find especially in bone substitutes is biodegradability. This is defined as the capacity of degradation of a particle by two mechanisms principally; through a passive chemical degradation or dissolution, and through active cellular activity mediated by osteoclast and/or macrophages. Moreover, the biological properties of bone substitute biomaterials are also influenced by their porosity, surface geometry and surface chemistry. The events leading to bone healing and regeneration are influenced by all the variables mentioned above. These properties are related to the biomaterial itself, however, host factors such as bone quality, vascularity of the graft bed and tobacco addiction may also influence the final outcome of a bone regeneration procedure with a bone substitute.

2. Biomaterials used for bone regeneration in implant dentistry

Bone graft materials can be divided in four large groups: Autografts, Allografts, Xenografts and Synthetic biomaterials.

2.1 Autograft

"Autograft" refers to bone tissue harvested from, and implanted in the same individual. Accordingly, autograft is a bone tissue that is separated from one site and implanted in other location in the same individual. The cellular component of trabecular bone graft includes few osteoblasts and a high number of precursor cells that survive the transplantation. These precursor cells explain the osteogenic potential of bone autograft. Autograft is considered the "gold standard" in bone regeneration due to its properties of osteoconduction, osteoinduction, osteogenicity and osteointegration. However there are major drawbacks to the use of this sort of ideal bone graft, namely the necessity of a second surgery to retrieve the bone graft at the donor site, with its associated morbidity; the increasing surgery time, the restrictions in quantity and shape of the bone graft, and the additional cost (Arrington, 1996; Giannoudis, 2005).
Autografts are subdivided in two groups: cancellous autografts and cortical autografts. *Cancellous autografts* are retrieved mainly from calcellous bone, and upon transaplantation, the majority of cells presnet in the grafts die as result of ischemia. However, the mesenchymal stem cells present in the bone marrow are resistant to ischemia and may survive the grafting procedure. The stem cells capacity of survival and proliferation after exposure to changes in the oxygen tension, pH and cytochine environment are the main reason behind the reliability of of cancellous bone autograft interventions. The incorporation of such type of autogrfraft is speed, about 8 weeks (Virolainen, 1995).
Cortical autografts are segments of cortical bone composed of necrotic bone that provides an osteoconductive support for bone formation, but does not supply significant amounts of living cells. For this reason, revascularization and integration of cortical autografts is slow. The main advantage of cortical autografts is the mechanical support that provides at the graft site (Bauer & Muchler, 2000), while its incorporation is slower than cancellous autografts.

Bone graft	Properties: Origin	Availability	Reabsorption	Graft´s form
Extraoral Autograft				
Calvaria	IM	+++	++	Block/Particulate
Iliac crest	EC	+++	+++	Block/Particulate
Tibia	EC	+++	+++	Particulate
Intraoral Autograft				
Ramus	IM	++	++	Block
Sinfisis	IM	+	++	Block/Particulate
Tuberosity	IM	+	+++	Particulate

IM: Intramembranous bone, EC: Endochondral bone

Table 1. Summary of bone autograft properties as a function of their anatomical origin

2.2 Allografts: Freeze dried bone allograft (FDBA) and demineralized freeze dried bone allograft (DFDBA)

Allograft is defined as tissue that has been harvested from one individual and implanted into another individual of the same species (Eppley, 2005).The use of cadaver bone for grafting is known as bone allograft and it is considered by some the best available alternative to autografts due its similarly characteristics. Despite the superior properties of autografts, allografts are usually preffered by patients as bone grafting material because they the problems associated to donor site surgery in autografts.. Allografts are obtained from cadaver tissue banks for mineralized freeze-dried (FDBA) or decalcified freeze-dried (DFDBA) bone.. Both FDBA and DFDBA are obtained from cortical bone of long bones due to its high content of bone inductive proteins and less antigenic activity than cancellous bone. Bone allografts come in various configurations, including powder, cortical chips, cancellous cubes, and cortical granules among others (Eppley, 2005). The granulated form is btained by milling the cortical bone under sterile conditions to obtain a particle size ranging from 250 to 750 μm. Moreover, allografts have been recently made available in different block forms; although their mechanical properties remains slightly lower than those of autograft cortical blocks.

Once the allograft is harvested they are processed through several methods including physical debridement to remove soft tissue and reduced cellular load, ultrasonic washing to remove remnant cells and blood, ethanol treatment in order to denaturalize proteins and viral deactivation, antibiotic wash to kill bacteria, and sterilization through gamma radiation and ethylene oxide for spore elimination (Khan, 2005). FDBA are washed in antibiotic twice for 1 hour, frozen at -70C° and dried up to 5% of water (Kao, 2007).During this process microfractures form along the allografts' collagen fibers, resulting in a decreased in its mechanical properties, for this reason it is advised to rehydrate allografts before use to regain some of the lost properties (Kao, 2007). Processed bone allografts do not include any living cells, and therefore, they lack osteogenic activity. Allografts are essentially osteoconductive, and depending how they are processes, they may have some osteoinductive properties (Stevenson, 1999).

FDBA: Mineralized bone matrix has no active bone morphogenetic proteins (BMPs) and therefore it lacks osteoinductive properties, although it has osteoconductive properties. Graft incorporation is qualitatively similar to autograft, but occur more slowly. Cortical allografts will incorporate and eventually resemble their autograft counterpart although with more unremodeled necrotic bone present in allografts (Stevenson, 1999). Milled forms present an open structure that facilitate invasion by blood cells, enhance graft incorporation and allows mixing with blood, platelet concentrates and other graft materials forming composites.

DFDBA: DFDBA forms are processed by acid demineralization in 0.5 to 0.6 molar hydrochloric acid as a result, 40% of the mineral content is removed leaving the organic matrix intact. This process preserves the BMPs present in bone, and therefore maintains some of the inherent osteoinductive properties (Khan, 2000). Moreover, the collagen matrix present in DFDBA acts as a scaffold that provides osteoconductive properties alone side the osteoinductive behavior. Osteoinductivity of DFDBA was first described by Urist et al, after observing endochondral bone formation on DFDBA when placed in soft tissue. It has since been discovered that BMPs are the factors responsible for the novo bone formation (Reddi, 1998). BMPs are associated with the organic matrix of bone and embedded within mineral content, so demineralised process increases its bioavailability. BMPs attract mesenchymal stem cells and induce them to differentiate into chondrocytes leading into endochondral bone formation. Endochondral bone formation is attributed to a osteoinductivity response, while intra-membranous bone formation is indicative of an osteoconductive response. Nevertheless, osteoinductivity of DFDBA has been recently questioned, since it seems that this property is highly dependent on the manufacturing procedures (Drosos, 2007)

The main advantage of allografts include easy availability, avoiding the need of harvesting a patient donor site, reduced costs in terms of anesthesia (general anesthesia is not needed) and reduced surgical time. However, the use of cadaver bone for grafting is avoided by many clinicians due to its potential risk of infectious disease. Nevertheless, allografts have been used for more than 25 years without any reported incidence of disease transmission. The risk of HIV infection through allograft implantation has been estimated to be 1 in 1.6 million, compared with the risk of 1 in 450.000 in blood transfusions (Khan, 2000). DFDBA forms may have even less risk of disease transmission than FDBA, because demineralization allows most affective removal of viruses and blood elements reducing immunological reactions (Eppley, 2005). Moreover the establishment of better equipped tissue banks has allowed an increase in the use of bone allografts, and there is a current tendency by many surgeons to replace autografts by bone allograft (Albert, 2006).

Allografts are available in the form of granules and blocks. Allograft granules' appearance is similar to other bone substitute granules, and they are ideal to fill bone cavities as alveolar bone defects and maxillary sinus. On the other hand, allograft blocks are especially useful in both vertical and horizontal bone augmentation procedures.

Bone graft	Properties			
	Structural stregth	Osteogenesis	Osteconductor	Osteoinductor
Autograft				
Cancellous	No	+++	+++	+++
Cortical	+++	++	++	++
Allograft				
Cancellous	No	No	++	+
Cortical	+++	No	++	No

Table 2. Comparison between bone autograft and allograft according to their properties

2.3 Xenografts: Anorganic bovine bone (ABB)

Bone xenograft is defined a bone tissue harvested from one species and implanted into a different species. One of the most commonly used xenografts is anorganic bovine bone (ABB). ABB is a biomaterial with major long-term success reports in the bone regeneration literature and it has been extensively used in the clinics for over 20 years (Frame et al., 1987). ABB has an ultrastructural composition similar to human bone, it is composed of almost pure hydroxyapatite, and it is chemically treated to remove all organic components so it can be used as a graft material without causing host immune response (Mish et al., 1993). ABB is thermally and chemically treated in order to extract organic constituents and thereby eliminating its antigenicity and potential inflammatory response by the host bone (Cohen et al., 1994). The structure consists of a wide interconnective pore system with a particle size of 0.25 to 1 mm that can easily be invaded by blood vessels resulting in osteoblastic migration. . ABB is up to 75% porous and has a high specific surface area of almost 100 m2/g that results in increased angiogenesis, enhances new bone growth (Hammerle et al., 1997; Rodriguez, 2003), and excellent osteoconduction properties. However, its highly porous consistency sometimes compromises its mechanical properties and its initial stability. ABB lacks osteoinductive properties, and its presentation in form of granules makes it difficult to hold on surgical sites. Moreover, it is non resorbable *in vivo*. Indeed, ABB might need several years (3-6 years) of implantation before showing some slow *in vivo* resorption through osteoclast activity, (Skoglung et al, reported that granules were present even after 44 months (Skoglund., 1997) . The presence of unresorbed granules within the newly formed bone is undesired because it affects the quality of the newly formed bone by interfering with its remodelling, compromising its osteointegration capacity with dental implants.

Although ABB is mostly used in form of granules, xenografts blocks design are also available. Xenogenic derived bone block have already been reported to achieve vertical bone augmentation in the mandible. However, these materials are quite brittle and fragile. This mechanical inconvenience not only complicates the surgical technique but it also hinders the bone graft healing process (Simion et al 2006; Felice et al., 2009). Other types of xenogenic (porcine) bone block seems to show better mechanical properties and low risk of fracture while screwing. (Simion et al., 2009). Generally speaking, the use of xenogenic bone blocks is still under evaluation and at this moment there is not sufficient information regarding its *in vivo* behaviour.

2.4 Synthetic calcium phosphates

Calcium phosphates constitute synthetic biomaterials that chemically resemble the bone mineral . Calcium phosphate biomaterials are widely selected to regenerate bone tissue due to thier biocompatibility, osteointegration and osteoconductivity (Alkhraisat et al., 2008). We can make a classification of calcium phosphates in order to its Ca^{2+} and P compounds.

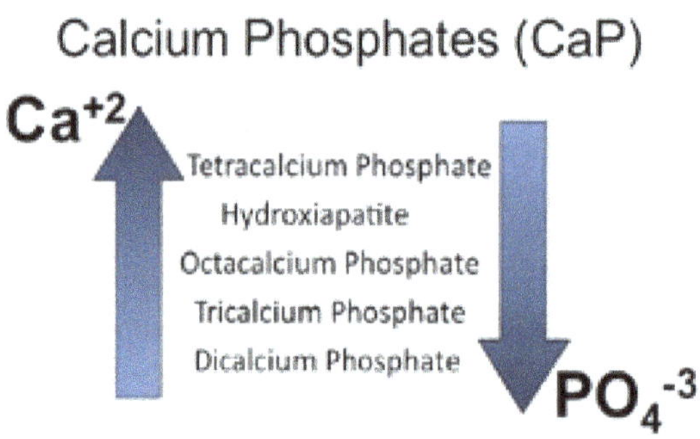

Calcium Phosphates (CaP)

CaP	Properties			
	Biocompatible	Reabsorbible	Osteoconductor	Osteoinductor
AP	+++	-	+++	-
CAP	+++	+	+++	-
β-TCP	++	++	+++	+
DCPD	++	+++	+++	-
BCP	+++	++	+++	+

Table 3. Summary of synthetic calcium phosphate bone substitutes arranged to their chemical composition and biological properties

Regarding this classification is interesting to know that materials which contains high levels of Ca^{2+} ions have alkaline Ph and therefore shows low resorption capability as hidroxiapatite (AP), while materials with low levels of Ca^{2+} ions have acid Ph and shows high resorption properties, as dicalcium phosphate forms.

According to their preparation, calcium phosphate could be divided into high temperature (ceramics of tricalcium phosphates, hydroxyapatite and biphasic calcium phosphate) and low temperature (cements) calcium phosphates. Such bone substitutes differ in the degradation rate in vivo, strength, alkalinity and acidity, and crystallographic structure. Generally, they are fragile materials and should be used in non-load bearing areas.

Hydroxyapatite and β-tricalcium phosphate (β-TCP) are the ceramics mostly recruited clinically to treat bone defects and voids. Biologicall, stoichiometric hydroxyapatite of Ca/P ratio of 1.67 is highly stable and its very slow degradation is mediated by phagocytosis [Constantino & Freidman, 1997). Such handicap is managed by introducing impurities like carbonate ions, silicon ions and other ionic species present in the bone mineral [Alkhraisat et al., 2008). Structurally, porous hydroxyapatite was introduced to resemble native bone architecture, improve the degradability and enhance tissue reaction of angiogenesis and new bone in-growth. This resulted in engineering apatite and calcium carbonate of live species to produce a hydroxypatite conserving the macro and microporous architecture of the source . An example of such technology is the anorganic bovine bone, coral apatite and algae apatite.

Since the experiments reported by Albee and Morrison (Albee, 1920), research and development projects have been dedicated to explore the potential of β-TCP ceramic bone substitute. β-TCP has Ca/P ratio of 1.5 and is more resorbable than hydroxyapatite. This higher degradability is related to higher solubility that aid phagocytosis to induce biomaterial replacement with new bone.

Biphasic calcium phosphate (BCP) is engineered to combine the advantages of both hydroxyapatite and β-TCP. A relation of 60% hydroxyapatite and 40% β-TCP is the most common among commercial biphasic calcium phosphate.

These ceramics are presented in porous granular and block forms and they are difficult to reshape. The granules have a size range between 0.2 mm and 1mm.

The lack of adaptability of calcium phosphate ceramics was solved by Brown and co-workers when they developed calcium phosphate cement (Brown & Chow, 1985). This cement is the mixture of calcium phosphate powders that upon reacting with aqueous phase produce new calcium phosphate. The chemical reaction that produce this new phase is termed setting reaction and the consistency of the cement is progressed from paste-like to solid structure by the entanglement of the setting product. This enable the cement to be moulded, adapt intimately to the bone defect borders and permits the development of injectable preparation for minimally invasive surgery. Such cements are biocompatable, degradable and osteoconductive (Figure 1) (Alkhraisat et al., 2008).

Calcium phosphate cements are classified according to the setting reaction end-product to hydroxyapatite and brushite cements. Hydroxyapatite cement is first developed by Brown and co-workers and since then variuos formulation have been developed and patented. Of such formulations are tetracalcium phosphate/dicalcium phosphate anhydrous (DCPA) system and α-TCP based system. The setting reaction of hydroxyapatite cement occurs at neutral pH which is biologically favourable. The hydroxyapatite as setting product is low-crystalline and the stoichiometry can be varied to produce calcium deficient-hydroxyapatite (Ca/P ratio less than 1.67). These features and the development of carbonated apatite cement improve the degradability of hydroxyapatite cement.

Since their development by Mirtchi and co-workers, brushite cements are recieveing much interest as bone substitute in the recent years [Mirtchi, 1990). These cements are obtained by various combinations, such as β-TCP + monocalcium phosphate monohydrate (MCPM) and β-TCP + phosphoric acid. The setting reaction of these cements is a continuous dissolution/precipitation mechanism at low pH values as brushite precipitates at pH <6 [Alkhraisat et al., 2010).. The relatively short setting time of brushite cements compared with hydroxyapatite forming pastes depends on both the higher solubility of the cement raw materials and the higher rate of brushite crystal growth (3.32×10^{-4} mol min^{-1} m^{-2}) [compared with hydroxyapatite (2.7×10^{-7} mol min^{-1} m^{-2}) (Zawackiet al., 1996).

The main advantage of brushite is its higher degradability compared to hydroxypatite that stems from higher solubility at physiological conditions. However, in vivo brushite transformation to hydroxyapatite is kinetically favourable and additives are patented to inhibit such transformation [Alkhraisat et al., 2010). This fact have raised the attention to the anhydrous form of brushite, monetite, that is prepared by drying brushite. Monetite is more stable than brushite due to its lower solubility and in vivo transformation to hydroxyapatite was not reported ensuring a predictable degradability (Tamimi et al., 2009).

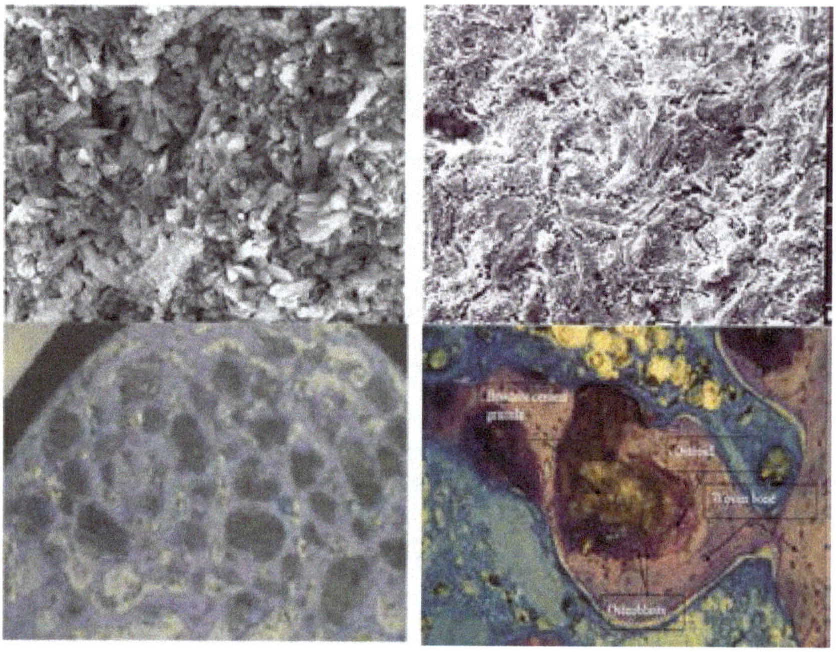

Fig. 1. The microcrystalline structure of dicalcium phosphate dihydrate cement provide support for osteoblasts growth and proliferation that permits bone formation on and between calcium phosphate granulate.

Recently, calcium phosphates are shown to be efficient as local drug and bioactives delivery system [Alkhraisat et al., 2010).and the technology is now available to prepare custom-made bone calcium phosphate based on patient's CT scan data to fit in a bone defect [Klammert et al., 2010). These biomaterials are the corner-stone in the development of 3D-porous scaffold in combination with organic components to resemble the inorganic-organic harmony of bone. Such scaffolds are designed to support the growth and differentiation of stem cells for their application in the emerging field of regenerative medicine.

2.5 Bio glass

Bioglass, also known as bioactive glass, is the commercial name for the first calcium substituted silicon oxide that was marketed as a bone regeneration material over 30 years ago. This material was developed by researchers working for the US army during the Vietnam War as a biomaterial for repairing bone loss in injured combat soldiers (Välimäki & Aro, 2006). In plain language bioglass is a glass similar to that in the windows of your house, but with a large portion of calcium in its chemical structure. It has a large surface area that is alkaline and highly reactive to serum ions. This feature enables it to interact with serum, allowing a very fast precipitation of hydroxyapatite on its surface once implanted *in vivo*. This phenomenon is called *bioactivity*, and is one of the unique characteristics of Bioglass that allows a quick integration to bone tissue.

Bioglass is suitable for bone regeneration in dental implant surgery; moreover, it is purely synthetic therefore it does not present problems regarding transmission of infectious diseases. However, its granule format is difficult to handle due to the repulsive charges between the highly charged surfaces the granules. This renders its clinical handling more demanding than other biomaterials (Välimäki & Aro, 2006).

The critical component of bioglass is SiO2 which constitutes 45-60% of its weigth. The first bioglass developed for bone regeneration was based on 4 components: SiO_2, Na_2O, CaO and P_2O_5.However, this composition tend to crystallize, and was modified to a more stable glass composed of: Na_2O-K_2O-MgO-CaO-B_2O_3-P_2O_5-SiO_2.In vivo experiments have shown that implantation of bioglass in bone defects causes an inhibition in bone formation during the early healing stages, but it eventually doubles the amount of bone formed when no biomaterial is used.
Moreover, bioglass experiences sever resorption during the first 2 weeks after implantation. However, beyond this point its resorption rate is stabilizes.
Upon implantation, the smaller ions present in bioglass (i.e. Na^+ and K^+) tend to leach to the extracellular fluids. This results in a rich Si layer coating the biomaterial. Ca^{2+} and PO_4^{3-} ions from the body fluids then react and precipitate on the Si rich layer, forming a thin coat of hydroxyapatite. The calcium phosphate layer adsorbs proteins. And these extracellular properties attract macrophages stem cells and osteoprogenitor cells (Välimäki & Aro, 2006).
Bioactive glass can be used in form of granules or as preformed cones designed for placement into fresh sockets to maintain the alveolar ridge (Stanley et al., 1997). It has shown clinical success in vertical bone augmentation procedures, in regeneration intra-bony defects and in the preservation of alveolar sockets (Gatti et al., 2006) .However, even though it is resorbable and promotes bone formation, its bone regeneration capacity in maxillofacial surgery has been shown to be lower than Calcium phosphate biomaterials (Santos et al., 2010).

3. Surgical procedures that require the use of bone substitutes

3.1 Sinus lift

Bone augmentation in sinus lifting procedures requires the use of bone regeneration biomaterials that would enable bone formation within the maxillary sinus. Ideally besides good osteoconductive properties, biomaterials used for sinus lifting should be easy to handle, and have a limited *in vivo* resorption. Underneath we discuss the main bone substitutes that have been employed in sinus lift bone augmentation procedures
Autograft: The use of bone autografts are recommended when treating large pneumatized sinuses and a short treatment period is required. The healing period in such situations is 3-4 months shorter than when other bone substitutes are used (7-9 months). Also the use of autografts is an option when patients reject the use of allograft or bovine bone. Several studies have reported high rate of success using autografts from either endochondral or intramembranous origin. (Daelemans et al., 1997). Intramembranous bone has been shown to resorb less readily than endochondral bone (Hardesty et al., 1990). Despite the excellent clinical results obtained with autografts, a high degree of morbidity has been reported in such procedures. In order to diminish the morbidity and also the high resorption rate of autografts, many clinicians use autografts in combination with other bone substitutes in different proportions, and obtaining promising results.
Autografts combined with ABB: Studies evaluating the use of bone autografts in combination with ABB, have shown great results in terms of percentage of newly formed bone in the sinus and subsequent implant success rate. Bone formation is higher when a major percentage of autograft is added (48%) and significantly lower amounts of vital bone forms when autograft is used in minimal propoprtions. Froum et al. observed a statistically significant increase in vital bone formation when as little as 20% autologous bone was added to ABB compared with ABB alone. Nevertheless, a high percentage of bone volume

formation within the sinus is not a crucial parameter regarding the subsequent success rate of the dental implants. Indeed, bone volumes as low as 24% have shown to be sufficient for successful osteointegration of dental implants placed in augmented maxillay sinuses (Esposito et al., 2010).

Vital bone formation with different types of graft in sinus augmentation			
Authors	*ABB:Autograft*	*Healing time (months)*	*Vital bone (%)*
Hallman et al 2002	*100 Autograft*	*6-9*	*37*
John et al 2004	*100 Autograft*	*3-8*	*53*
Mish & Krauser 2003	*20:80*	*4-9*	*48*
Mish & Krauser 2003	*40:60*	*4-9*	*36*
Mish & Krauser 2003	*60:40*	*4-9*	*38*
Galindo et al 2010	*80:20*	*6-9*	*46*
Hallman et al 2002	*80:20*	*6-9*	*41*
Froum et al 2008	*100 ABB*	*6*	*22*
Hallman et al 2002	*100 ABB*	*6-9*	*39*
John et al 2004	*100 ABB*	*3-8*	*29*

Table 4. Overview of different composite graft material in sinus lift technique

Allografts: Despite the risk of disease transmission associated with its use, approximately 350.00 to 400.000 bone allografts procedures are performed in the United States, Out of which 100.000 are dental related. The use of Allografts in sinus augmentation procedures has shown high success rates. (Avila et al., 2010). The percentage of bone volume obtained with FDBA in sinus lifting procedures is 23%. Moreover, the success rate of implants placed in the maxillary sinuses following bone augmentation with solely applied allograft has been shown to be a 97.7% in three years follow up (Minichetti et al., 2008). On the other hand, Peleg et al reported a 100% success rate over 160 implants placed in 63 grafted sinuses using as graft material autogenous graft harvested from symphysis with DFDBA combined in 1:1 ratio after a 4 year follow up (Peleg et al., 1999).

DFDBA was compared with autograft in sinus augmentation procedures; DFDBA showed 29% of new bone formation compared to a 40% achieved with autograft (Kao 11). Froum also studies the differences between FDBA and ABB, observing a high vital bone formation (28%) in FDBA grafted sinuses compared to a 12% in ABB grafted ones'. (Froum et al., 2006). No differences have been observed between DFDBA and FDBA in terms of percentage of vital bone formation in the maxillary sinus.

Anorganic bovine bone (ABB): ABB is a biocompatible and osteoconductive anorganic bovine bone (ABB), that provides an ideal scaffold for new bone formation (Hammerle et al., 1998, Piatelli et al., 1999). It has been extensively used in maxillary sinus floor augmentation (Valentini et al., 2003, Wallace et al., 2005) with high clinical success rates (Carmagnola et al., 2003). Comparative studies by Hallman et al and Valentini and Abensur observed higher survival rates for implants placed in sinuses grafted with 100% ABB compared with sinuses grafted with 100% autograft (Hallman., 2002, Valentini., 2003). Also Froum reports higher implant survival rate in sinuses grafted with ABB alone than those grafted with a composite of ABB+DFDBA (Froum et al., 2006). In a recent study Torres et al observed a 97% implant success rate in 286 implants placed in 144 sinuses grafted with ABB alone or ABB+PRP. Overall, 96.2% of ABB and 98.6% of ABB+PRP implant success was obtained during the monitoring period and differences were not found between sites grafted with and without

PRP in the 87 patients studied. (Torres et al., 2009). Regarding vital bone formation achieved with ABB in maxillary sinuses, Scarano et al compared ABB to autograft bone in maxillary sinus augmentation procedures. In this study, 6 months after the initial intervention, ABB resulted in 39% new bone formation compared to 40% with autograft. Although the results of new bone generation were very similar, 31% of the grafted Bio-Oss was still present at the graft site compared to only 18% of autograft (Scarano et al., 2006).(Fig 2)

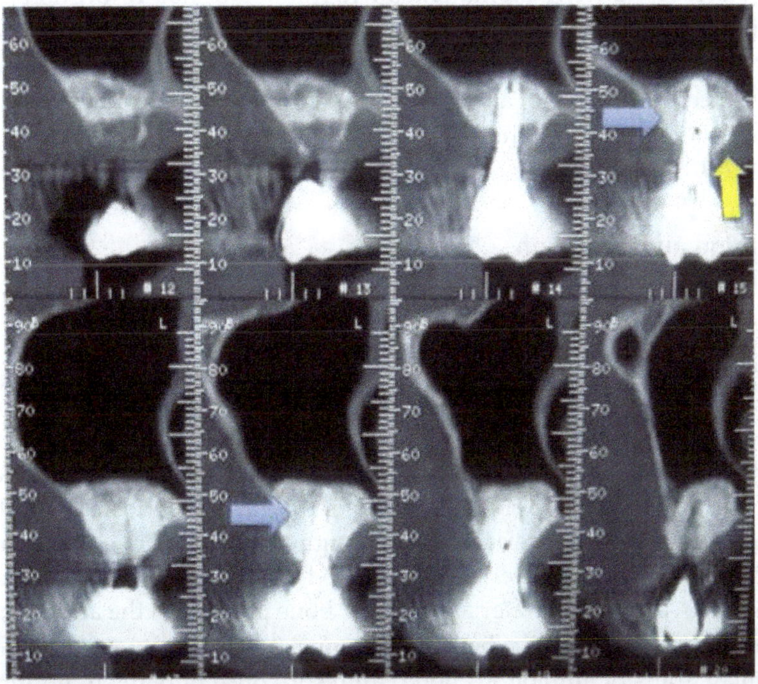

Fig. 2. Slow resorption of ABB particles could be observed after 24 months of implant´s placement. Blue arrow shows remanent ABB graft. Yellow arrow shows residual host bone

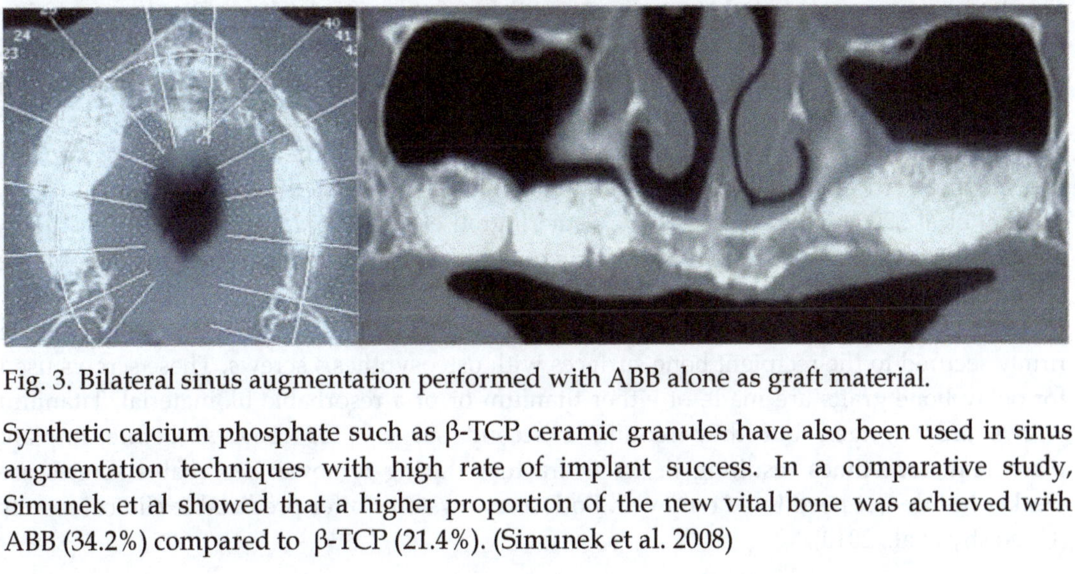

Fig. 3. Bilateral sinus augmentation performed with ABB alone as graft material.

Synthetic calcium phosphate such as β-TCP ceramic granules have also been used in sinus augmentation techniques with high rate of implant success. In a comparative study, Simunek et al showed that a higher proportion of the new vital bone was achieved with ABB (34.2%) compared to β-TCP (21.4%). (Simunek et al. 2008)

However Szabó et al in another comparative study between β-TCP ceramic granules versus autograft observe that vital bone areas were 36% and 38%, respectively.(Szabó et al. 2005)
Rapidly resorbable biomaterials are not recommended for sinus lift procedures since the maxillary sinus is a non functional site for bone to form, and in the absence of mechanical load any bone augmentation achieved is likely to be lost if the scaffold provided by the biomaterial resorbs. For these reasons the most suitable biomaterials for sinus lifting procedures are osteoconductive biomaterials with limited or non resorption properties such as granules of ABB, β-TCP, hydroxyapatite, biphasic calcium phosphate and Bioglass.
In a recent systematic review performed by Esposito, it was concluded that ABB and β-TCP might be as effective as bone autografts for augmenting atrophic maxillary sinuses. Therefore these biomaterials might be used as replacement for autogenous bone grafting (Esposito et al. 2010).(Fig 3)

3.2 Alevolar ridge augmentation
3.2.1 Onlay bone grafts

Onlay bone grafts

Onlay bone grafting is the most predictable technique available for bone augmentation of the alveolar ridge. This procedure is used to augment bone before or at the time of implant placement to ensure proper implant osteointegration (Rocchietta et al. 2008)
Onlay bone grafting is achieve by fixing a biomaterial in the shape of a block directly onto the bone surface of the alveolar ridge, and covered with the periosteum and oral mucosa. This procedure requires a biomaterial strong enough to bear direct occlusal forces and allow screw fixation. Besides, the biomaterial should also be bioresorbable and osteconductive.
Currently the best available biomaterial for onlay bone grafting is the autologous bone graft. Autologus onlay bone grafts can be harvested from extra-oral or intra-oral bones (Rocchietta et al., 2008).Onlay grafts of autologous bone can resorb once implanted, limiting the amount of bone volume available for dental implant stabilization. In this sence, intra-oral grafts are always preferred, since they tend resorb less than extra-oral bone grafts after implantation (Rocchietta et al., 2008).
The limited amount of autlogous bone available for grafting alongside the morbidity associated to the donor site has driven the need for developing alternative materials. Accordingly, alloplastic, allogenic and xenogenic onlay blocks have been recently developed and tested showing promising results. Several animals studies have shown that blocks made of either allogenic materials, hydroxyapatite, tricalcium phosphate or monetite are capable of achieving vertical bone augmentation in onlay bone graft procedures (Tamura et al., 2007, Tamimi et al .,2009, Fujita et al., 2003, Hetherington et al., 1996).Moreover, clinical studies have confirmed the great potential of allogenic bone blocks as biomaterials for onlay bone augmentation (Waasdorp et al., 2010)
In order to achieve succes with an onlay bone graft procedure, the onlay blocks have to be firmly secured to the recipient bone surfaces with osteosynthesis screws. These screws used for onlay bone grafts are made of either titanium or of a resorbable biomaterial. Titanium screws are stronger, but they require a second surgery for removal before implant placement, sometimes resulting in screw fracture during removal. Resorbable screws are weaker but do not need to be removed. Both screw systems offer predictable clinical results (Quereshy et al., 2010).

Usually, onlay bone grafts are placed without the use of barrier membranes. This fact renders the onlay sensitive to masticatory forces, and requires the patients not to wear any removable prosthesis after the regeneration procedure for a period of at least 2 months (Rocchietta et al., 2008).For this reason, recent studies have tested the benefits of covering onlay bone grafts with resorbable membranes. This novel procedure, been shown to be beneficial in preventing grafts resorption due to masticatory forces (Rocchietta et al., 2008).(Fig 4,5)

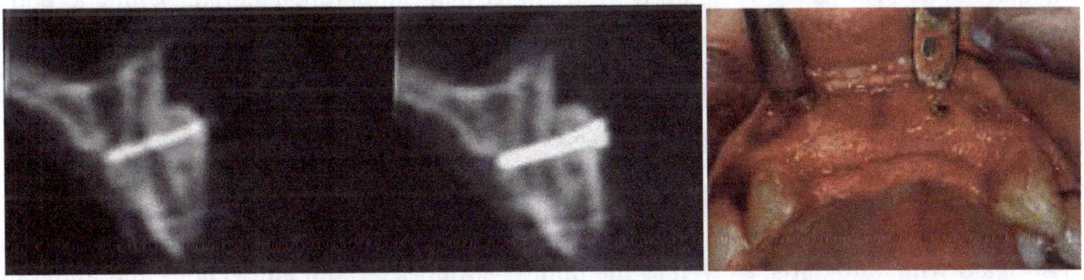

Fig. 4. Slightly resorption with autogenous intraoral bone in the most coronal part of the graft is observed in a patient where no membrane was used.

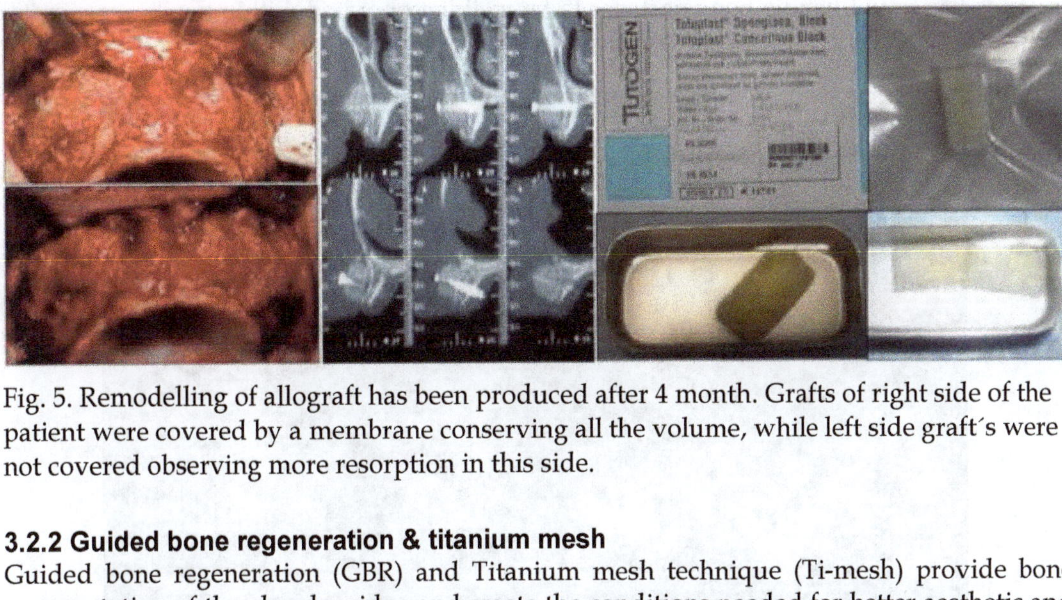

Fig. 5. Remodelling of allograft has been produced after 4 month. Grafts of right side of the patient were covered by a membrane conserving all the volume, while left side graft´s were not covered observing more resorption in this side.

3.2.2 Guided bone regeneration & titanium mesh

Guided bone regeneration (GBR) and Titanium mesh technique (Ti-mesh) provide bone augmentation of the alveolar ridge and create the conditions needed for better aesthetic and higher rate of dental implants success. In order to achieve high rates of success in GBR and Ti-mesh procedures, there are three major issues that need to be addressed: coagulum maintenance, free tension flap closure and an adequate biomaterial selection.

In the treatment of large defects autografts are considered the gold standard, since they have osteoinductive, osteoconductive, osteogenic properties and no risk of immunologic rejection. In view of mechanical properties, cancellous bone grafts still clearly surpassed by ABB, coral, or synthetic bone substitute. However, it provides a high amount of vital stem cells and proteins, such as BMPs, that result in osteogenesis and osteoinduction, therefore GBR with particulated autografts is a safe and predictable treatment (Urban et al., 2009).

Autografts combined with ABB have been used with success in GBR (Table 5). However in the last years different studies have shown that even allografts alone offer reliable results in large defects, with less cost on the patient. In a study performed by Dahlin they conclude that reconstruction of atrophic maxillae with DFDB using the GBR technique can be performed with an equal success as iliac crest autografts (Dahlin., 2010)

Allografts, alloplasts or xenografts are considered appropriate candidates for small defects (Fig 6, 7). Allograft bone, is the most popular alternative to autogenous bone. It offers the substantial advantage of allowing the patient to avoid a second surgical procedure, with the attendant risks of pain, complications, and morbidity. Available in various shapes and sizes, allograft bone also has fewer supply restrictions than autograft material. Synthetic bone graft materials (alloplasts) constitute a third category of widely used bone-grafting materials, including such non-human, artificially produced materials as calcium sulfate, calcium phosphate, hydroxyapatite, and bioactive glass. Their advantages consist on their abundant supply, long shelf lives, and lack of potential disease transmission. Their capacity to predictably regenerate bone has not yet been demonstrated consistently. Xenografts constitute the final category of bone-grafting materials in common use. Derived from animal sources, xenografts have been developed largely in response to the donor site complications associated with autografts, as well as the limited supplies of both autogenous and allograft material. Porous bovine-derived material is by far the most common variety of xenograft in use today. Such material has been demonstrated to be highly biocompatible. Histologic analysis has found bovine bone particles to be well incorporated within newly regenerated grafted bone and a high degree of osseoconductivity

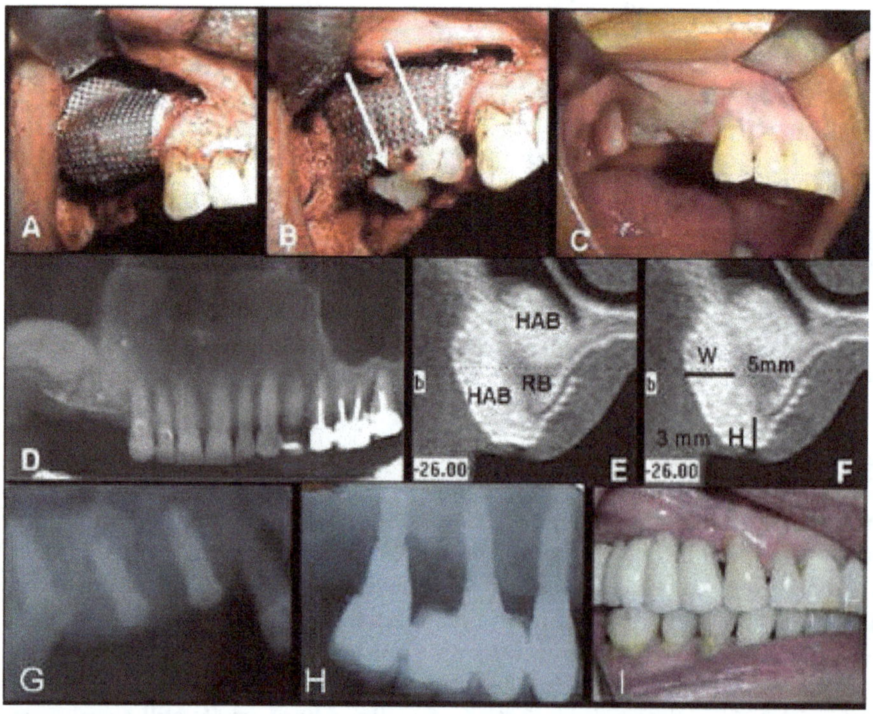

Fig. 6. A. Ti mesh augmentation procedure in upper maxilla using ABB alone as graft material. B. PRP covering Ti mesh in order to enhance soft tissue healing. C. Soft tissue healing after six month of surgery. D,E, F. TC scan images showing horizontal (5 mm) and vertical (3 mm) bone augmentation achieved.G,H,I. Implant´s placement and prosthesis evaluation radiography. I. Image of prosthesis rehabilitation.

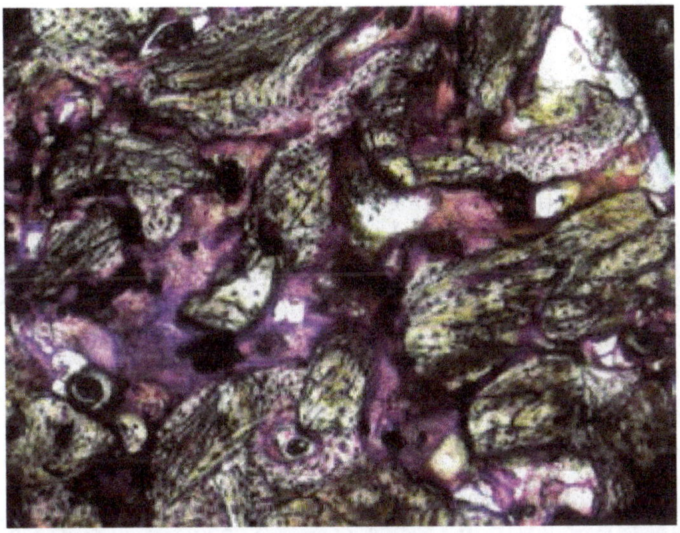

Fig. 7. ABB particles surrounded by newly formed bone in a Ti-mesh bone augmentation procedure where ABB alone was used as graft material.

Type of Graft (%)	ABW (mm)	ABH (mm)	Survival (%)	Success (%)	References
AB (100)	ID	ID	ID	ID	Von Arx et al 1996
AB (100)	5.65	ID	ID	100	Malchiodi et al 1998
AB (100) *	ID	5	ID	ID	Rocuzzo et al 2004
AB (100) *	ID	4.8	100	100	Rocuzzo et al 2007
AB/ABB (50/50)	ID	ID	98.3	ID	Maiorana et al 2001
AB/ABB (70/30)	4.16	3.71	100	100	Pieri et al 2008
AB/ABB (70/30)	ID	ID	100	100	Corinaldesi et al 2007
AB/ABB (ID)	3.71	2.86	ID	ID	Profusaefs & Lozana 2006
ABB (100)	ID	5.2	100	ID	Artzi et al 2003

Pts: patients; BAP: bone augmentation procedures; ABW: average bone width gained; ABH: average bone height gained; AB: autologous bone; ID: insufficient data;: block grafts.*

Table 5. Summary of clinical studies reporting the amount bone gained, type of graft and complications rate using the Ti-mesh technique. (Modified from Torres et al 2010)

3.3 Treating fenestrations and dehiscence

Particulate autogenous bone, anorganic bovine bone and FDBA have been proposed for treatment such defects in combination with GBR technique.

4. Summary

Since the introduction of dental implants, bone grafting has become an important procedure required for the treatment of patients with limited bone availability. Bone autograft, alone or together with other bone substitutes, has been the biomaterial of choice for clinicians worldwide. However different xenogenic, allogenic and synthetic biomaterials have shown promising results in many bone augmentation procedures.

The bone substitute needed for each bone regeneration procedure must be selected based on the individual´s characteristics, and the surgical procedure it self. Factors such as the osteogenic potential of the host residual bone, systemic health of patients, and morphology of the defects, will delimit the ideal bone substitute for each situation. For example in sinus augmentation, allografts, xenografs and synthetic calcium phosphates have been used as alternative to autografts with high rate of implants success and survival. On the other hand, when major alveolar ridge augmentations are required autograft onlay block are the most predictable biomaterials, although autograft granules mixed in different proportions with ABB in GBR procedures have also a high rate of success.

5. References

Albee FH. (1920). *Ann Surg.*;71(1):32-9.

Albert A, Leemrijse T, Druez V, Delloye C. & Cornu O. (2006). *Acta Orthop Belg*; 72(6):734-40.

Alkhraisat MH, Rueda C, Jerez LB, Tamimi Mariño F, Torres J, Gbureck U & Lopez Cabarcos E. (2010).. *Acta Biomater*;6:257-65.].

Alkhraisat MH, Moseke C, Blanco L, Barralet JE, Lopez-Carbacos E. & Gbureck U. (2008). *Biomaterials*;29:4691-7.

Alkhraisat MH, Mariño FT, Retama JR, Jerez LB. &López-Cabarcos E.(2008). *J Biomed Mater Res*;84:710-7

Artzi, Z ., Dayan, D., Alpern, Y. & Nemcovsky C.E. (2003). *International Journal Oral Maxillofacial Implants* 18,440-446

Arrington ED, Smith WJ, Chambers HG, Bucknell AL. & Davino NA.(1996). *Clin Orthop Relat Res*;(329):300-9.

Avila G, Neiva R, Misch CE, Galindo-Moreno P, Benavides E, Rudek I & Wang HL. (2010).*Implant Dent*;19(4):330-41.

Bauer TW. & Muschler GF.(2000).. *Clin Orthop Relat Res*;(371):10-27. .

Brown W. & Chow L. (1985). Dental restorative cement pastes. US Patent No. 4518430

Cammack GV 2nd, Nevins M, Clem DS 3rd, Hatch JP & Mellonig JT. (2005). *Int J Periodontics Restorative Dent*;25(3):231-7.

Cohen RE, Mullarky RH, Noble B, Comeau RL. & Neiders ME. (1994) *J Periodontol*; 65; 1008-15

Constantino PD & Freidman CD. (1997).. *Otalaryngol Clin North Am*;27:1037-1073

Carmagnola, D., Adriaens, P. & Berglundh, T. (2003). *Clinical Oral Implants Research* 14, 137-143

Corinaldesi G., Pieri F., Marchetti C., Fini M., Aldini N. N. & Giardino R. (2007). *Journal of Periodontology* 78,1477-1484.

Daelemans P, Hermans M, Godet F. & Malevez C.(1996). *Clin Oral Implants Res*;7(2):162-9.

Dahlin C, Simion M. & Hatano N.(2010). *Clin Implant Dent Relat Res*;12(4):263-70

Drosos GI, Kazakos KI, Kouzoumpasis P & Verettas DA.(2007). *Injury*;38 Suppl 4:S13-21.

Eppley BL, Pietrzak WS. & Blanton MW.(2005). *J Craniofac Surg*;16(6):981-9.

Esposito M, Piattelli M, Pistilli R, Pellegrino G. & Felice P.(2010). *Eur J Oral Implantol*;3(4):297-305.

Felice P, Marchetti C, Iezzi G, Piattelli A, Worthington H, Pellegrino G. & Esposito M (2009).. *Clinical Oral Implants Research*; 20;1386-93

Frame JW, Rout PG. & Browne RM.(1987). *J Oral Maxillofac Surg*;45(9):771-8.

Froum SJ, Wallace SS, Elian N, Cho SC & Tarnow DP.(2006). *Int J Periodontics Restorative Dent*;26(6):543-51.

Froum SJ, Wallace SS, Cho SC, Elian N & Tarnow DP.(2008).. *Int J Periodontics Restorative Dent.*;28(3):273-81.

Fujita R, Yokoyama A, Kawasaki T & Kohgo T.(2003).. *J Oral Maxillofac Surg*;61(9):1045-53.

Galindo-Moreno P, Moreno-Riestra I, Avila G, Fernández-Barbero JE, Mesa F, Aguilar M, Wang HL. & O'Valle F.(2010).. *Clin Oral Implants Res.*;21(1):122-8.

Gatti AM, Simonetti LA, Monari E, Guidi S. & Greenspan D.(2006). *J Biomater Appl*;20(4):325-39.

Giannoudis PV, Dinopoulos H. & Tsiridis E.(2005). *Injury*;36 Suppl 3:S20-7.

Hallman M, Sennerby L. & Lundgren S.(2002). *J Oral Maxillofac Surg*;60(3):277-84.

Hämerle, C.H., Chiantella, G.C., Karring, T. & Lang, N.P. (1998) *Clinical Oral Implants Research;* 9: 151-162

Hämmerle CH, Olah AJ, Schmid J, Flückiger L, Gogolewski S, Winkler JR. & Lang NP.(1997). *Clin Oral Implants Res*;8(3):198-207

Hetherington HE, Hollinger JO, Morris MR. & Panje WR.(1996). *Ann Otol Rhinol Laryngol.*;105(7):568-73.

John HD. & Wenz B.(2004). *Int J Oral Maxillofac Implants*;19(2):199-207.

Khan SN, Tomin E. & Lane JM.(2000). *Orthop Clin North Am*;31(3):389-98

Kao ST. & Scott DD.(2007). *Oral Maxillofac Surg Clin North Am*;19(4):513-21

Klammert U, Gbureck U, Vorndran E, Rödiger J, Meyer-Marcotty P. & Kübler AC. (2010).. *J Craniomaxillofac Surg*;38:565-70.

Maiorana C., Santoro F., Rabagliati M.& Salina S. (2001). *International Journal Oral Maxillofacial Implants* 16,427-432.

Malchiodi L., Scarano A., Quaranta M. & Piattelli A. (1998). *International Journal Oral Maxillofacial Implants* 13,701-705.

Minichetti JC, D'Amore JC. & Hong AY.(2008). *J Oral Implantol.*;34(3):135-41.

Mirtchi AA, Lemaitre J & Terao N.(1990).. *Biomaterials*:10:475-480

Misch CE. & Dietsh F.(1993). *Dent Implantol Update*;4(12):93-7

Moore WR, Graves SE. & Bain GI.(2001). *ANZ J Surg*;71(6):354-61

Peleg M, Mazor Z. & Garg AK.(1999). *Int J Oral Maxillofac Implants*;14(4):549-56.

Petersson K, Pamenius M, Eliasson A, Narby B, Holender F, Palmqvist S. & Håkansson J.(2006). *Swed Dent J.*;30(2):77-86

Piattelli, M., Favero, G.A., Scarano, A., Orsini, G. & Piattelli, A. (1999) *International Journal of Oral and Maxillofacial Implants* 14, 835-840.

Pieri F., Corinaldesi G., Fini M, Aldini N. N., Giardino R. & Marchetti C. (2008). *Journal of Periodontology* 79,2093-2103.

Proussaefs P. & Lozada J. (2006). *Journal of Oral Implantology* 32,237-247.

Reddi AH.(1998). *Clin Orthop Relat Res*;(355 Suppl):S66-72.

Quereshy FA, Dhaliwal HS, El SA, Horan MP. & Dhaliwal SS.(2010). *J Oral Maxillofac Surg*;68(10):2497-502.

Rocchietta I, Fontana F. & Simion M.(2008). *J Clin Periodontol*;35(8 Suppl):203-15.

Roccuzzo M., Ramieri G., Spada M. C., Bianchi S. D. & Berrone S. (2004). *Clinical Oral Implants Research* 15,73-81

Roccuzzo, M., Ramieri, G., Bunino, M. & Berrone S. (2007). *Clinical Oral Implants Research.* 18,286-294

Rodriguez A, Anastassov GE, Lee H, Buchbinder D. & Wettan H.(2003). *J Oral Maxillofac Surg.*;61(2):157-63

Santos FA, Pochapski MT, Martins MC, Zenóbio EG, Spolidoro LC. & Marcantonio E Jr.(2010). *Clin Implant Dent Relat Res*;12(1):18-25.

Scarano A, Degidi M, Iezzi G, Pecora G, Piattelli M, Orsini G, Caputi S, Perrotti V, Mangano C.& Piattelli A.(2006). .*Implant Dent*;15(2):197-207.

Simunek A, Kopecka D, Somanathan RV, Pilathadka S. & Brazda T.(2008). Int *J Oral Maxillofac Implants*;23(5):935-42.

Simion M, Rocchietta I, Kim D, Nevins M. & Fiorellini (2006). *International Journal Periodontics and Restorative Dentistry*;26: :415-23

Simion M, Nevins M, Rocchietta I, Fontana F, Maschera E, Schupbach P & Kim DM (2009).. *International Journal Periodontics and Restorative Dentistry*;29: 245-55.

Simunek A, Kopecka D, Somanathan RV, Pilathadka S. & Brazda T.(2008). Int *J Oral Maxillofac Implants*;23(5):935-42.

Skoglund A, Hising P. & Young C.(1997). *Int J Oral Maxillofac Implants*;12(2):194-9.

Stanley HR, Hall MB, Clark AE, King CJ 3rd, Hench LL. & Berte JJ.(1997). *Int J Oral Maxillofac Implants*;12(1):95-105

Stevenson S.(1999). *Orthop Clin North Am.*;30(4):543-52.

Szabó G, Huys L, Coulthard P, Maiorana C, Garagiola U, Barabás J, Németh Z, Hrabák K,. & Suba Z.(2005). *Int J Oral Maxillofac Implants*;20(3):371-81.

Tamimi F, Torres J, Gbureck U, Lopez-Cabarcos E, Bassett DC, Alkhraisat MH,. & Barralet JE.(2009). *Biomaterials*;30(31):6318-26.

Tamura K, Sato S, Kishida M, Asano S, Murai M. & Ito K.(2007).. *J Periodontol*;78(2):315-21.

Torres, J., Tamimi, F., Martinez, P.P., Alkhraisat, M.H., Linares, R., Hernández, G., Torres-Macho, J. & López-Cabarcos, E. (2009). *Journal of Clinical Periodontology* 36, 677-687.

Urban IA, Jovanovic SA. & Lozada JL.(2009). *Int J Oral Maxillofac Implants*;24(3):502-10.

Valentini, P. & Abensur, D.J. (2003) *International Journal of Oral and Maxillofacial Implants* 18, 556-560.

Välimäki VV. & Aro HT.(2006). *Scand J Surg*;95(2):95-102.

Virolainen P, Perälä M, Vuorio E. & Aro H.(1995). *Clin Orthop Relat Res*;(317):263-72.

Von Arx T., Hardt N. & Wallkamm B. (1996 *International Journal Oral Maxillofacial Implants* 11,387-394.

Waasdorp J. & Reynolds MA.(2010). *Int J Oral Maxillofac Implants*;25(3):525-31.

Wallace RH. (2000). *The European Journal of Prosthodonthic and Restorative Dentistry* 8, 103-106

Zawacki SJ, Koutsoukos PB, Salimi NH. & Nancollas GH.(1996). vol. (323). Am Chem Soc Symp Series;. p. 650–62.

7

Oral Bacterial Adhesion and Biocompatibility of Silver-Amorphous Carbon Films: A Surface Modification for Dental Implants

Argelia Almaguer-Flores[1], Sandra E. Rodil[1]
and René Olivares-Navarrete[2]
Universidad Nacional Autónoma de México, México City
[2]Georgia Institute of Technology, Atlanta, GA,
USA

1. Introduction

Bacterial adhesion and the subsequent biofilm formation on dental implants is a persistent problem that can cause implant failure. Once biofilm is formed, bacterial cells become highly resistant to antibiotics and host defences (Costerton et al., 1999, Patel, 2005), and clinical experience has shown that biofilms must be removed physically before the infection can be resolved (Costerton, 2005).

There is an apparent clinical and microbiological similarity between peri-implantitis and periodontitis (Listgarten and Lai, 1999, Papaioannou et al., 1996). The first indication of the specific role of bacteria in peri-implant infections was originated from microscopic analysis of samples taken from failing implants that shown an abundance of motile rods, fusiform bacteria and spirochetes, whereas samples from successful implants contained only a small number of coccoid cells and very few rods (Mombelli, 2002, Mombelli et al., 1987, Rams and Link, 1983). These findings revealed a site-specific disease process with microorganisms associated in patterns known from chronic periodontitis of natural teeth. The term peri-implantitis introduced in the 1980s, describe a destructive inflammatory process affecting the soft and hard tissues around osseointegrated implants, leading to the formation of a peri-implant pocket and loss of supporting bone (Mombelli et al., 1987).

Adhesion to a surface is the essential first step in the development of a biofilm and the sequential colonization and formation of the dental plaque is highly orchestrated (Xie et al., 2000). The association of bacteria within mixed biofilms is not random; it has been shown that there are specific associations (complexes) among bacteria in dental biofilms (Socransky and Haffajee, 2005, Socransky et al., 1998, Kolenbrander et al., 2006). In addition, these microbial complexes, can be used to describe the sequential colonization of the subgingival plaque. Some bacterial strains, mainly belonging to the genus *Actinomyces* (blue complex) and *Streptococcus* (yellow complex) have been identified as early colonizers of the dental surface, attaching and proliferating at an early stage. A second group of bacteria that functions as bridge between the early and late colonizers are formed by species belonging to the green, purple and orange complexes (i.e. *Fusobacterium nucleatum, Capnocytophaga sputigena, Eikenella corrodens*). Finally, the third group of species that appears at late stages in

biofilm development and that are considered true periodontal pathogens are species of the red complex (*Porphyromonas gingivalis, Tannerella forsythia* and *Treponema denticola*).
This biomaterial-related infection is characterized by chronicity, persistence and lack of susceptibility to antimicrobial agents. This information suggests that the first steps on the biofilm formation on implant surfaces such as titanium (Ti) or stainless steel (SS) can be similar to the process on teeth. In fact, the experimental gingivitis model described by Löe et al. that demonstrated the cause and effect relationship between biofilm formation on teeth and gingivitis (Loe et al., 1965), has been also used to explain the implant and peri-implant mucositis (Pontoriero et al., 1994, Zitzmann et al., 2001). Studies about the peri-implant microbiota *in vivo* have examined the influence of oral health status on the presence of specific bacterial species. Some of these studies reported similar supra and subgingival microbiota on teeth and Ti implants (Shibli et al., 2008, Furst et al., 2007, Groessner-Schreiber et al., 2004). In contrast, other studies found an absence of periodontal pathogens like *Aggregatibacter* (formerly *Actinobacillus*) *actinomycetemcomitans* and *Porphyromonas gingivalis* (Heuer et al., 2007) or sporadic high numbers of *Parvimonas micra* (formerly *Peptostreptococcus micros*), *Staphylococcus aureus* and *Staphylococcus epidermidis* (Furst et al., 2007, Salvi et al., 2008).
The biofilm formation process is extremely complicated and this is particularly true when multiple species are present in the biofilm as in dental plaque. This process is affected by many factors including environment, bacterial properties and material surface characteristics, such as chemical composition, surface energy, hydrophilicity and topography (Katsikogianni and Missirlis, 2004, An and Friedman, 1998, Merritt and Chang, 1991). In addition, for *in vitro* studies, the media play an important role as well, as was shown in a previous work comparing the influence of two different media on the bacterial adhesion and the initial biofilm formation (*Mycoplasma* media, a standard bacterial culture media, and sterilized human saliva); revealing different patterns of adhesion on the same surface when bacteria were cultured with different media (Almaguer-Flores et al., 2010).

2. Surface modifications to prevent bacterial adhesion and biofilm formation on dental implants

Surfaces are critical in the field of biomaterials; the nature of an implant surface determines their interaction with the biological environment. Surface modifications can be classified as physical modifications (sandblasting, patterning, etching, lithography, etc) or chemical modifications (deposition, thin films, polymer coating, etc). Often these techniques are applied in combination to alter both topography and surface energy. Surface modifications can be classified on basically three classes: (a) topographic modifications; such as size and porous distribution and roughness, (b) chemical modifications of the surface; which involve controlled cleaning and oxidation by glow discharge plasma techniques, thin film growth, and deposition of organic overlayers such as polymers, proteins and antimicrobial substances and (c) micromechanical or viscoelastic modifications of the surface, which can affect (enforce or reduce) the mechanical stress-strain fields at the interface (Bagno and Di Bello, 2004, Kasemo and Gold, 1999). These modifications offers the possibility of combining ideal bulk properties with desired properties such as increased bioactivity or prevent bacterial adhesion.
Antibacterial surface modifications have been created in order to prevent bacterial contamination and resulting infections, which can lead to the loss of the implant. These surface modifications must be designed to retard bacterial colonization or can function as

antimicrobial agents without affecting the cells and tissues adjacent to the implant; in other words, they need to be biocompatible.

Some studies have explored the *in vitro* biofilm formation on modified titanium implant surfaces; unfortunately, most of these biofilm models have only included one or two oral bacterial strains (Table 1). In the oral cavity however, the microbial ecology is complex and consists of hundreds of species (Socransky and Haffajee, 2005). For this reason, these models are good tools in order to study species-specific infections or mono-infections, but not very useful to study mixed anaerobic infections such as peri-implantitis.

Strain	Surface	Ref.
S. sanguis *S. mutans*	Ti, and TiN, ZrN, TiO_2	(Grossner-Schreiber et al., 2001)
P. gingivalis	Ti with ion implantation (Ca+, N+, F+), oxidation (anode oxidation, titania spraying), ion platting (TiN, alumina) and ion beam mixing (Ag, Sn, Zn, Pt)	(Yoshinari et al., 2001)
E. coli *P. aeruginosa* *B. cepacia* *B. subtilis*	11 different glass and metal oxide-coated glass surfaces	(Li and Logan, 2004)
S. sanguis	Ti with different roughness	(Pereira da Silva et al., 2005)
S. aureus *P. aeruginosa*	Ti coated with albumin	(Kinnari et al., 2005)
P. gingivalis	Ti and TiN thin films	(Jeyachandran et al., 2007)
S. aureus *S. epidermidis* *S. mutans* *P. aeruginosa*	Ti with bioactive polymers layers	[Maddikeri, 2008 #56]
S. sanguinis	Ti, Au, and ceramic and composite dental materials	(Hauser-Gerspach et al., 2007)
S. aureus	Ti with polyelectrolyte multilayers	(Chua et al., 2008)
S. aureus *S. epidermidis*	Ti with (P(MAA)) followed by immobilization of silk sericin	(Zhang et al., 2008)
S. aureus	Ti, Ta, Cr and DLC surfaces	(Levon et al., 2009)
S. sanguinis	Ti with two modified different roughness	(Burgers et al., 2010)
S. aureus *P. aeruginosa*	Ti with micro and nano scale surface roughness	(Truong et al., 2010)
S. epidermidis	Ti with four modified different roughness	(Wu et al., 2011)

Table 1. *In vitro* bacterial adhesion studies on Ti modified implant surfaces.

2.1 Amophous carbon films

It has been shown that all the different forms of amorphous carbon can be considered as biocompatible (Das et al., 2007, Hauert, 2003, Lettington, 1998, Du et al., 1998) and might be adequate as a surface modification for biomedical applications, such as, dental and orthopaedic implants (Santavirta, 2003, Affatato et al., 2000). Amorphous carbon films are nanostructured materials deposited as thin films which consist of sp^2 hybridized carbon atoms, clustered within a typical size of a few nanometers, and connected among them by sp^3 hybridized carbon atoms. Depending on the fraction of sp^2 to sp^3 hybridized C atoms, the films have been name as diamond-like carbon (DLC), graphite-like carbon (GLC) or when highly hydrogenated as polymer-like carbon (PLC). The fundamental difference between graphite and diamond-like is the amount of sp^3 hybridized carbon atoms, which is very low in the first group and above 40-50% for DLC. This leads to strong differences in many of the physical properties, such as, optical gap, conductivity, surface energy, etc. (Robertson, 2002).

2.1.1 Biocompatibility

Biomaterials must satisfy certain criteria in order to be used as implants or medical devices. The most important requirement for biomaterials is that they need to be biocompatible. Several definitions of biocompatibility have been established, but in general, biocompatibility can be defined as the ability of the material, intentionally in contact or implanted into the body tissues, to perform as designed without inducing any local effect in the cells or tissue or a systemic response that elicits an immunological reaction. In addition, the biomaterial should not cause denaturalization of the proteins adsorbed on the surface or leach any substance that can induce toxicity to the cells or tissues adjacent to the implant.

In dental and orthopaedic implants, de novo bone formation in direct contact with the bone, also known as osseointegration, is desired. In order to achieve successful osseointegration, progenitor cells and osteoblasts must attach to the implant surface, differentiate into mature osteoblasts, produce an organized extracellular matrix, and finally mineralize the extracellular matrix. Several biomaterials have been applied with a broad range of success in orthopaedic and dental implants. Metallic biomaterials generally have been used for dental and orthopaedic application due to their mechanical properties. Several publications have addressed *in vitro, in vivo,* and clinically that metallic implant surface modifications improve osseointegration, increase bone to implant contact, decrease healing time, and are clinically successful (Schwarz et al., 2010, Stanford, Li et al., 2010, Dohan Ehrenfest et al., 2010, Karabuda et al., 2010, Schatzle et al., 2009).

During the last years, we have been investigating different aspects of the interaction between human cells (osteoblasts) and graphite-like carbon films (GLC) as possible candidates for coating dental implants. Contrary to many other research groups, we choose GLC instead of DLC films because the main interest was on the osseointegration and not on the tribological properties and graphite itself has been established as a good osteoinductor material (Rodil et al., 2003, Rodil et al., 2005). Graphite-like amorphous carbon films were produced by a hollow cathode DC magnetron sputtering system attached to a high vacuum chamber. We have obtained good results concerning the interaction to human osteoblasts and also good osteoconductive properties (Rodil et al., 2006, Olivares et al., 2004).

2.1.2 Bacterial adhesion

Nevertheless, another important factor for the success of implants (included dental implants) is to avoid formation of biofilms that might lead to implant failure or strong inflammatory process (infection). Limited studies regarding bacterial adhesion on the different carbon films have been published before (Wang et al., 2004, Ishihara et al., 2006,

Jones et al., 2006, Katsikogianni et al., 2006, Morrison et al., 2006, Kwok et al., 2007, Zhao et al., 2007, Zhou et al., 2008, Kinnari et al., 2008). These works included mainly DLC or modified-DLC films and concluded that the carbon surface has great biocompatibility properties and good resistance to microbial adhesion. However, these results could not be extrapolated to the GLC films due to the strong differences between DLC and GLC physical properties, which are known to affect the bacterial adhesion. Moreover, none of these studies include oral bacteria and in any case no more than three bacterial strains were used.
We have developed a biofilm model using nine selected species representative of all the complexes of the subgingival dental plaque, described by Socransky et al. (Socransky et al., 1998) (Table 2). We used *A. israelii* and *S. sanguinis* as early colonizers. A second group of bacteria included *F. nucleatum, C. rectus, E. corrodens, P. micra* and *P. intermedia,* these species are known because functions as a bridge between the early and late colonizers. *P. gingivalis* was used as a representative of the third group of species that appears at late stages of biofilm development and *A. actinomycetemcomitans* was used due to the role that seems to have in periodontal infections (Wilson and Henderson, 1995). All strains were grown under anaerobic conditions (80% N_2, 10% CO_2 and 10% H_2).
In a first study, the bacterial adhesion of these microorganisms was evaluated on amorphous carbon (a-C) films in comparison to titanium (Ti) and stainless steel (SS) control surfaces. The results showed that the oral bacterial adhesion on these GLC films was relative high in comparison to standard surfaces (Ti and SS) (Almaguer-Flores et al., 2009).
In a second experiment, (Almaguer-Flores et al., 2010), the influence of the surface roughness and culture media was investigated comparing carbon and titanium films. The surface roughness was modified by deposition of films on both rough stainless steel and silicon substrates, the roughness of the stainless steel was significantly larger than the silicon (1.89 ± 0.5 μm and 0.028 ± 0.003 μm, respectively) therefore two different roughness were compared. In addition, the study was done comparing two different media; *Mycoplasma* media (MM), which is an standard bacterial culture media, and sterilized human saliva (HS) because is the major bulk fluid in the oral cavity.

Specie	ATCC*
Aggregatibacter actinomycetemcomitans serotipe b	43718
Actinomyces israelii	12102
Campylobacter rectus	33238
Eikenella corrodens	23834
Fusobacterium nucleatum subsp. *nucleatum*	25586
Parvimonas micra	33270
Porphyromonas gingivalis	33277
Prevotella intermedia	25611
Streptococcus sanguinis	10556

* American Type Culture Collection, Rockville, MD

Table 2. Reference strains employed for the adhesion and biofilm formation assays.

AFM images of the samples presented in Figure 1 (a,b,c and d), showed that not only the roughness values were modified, but also the topographical features of the samples were different. The samples deposited on silicon showed a spiky homogeneous topography but the maximum height of the peaks is in the nanometer scale. While for the rough surfaces, the topography is like a series of non-homogeneous hills and valleys, reaching heights in the micrometer scale.

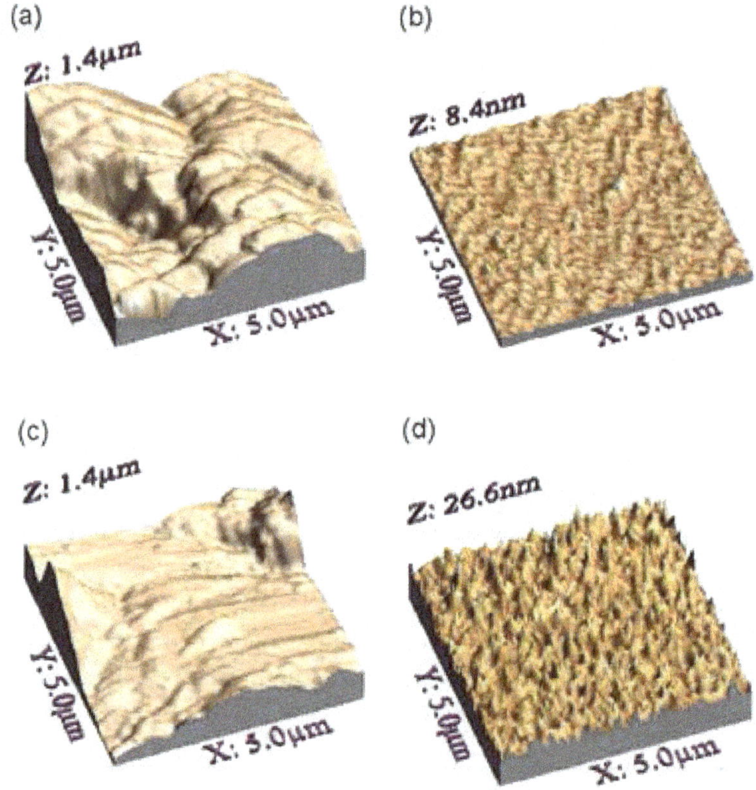

Fig. 1. AFM images of the test substrates. Vertical scale has been normalized, Z value indicate maximum height in each film. (a) a-C film deposited on the stainless steel sandblasted substrate (a-C r). (b) a-C film deposited on silicon substrate (a-C s). (c) Ti film deposited on the stainless steel sandblasted substrate (Ti r). (d) Ti film deposited on silicon substrate (Ti s).

Bacterial adhesion on the test samples varied depending on the media used, the surface roughness and the surface chemistry, data are presented in Figure 2A as the number of CFUs/cm^2 x 10^5. There were consistently more bacteria on the rough surfaces and in the surfaces cultivated with *Mycoplasma* media. The number of CFU´s was reduced on the Ti surfaces compared with the a-C surfaces. Significant differences were observed between Ti s and Ti r ($p < 0.05$) and Ti s and a-C s ($p < 0.05$). When human saliva was used, lower bacterial counts were detected on all surfaces compared to the *Mycoplasma* media. Indeed, the number of CFU's was highly reduced on the a-C s surfaces, and statistical differences were found comparing a-C s vs a-C r and a-C s vs Ti s ($p < 0.05$).

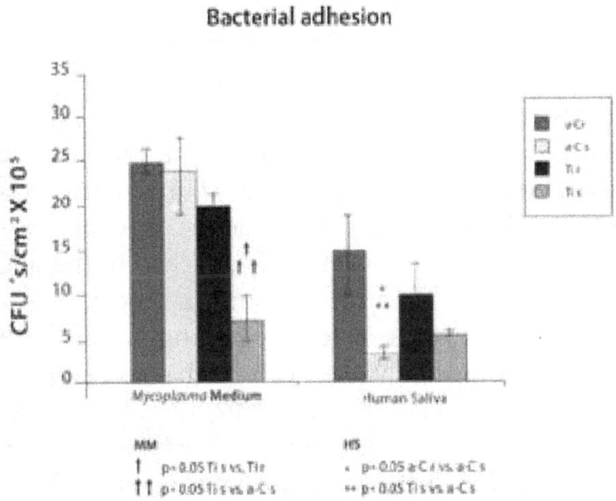

A

Fig. 2A. Bacterial adhesion (CFU's x 10^5) on rough (r) and smooth (s) a-C and Ti films, after 24h of anaerobic incubation with *Mycoplasma* medium (MM) or Human Saliva (HS).

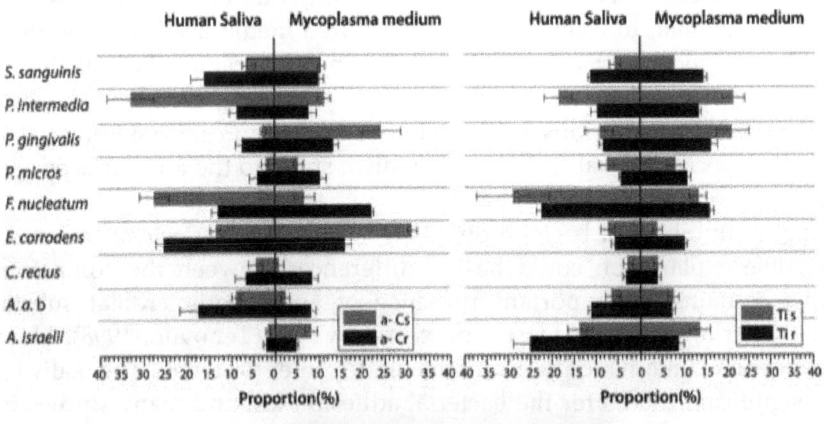

p> 0.05
NS= no significant

a-C r vs. a-Cs		Ti r vs. Ti s	
Saliva	*Mycoplasma*	Saliva	*Mycoplasma*
E. corredens *S. sanguinis* *F. nucleatum*	*E. corredens* *F. nucleatum* *C. rectus*	*S. sanguinis*	*E. corredens* *S. sanguinis*

Roughness (r vs. s)		Surface chemistry (a-C VS. ti)		Incubation Media (Saliva vs. Mycoplasma)			
Saliva	*Mycoplasma*	Saliva	*Mycoplasma*	r	s	a-C	Ti
P. intermedia *S. sanguinis*	NS	*E. corrodens* *A. israelii*	*E. corrodens*	*P. micros* *P. gingivalis*	NS	*P. gingivalis* *A. israelii*	NS

Fig. 2B. Proportion of the nine bacterial strains in the biofilms formed on rough (r) and smooth (s) a-C and Ti films, after 24h of anaerobic incubation with *Mycoplasma* medium (MM) or Human Saliva (HS). Table at the bottom shows the statistical analysis divided according to the factors that influence the bacterial colonization. Where the bacteria name is shown, it indicates a significance of $p<0.05$ for that strain and NS means no statistical difference.

The influence of roughness was clearly observed in the number of bacteria attached to the rough surfaces (number of CFU's). Similarly, a positive correlation between surface roughness and bacterial attachment *in vitro* has been shown (Quirynen et al., 1996). The proportions of the bacterial strains were also affected by the surface roughness and this effect seems to be more pronounced when saliva was used. The proportion of *S. sanguinis* was significantly higher ($p < 0.05$) on rough surfaces for both a-C and Ti, i.e. independently of the surface chemistry. Meanwhile, *P. intermedia* showed a higher proportion on the smooth surfaces ($p < 0.05$). Nevertheless, other studies have suggested that regarding to bacterial adhesion or initial biofilm formation; roughness appears to be a minor factor (Bos et al., 1999).

Regarding the surface chemistry, higher numbers of attached bacteria (CFU´s) were detected on amorphous carbon than on the Ti samples, confirming the results from the initial study that indicate large affinity of oral bacteria for the carbon surface (Almaguer-Flores et al., 2009). These results differ with other published papers that have reported that carbon-based films can inhibit bacterial adhesion (Wang et al., 2004, Liu et al., 2008, Zhou et al., 2008).In addition, it has been suggested that Ti has some antibacterial properties explained due to the formation of peroxides at the surface (Jeyachandran et al., 2007). Although, another study suggested that pure Ti was more colonized by two oral bacteria strains in comparison to other surfaces like TiN, ZrN or TiO_2, (Grossner-Schreiber et al., 2001).

An interesting finding was the proportion of *E. corrodens* on the biofilms formed on the a-C surfaces. This strain was found in higher proportions on the a-C samples on both, rough and smooth surfaces, for both media MM or HS, suggesting that *E. corrodens* was more sensitive to surface chemistry than to roughness or the cultured media used. This finding supported the notion that chemical surface is directly affecting the colonization of the oral bacteria (Groessner-Schreiber et al., 2004). *E. corrodens* posses an specific lectin-like substance that mediates its adherence to various host tissue cell surfaces (Yamazaki et al., 1988), so it is possible that the specificity that this microorganism show to the a-C surfaces has to be with some specific adhesion properties of this strain.

We found higher numbers of bacteria on all surfaces when *Mycoplasma* culture media was used. A possible explanation could be the differences between the components of both media; saliva contains an important presence of some antimicrobial substances, such lysozyme, lactoferrin, lactoperoxidase, and secretory IgA (Tenovuo, 1998). Meanwhile, the *Mycoplasma* media contains only nutrients and some proteins. The saliva is a more biologically significant media for the bacterial adhesion test and many studies indicate that the saliva is critical for the colonization of certain taxa (Gibbons, 1996, De Jong and Van der Hoeven, 1987), and it is determinant for the type and amount of bacteria that will attach on a surface (Gibbons, 1996, Sela et al., 2007). However, human saliva is a very complex and non-homogeneous media in comparison to the MM, and actually changes in the composition can be found from donor to donor. So, in order to study the surface-bacteria interactions, a more homogeneous media could be more convenient.

2.2 Silver – amorphous carbon films (a-C:Ag)

Searching for reducing implant infections different modifications have been proposed such as functionalization of the surface with bactericidal polycationic groups (Tiller et al., 2001, Cen et al., 2004), developing delivery systems to coating the surface with polymers loaded with antibiotic or antimicrobial substances (Shi et al., 2006, Schmidmaier et al., 2006) or covering the implant surface with quaternary ammonium compounds or silver and iodine ions (Yorganci et al., 2002, Nohr and Macdonald, 1994, Tyagi and Singh, 1997, Ewald et al., 2006).

Silver antimicrobial properties have been recognized since historic times (Klasen, 2000, Burrell, 2003), and the coating of medical devices with silver coatings (Ewald et al., 2006,

Bosetti et al., 2002, Darouiche, 1999, Schierholz et al., 1998) or the addition of silver nanoparticles (Chen et al., 2006, Kwok et al., 2007, Jung et al., 2009, Rai et al., 2009) into the material's surface might be a good method to prevent device-associated infections by physical routes instead of the chemical routes mentioned above. Silver exhibits a rather broad-spectrum antimicrobial activity *in vitro* by binding both to microbial DNA, preventing bacterial replication, and to the sulfhydryl groups of the metabolic enzymes of the bacterial electron transport chain, causing their inactivation (Darouiche, 1999).
Considering the well-known silver antibacterial activity, amorphous carbon films with silver nanoparticles inclusions were produced and the biocompatibility and antibacterial properties of such films was evaluated. Details concerning the deposition conditions and properties of the films can be found somewhere else (Garcia-Zarco et al., 2009).

2.2.1 Biocompatibility

Several assays are used to test biocompatibility; however, due to the scope of this chapter focus on common assays that we perform to test the biocompatibility of our surface modifications.
To test biocompatibility of a-C:Ag surfaces, we perform the following assays.

MTT Assay

The MTT is a colorimetric assay that measures the reduction of a tetrazolium component (MTT, 3-(4,5-Dimethylthiasol-2-yl)-2,5-diphenyltetrazolium bromide) into a insoluble purple formazan product by the cell mitochondria. This reaction only occurs in viable cells, which have metabolic activity are capable to reduce the MTT. This assay is commonly used to determine the cytotoxicity of potential medical agents and biomaterials since released molecules can cause metabolic dysfunction that decreases or abolishes MTT reduction in the mitochondria and result in cell toxicity (Mosmann, 1983, Denizot and Lang, 1986). Thus, MTT reduction is proportional to cellular metabolic activity, and decreased MTT reduction infers a possible toxicity of the biomaterial or drug tested (Chen et al., 2011, Niu et al., 2011, Sahithi et al., 2010, Bispo et al., 2010).

Cell culture

Human MG63 osteoblast-like cells are commonly used in testing metallic biomaterials. MG63 cells present an immature osteoblast phenotype, which gives them the potential to be studied as a model of osteoblastic differentiation (Bachle and Kohal, 2004) (Schwartz et al., 1999). MG63 cells were purchased from the American Type Culture Collection (ATCC, Manassas, VA). Cells were cultured in Dulbecco's Modification of Eagle's Medium (DMEM, cellgro ®, Manassas, VA) supplemented with 10% fetal bovine serum (Gibco, Carlsbad, CA) and 1% penicillin-streptomycin (Gibco) at 37°C in 5% CO2 and 100% humidity.

Cell viability

MG63 cells were plated at a density of 10,000 cells/cm2 on tissue culture polystyrene (TCPS) or substrates coated with amorphous carbon (a-C) or amorphous carbon/silver (a-C:Ag). Cell viability was measured using Methylthiazolyldiphenyl-tetrazolium bromide (MTT) dye after 1, 3, or 7 days in culture. MTT dye was dissolved in water to yield a 5 mg/mL solution. MTT dye was then added to culture media of each well to a final concentration of 1 mg/mL and incubated for 4 hours. The media was then removed, the monolayer rinsed twice with PBS, and formazan crystals dissolved in 500 µL DMSO. 200 µL of the resulting solution was aliquoted into a 96 well microplate and read in an absorbance plate reader using a test wavelength of 570 nm and a reference wavelength of 630 nm.

Viability of MG63 cells cultured on a-C or a-C:Ag thin films was measured using MTT. One day after plating, cells cultured on both a-C and a-C:Ag had similar MTT activity to cells cultured on TCPS (Fig. 4). Viability at day 3 and day 7 was also similar in cells cultured on thin films than cells on TCPS. These results indicate that thin film coatings analyzed in this experiment did not affect cellular metabolism, indicating that they are not cytotoxic.

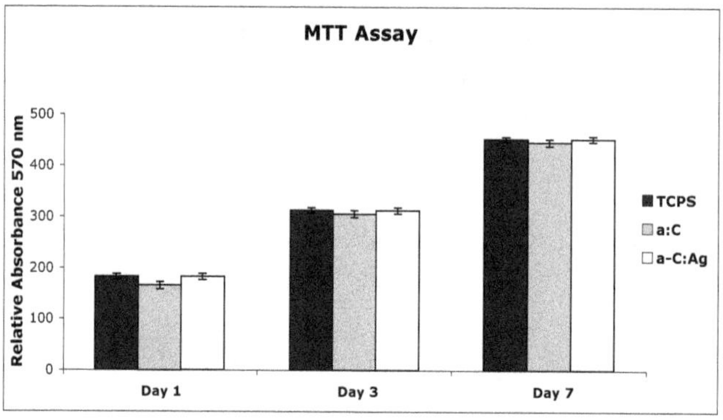

Fig. 4. Effect of thin films on MG63 cell viability. MG63 cells were cultured on tissue culture polystyrene (TCPS) or amorphous carbon (a-C) or amorphous carbon-silver (a-C:Ag) thin films. MTT activity was measured after 1 day, 3 days, or 7 days in culture. No significant differences were detected between the surfaces.

Osteoblast phenotype

MG63 cells were plated at a density of 10,000 cells/cm2 on tissue culture polystyrene (TCPS) or substrates coated with amorphous carbon (a-C) or amorphous carbon/silver (a-C:Ag). At confluence, cells were incubated with fresh media for 24h. Conditioned media was harvested and levels of secreted osteocalcin measured using a commercially available radioimmunoassay (Biomedical Technologies, Inc., Stoughton, MA). Cells were detached from the surface using two sequential incubations in 0.25% trypsin-EDTA and cell number determined using a Z2 Particle Counter (Beckman Coulter, Hialeah, FL). Cells were lysed in 0.05% Triton X-100 and homogenized by sonicating each sample for 10 s. Alkaline phosphatase specific activity was measured in cell lysates as a function of the release of p-nitrophenol from p-nitrophenylphosphate at pH 10.2 (Martin et al., 1996, Bretaudiere, 1984) and normalized to the total protein concentration (BCA Protein Assay, Pierce Chemical Co., Rockford, IL).

Whether surface modifications enhance osteoblast maturation can be assessed using three specific outcomes: cell number, alkaline phosphatase specific activity, and osteocalcin levels. Cells attach to biomaterials through the proteins adsorbed in the surface of the material. After this event, cell undergo proliferation and extracellular matrix production. It has been demonstrated that proliferation is reduced when cells undergo differentiation (Stein et al., 1990). In our experiment, cell number was lower on a-C and a-C:Ag thin films than on TCPS (Fig. 5A). Alkaline phosphatase specific activity, an early marker of osteoblast differentiation, is commonly used as a marker of bone formation. Alkaline phosphatase is an enzyme that acts on the phosphate groups of various molecules and generates a microenvironment rich in phosphate ions, which, in concert with calcium, mineralize the extracellular matrix to form bone. In osteoblasts, alkaline phosphatase increases when proliferation is inhibited during differentiation. Our results show that alkaline phosphatase was higher in cells grown on a-C and a-C:Ag than on TCPS (Fig. 5B). However, alkaline phosphatase specific activity increases in early differentiation, reaches a maximum, and begins to decrease as mineralization is initiated (Stein et al., 1990). To establish the specific stage of osteoblast maturation, osteocalcin was measured in the conditioned media. Osteocalcin is considered a later marker of osteoblast maturation, is present in all mineralized tissues in our body, and increases in relation to total mineralization during bone formation. In our experiments, cells cultured on a-C and a-C:Ag secreted more osteocalcin than cells on TCPS (Fig. 5C). The combination of these factors allows us to gauge more precisely the stage of osteoblast maturation, and the ability of surface modifications to enhance this, than any one factor alone. Taken together, our results establish that both a-C and a-C:Ag are not toxic, and promote osteoblast maturation increasing two main factors needed for bone formation, alkaline phosphatase activity and osteocalcin.

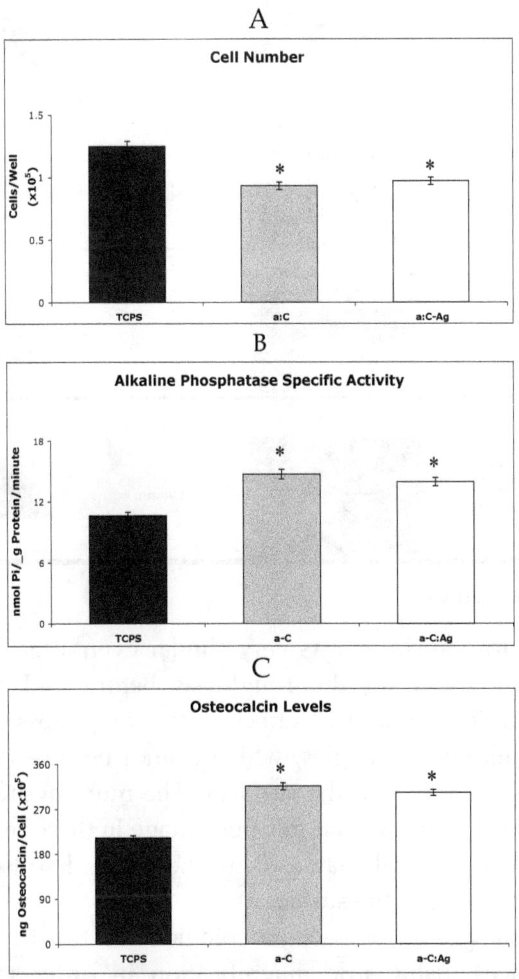

Fig. 5. Osteoblast phenotype in response to culture on thin films. MG63 cells were cultured on tissue culture polystyrene (TCPS) or amorphous carbon (a-C) or amorphous carbon-silver (a-C:Ag) thin films. At confluence, cell number (A), alkaline phosphatase specific activity in cell lysates (B), and secreted osteocalcin (C) were measured. *$p<0.05$, vs. TCPS.

2.2.2 Antibacterial effect

The oral bacterial adhesion and the initial biofilm formation on the amorphous carbon films modified with the Ag nanoparticles, was evaluated using our standard protocol for the oral bacteria. All surfaces (Table 3) were were incubated for 24 hours, 3 and 7 days with a mixture of the nine bacterial strains. One set of surfaces was used for determining the total counts of bacteria attached to each surface, by counting the colony forming units (CFU's) from each sample. In order to observe biofilm morphology and the surface coverage by bacteria, an additional set of samples was prepared for Scanning Electron Microscopy (SEM) following standard procedures.

Surface	SEM image (scale 5 μm) and Ra profilometer (Scan 5 mm)	Film thickness	Contact angle
Stainless steel medical grade 316L sandblasted substrate	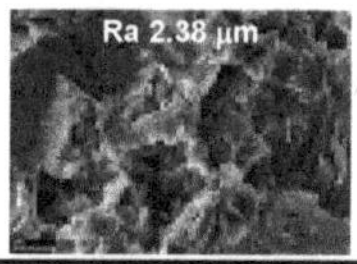	NA	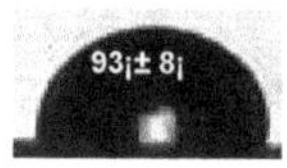
a-C film stainless steel medical grade 316L sandblasted substrate	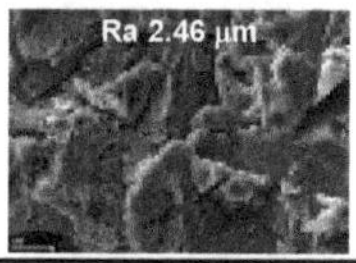	53.8 nm	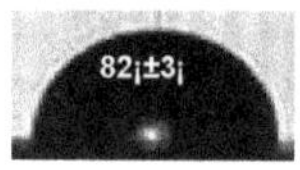
a-C:Ag film stainless steel medical grade 316L sandblasted substrate	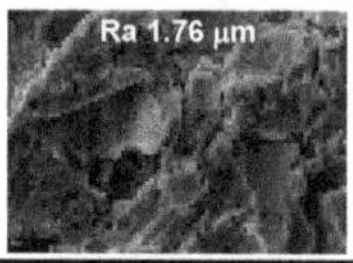	82.5 nm	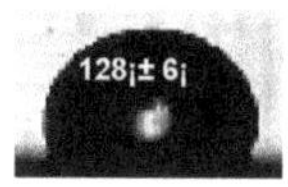
Ti film on stainless steel medical grade 316L sandblasted substrate	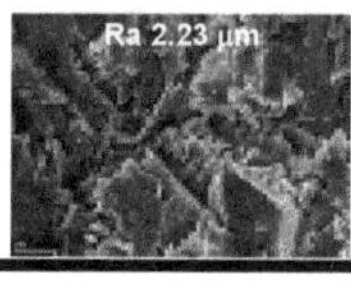	190 nm	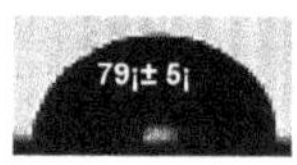

Table 3. Surface characterization.

The morphology of the four surfaces was very similar even after the film deposition. This was also confirmed by measuring the roughness before and after deposition, which remained close to 2 μm. The combined effect of the roughness value and the chemical composition lead to water contact angles, which cannot be directly related to the surface energy, but reflects the wettability of the surfaces. The more hydrophobic surface was the silver modified carbon film. The silver atomic percentage in these samples was around 6 at% and the average particle size as calculated using the Image J software (Collins, 2007) was 63.5 nm corresponding to ~10% of the surface area.

Figure 6 shows the BE images of the bacteria colonies as a function of the incubation time and for the four surfaces, using low magnification in order to observe the bacterial distribution among a large area of the surfaces (1.76 mm2). At the first day, mainly isolated attached bacteria were observed, as time went on, the formation of the biofilm was clearly observed and represents the large dark areas in the image, where the thick glycoprotein matrix was developing.

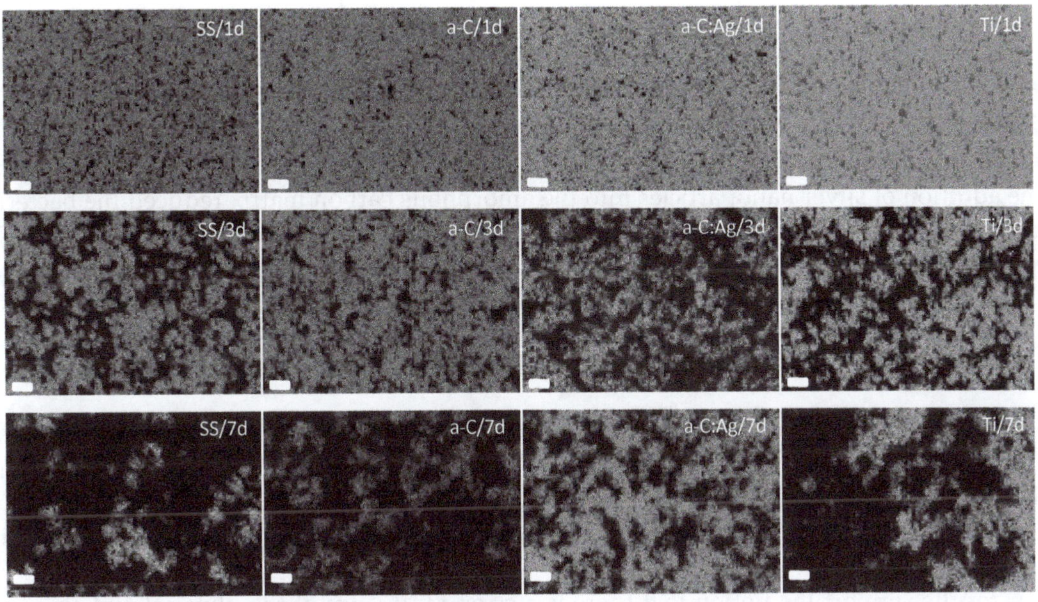

Fig. 6. Backscattering SEM images of the biofilms formed on the SS, a-C, a-C:Ag and Ti surfaces after 1, 3 and 7 days of anaerobic incubation. The scale bar corresponds to 100 μm and the magnification used was 250X.

The increment in the percentage of the surface covered by bacteria (or bacteria surface growth, BSG) as a function of time is clearly observed in figure 7, which also included the statistical analysis. Six different zones were analyzed and the area quantification was done at least three times for each zone, therefore it is possible to describe statistically the variations in the BSG. At the first day, less than 10 % of the total area was covered; actually, the bacteria were observed forming small groups (figure 6). However, at this time, a large amount of bacteria were found in the a-C:Ag films and less number was observed on the metallic surfaces. At three days, the larger number was found on the a-C films, while the other surfaces present similar coverage (~20 %). At 7 days, the amount of bacteria was highly reduced in the a-C:Ag films compared to the other surfaces.

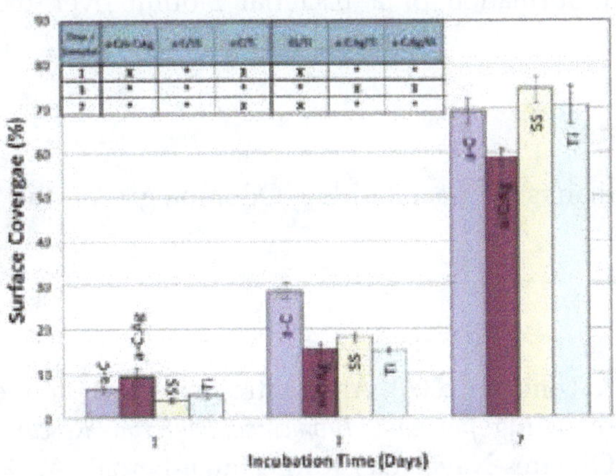

Fig. 7. Surface coverage estimated as the percentage of area covered by bacteria in the images shown in figure 6, using the ImageJ particle analyzer function. Statistically significant data are included in the table (* $p < 0.05$).

The reduction in surface coverage obtained for the a-C:Ag films after 7 days of incubation was significant lower than in the other surfaces. This is in agreement with the antimicrobial mechanism of the silver, where the active agents are really silver ions or radicals that in our samples will be produced via an erosion/corrosion process, taking place as the sample is immersed in the medium.

The addition of silver nanoparticles into the amorphous carbon matrix reduced the bacterial surface growth approximately 10% in comparison to the pure carbon matrix. The results indicated that the action of silver ions occurs in time, therefore not immediate response was observed for the bacterial adhesion.

3. Conclusions

The use of different bacterial strains from the oral cavity to study the bacteria adhesion profile on amorphous carbon have shown that it is not straightforward to reach conclusions about the anti-bacterial properties of any surface. When bacterial adhesion was tested using individual species, the adhesion profiles varied on the same surface depending of the bacterial strain.

Our results support the notion that there is a strong influence of the physical and chemical properties of the substrate in the colonization of oral bacteria, moreover when using human saliva, significantly reduced levels of bacteria were found on the a-C smooth surfaces.

In summary, it seems that Graphite-like amorphous carbon is not a suitable surface to prevent adhesion from the oral media but a-C:Ag films seems to inhibit bacteria adhesion after seven days of incubation. However, a-C films seem to be good to repel bacteria from certain oral strains, such as, *A. israelii*, *P. gingivalis* and *P. intermedia*. Although *E. corrodens* was capable to colonize in very high rates the a-C surfaces despite of their roughness or the culture media used.

Therefore, the determination of bacterial adhesion properties on biomaterials using only one or two bacterial strains is not accurate and cannot lead to general conclusions about the anti-bacterial properties of the biomaterial, at least when strains from the oral cavity are use.

Further studies are required in order to evaluate other physical, chemical and biological properties of the a-C:Ag films in order to understand the observed differences and also to analyze the sequential formation of a bacterial biofilm over these and other implant surfaces.

4. Acknowledgments

A. Almaguer-Flores thanks to Facultad de Odontología of the Universidad Nacional Autónoma de México.

5. References

Affatato, S., Frigo, M. & Toni, A. (2000). An in vitro investigation of diamond-like carbon as a femoral head coating. *Journal of Biomedical Materials Research* 53, 221-226.

Almaguer-Flores, A., Olivares-Navarrete, R., Lechuga-Bernal, A., Ximenez-Fyvie, L. A. & Rodil, S. E. (2009). Oral bacterial adhesion on amorphous carbon films. *Diamond and Related Materials* 18, 1179-1185.

Almaguer-Flores, A., Ximenez-Fyvie, L. A. & Rodil, S. E. (2010). Oral bacterial adhesion on amorphous carbon and titanium films: effect of surface roughness and culture media. *J Biomed Mater Res B Appl Biomater* 92, 196-204.

An, Y. H. & Friedman, R. J. (1998). Concise review of mechanisms of bacterial adhesion to biomaterial surfaces. *J Biomed Mater Res* 43, 338-348..

Bachle, M. & Kohal, R. J. (2004). A systematic review of the influence of different titanium surfaces on proliferation, differentiation and protein synthesis of osteoblast-like MG63 cells. *Clin Oral Implants Res* 15, 683-692.

Bagno, A. & Di Bello, C. (2004). Surface treatments and roughness properties of Ti-based biomaterials. *J Mater Sci Mater Med* 15, 935-949.

Bispo, V. M., Mansur, A. A., Barbosa-Stancioli, E. F. & Mansur, H. S. (2010). Biocompatibility of nanostructured chitosan/ poly(vinyl alcohol) blends chemically crosslinked with genipin for biomedical applications. *J Biomed Nanotechnol* 6, 166-175.

Bos, R., van der Mei, H. C. & Busscher, H. J. (1999). Physico-chemistry of initial microbial adhesive interactions--its mechanisms and methods for study. *FEMS Microbiol Rev* 23, 179-230.

Bosetti, M., Masse, A., Tobin, E. & Cannas, M. (2002). Silver coated materials for external fixation devices: in vitro biocompatibility and genotoxicity. *Biomaterials* 23, 887-892.

Bretaudiere, J. (1984) Alkaline Phosphatases. In: *Methods of Enzymatic Analysis,* (ed.) V. Chemie, pp. 75-92. Weinheim, Germany.

Burgers, R., Gerlach, T., Hahnel, S., Schwarz, F., Handel, G. & Gosau, M. (2010). In vivo and in vitro biofilm formation on two different titanium implant surfaces. *Clin Oral Implants Res* 21, 156-164.

Burrell, R. E. (2003). A scientific perspective on the use of topical silver preparations. *Ostomy Wound Manage* 49, 19-24.

Cen, L., Neoh, K. G. & Kang, E. T. (2004). Antibacterial activity of cloth functionalized with N-alkylated poly(4-vinylpyridine). *J Biomed Mater Res A* 71, 70-80.

Chen, W., Liu, Y., Courtney, H. S., Bettenga, M., Agrawal, C. M., Bumgardner, J. D. & Ong, J. L. (2006). In vitro anti-bacterial and biological properties of magnetron co-sputtered silver-containing hydroxyapatite coating. *Biomaterials* 27, 5512-5517.

Chen, Z. F., Tan, M. X., Liu, Y. C., Peng, Y., Wang, H. H., Liu, H. G. & Liang, H. (2011). Synthesis, characterization and preliminary cytotoxicity evaluation of five Lanthanide(III)-Plumbagin complexes. *J Inorg Biochem* 105, 426-434.

Chua, P. H., Neoh, K. G., Kang, E. T. & Wang, W. (2008). Surface functionalization of titanium with hyaluronic acid/chitosan polyelectrolyte multilayers and RGD for promoting osteoblast functions and inhibiting bacterial adhesion. *Biomaterials* 29, 1412-1421.

Collins, T. J. (2007). ImageJ for microscopy. *Biotechniques* 43, 25-30.

Costerton, J. W. (2005). Biofilm theory can guide the treatment of device-related orthopaedic infections. *Clin Orthop Relat Res*, 7-11.

Costerton, J. W., Stewart, P. S. & Greenberg, E. P. (1999). Bacterial biofilms: a common cause of persistent infections. *Science* 284, 1318-1322.

Darouiche, R. O. (1999). Anti-infective efficacy of silver-coated medical prostheses. *Clin Infect Dis* 29, 1371-1377.

Das, T., Ghosh, D., Bhattacharyya, T. K. & Maiti, T. K. (2007). Biocompatibility of diamond-like nanocomposite thin films. *Journal of Materials Science-Materials in Medicine* 18, 493-500.

De Jong, M. H. & Van der Hoeven, J. S. (1987). The growth of oral bacteria on saliva. *J Dent Res* 66, 498-505.

Denizot, F. & Lang, R. (1986). Rapid colorimetric assay for cell growth and survival. Modifications to the tetrazolium dye procedure giving improved sensitivity and reliability. *J Immunol Methods* 89, 271-277.

Dohan Ehrenfest, D. M., Coelho, P. G., Kang, B. S., Sul, Y. T. & Albrektsson, T. (2010). Classification of osseointegrated implant surfaces: materials, chemistry and topography. *Trends Biotechnol* 28, 198-206.

Du, C., Su, X. W., Cui, F. Z. & Zhu, X. D. (1998). Morphological behaviour of osteoblasts on diamond-like carbon coating and amorphous C-N film in organ culture. *Biomaterials* 19, 651-658.

Ewald, A., Gluckermann, S. K., Thull, R. & Gbureck, U. (2006). Antimicrobial titanium/silver PVD coatings on titanium. *Biomed Eng Online* 5, 22.

Furst, M. M., Salvi, G. E., Lang, N. P. & Persson, G. R. (2007). Bacterial colonization immediately after installation on oral titanium implants. *Clin Oral Implants Res* 18, 501-508.

Garcia-Zarco, O., Rodil, S. E. & Camacho-Lopez, M. A. (2009). Deposition of amorphous carbon-silver composites. *Thin Solid Films* 518, 1493-1497.

Gibbons, R. J. (1996). Role of adhesion in microbial colonization of host tissues: a contribution of oral microbiology. *J Dent Res* 75, 866-870.

Groessner-Schreiber, B., Hannig, M., Duck, A., Griepentrog, M. & Wenderoth, D. F. (2004). Do different implant surfaces exposed in the oral cavity of humans show different biofilm compositions and activities? *Eur J Oral Sci* 112, 516-522.

Grossner-Schreiber, B., Griepentrog, M., Haustein, I., Muller, W. D., Lange, K. P., Briedigkeit, H. & Gobel, U. B. (2001). Plaque formation on surface modified dental implants. An in vitro study. *Clin Oral Implants Res* 12, 543-551.

Hauert, R. (2003). A review of modified DLC coatings for biological applications. *Diamond and Related Materials* 12, 583-589.

Hauser-Gerspach, I., Kulik, E. M., Weiger, R., Decker, E. M., Von Ohle, C. & Meyer, J. (2007). Adhesion of Streptococcus sanguinis to dental implant and restorative materials in vitro. *Dent Mater J* 26, 361-366.

Heuer, W., Elter, C., Demling, A., Neumann, A., Suerbaum, S., Hannig, M., Heidenblut, T., Bach, F. W. & Stiesch-Scholz, M. (2007). Analysis of early biofilm formation on oral implants in man. *J Oral Rehabil* 34, 377-382.

Ishihara, M., Kosaka, T., Nakamura, T., Tsugawa, K., Hasegawa, M., Kokai, F. & Koga, Y. (2006). Antibacterial activity of fluorine incorporated DLC films. *Diamond and Related Materials* 15, 1011-1014.

Jeyachandran, Y. L., Venkatachalam, S., Karunagaran, B., Narayandass, S. K., Mangalaraj, D., Bao, C. Y. & Zhang, C. L. (2007). Bacterial adhesion studies on titanium, titanium nitride and modified hydroxyapatite thin films. *Materials Science & Engineering C-Biomimetic and Supramolecular Systems* 27, 35-41.

Jones, D. S., Garvin, C. P., Dowling, D., Donnelly, K. & Gorman, S. P. (2006). Examination of surface properties and in vitro biological performance of amorphous diamond-like carbon-coated polyurethane. *J Biomed Mater Res B Appl Biomater* 78, 230-236.

Jung, R., Kim, Y., Kim, H. S. & Jin, H. J. (2009). Antimicrobial properties of hydrated cellulose membranes with silver nanoparticles. *J Biomater Sci Polym Ed* 20, 311-324.

Karabuda, Z. C., Abdel-Haq, J. & Ariotasan, V. (2010). Stability, marginal bone loss and survival of standard and modified sand-blasted, acid-etched implants in bilateral edentulous spaces: a prospective 15-month evaluation. *Clin Oral Implants Res.* doi:10.1111/j.1600-0501.2010.02065.x.

Kasemo, B. & Gold, J. (1999). Implant surfaces and interface processes. *Adv Dent Res* 13, 8-20.

Katsikogianni, M. & Missirlis, Y. F. (2004). Concise review of mechanisms of bacterial adhesion to biomaterials and of techniques used in estimating bacteria-material interactions. *Eur Cell Mater* 8, 37-57.

Katsikogianni, M., Spiliopoulou, I., Dowling, D. P. & Missirlis, Y. F. (2006). Adhesion of slime producing Staphylococcus epidermidis strains to PVC and diamond-like carbon/silver/fluorinated coatings. *J Mater Sci Mater Med* 17, 679-689.

Kinnari, T. J., Peltonen, L. I., Kuusela, P., Kivilahti, J., Kononen, M. & Jero, J. (2005). Bacterial adherence to titanium surface coated with human serum albumin. *Otol Neurotol* 26, 380-384.

Kinnari, T. J., Soininen, A., Esteban, J., Zamora, N., Alakoski, E., Kouri, V. P., Lappalainen, R., Konttinen, Y. T., Gomez-Barrena, E. & Tiainen, V. M. (2008). Adhesion of staphylococcal and Caco-2 cells on diamond-like carbon polymer hybrid coating. *J Biomed Mater Res A* 86, 760-768.

Klasen, H. J. (2000). Historical review of the use of silver in the treatment of burns. I. Early uses. *Burns* 26, 117-130.

Kolenbrander, P. E., Palmer, R. J., Jr., Rickard, A. H., Jakubovics, N. S., Chalmers, N. I. & Diaz, P. I. (2006). Bacterial interactions and successions during plaque development. *Periodontol 2000* 42, 47-79.

Kwok, S. C. H., Zhang, W., Wan, G. J., McKenzie, D. R., Bilek, M. M. M. & Chu, P. K. (2007). Hemocompatibility and anti-bacterial properties of silver doped diamond-like carbon prepared by pulsed filtered cathodic vacuum arc deposition. *Diamond and Related Materials* 16, 1353-1360.

Lettington, A. H. (1998). Applications of diamond-like carbon thin films. *Carbon* 36, 555-560.

Levon, J., Myllymaa, K., Kouri, V. P., Rautemaa, R., Kinnari, T., Myllymaa, S., Konttinen, Y. T. & Lappalainen, R. (2009). Patterned macroarray plates in comparison of bacterial adhesion inhibition of tantalum, titanium, and chromium compared with diamond-like carbon. *J Biomed Mater Res A* 92, 1606-1613.

Li, B. & Logan, B. E. (2004). Bacterial adhesion to glass and metal-oxide surfaces. *Colloids Surf B Biointerfaces* 36, 81-90.

Li, Y., Zou, S., Wang, D., Feng, G., Bao, C. & Hu, J. (2010). The effect of hydrofluoric acid treatment on titanium implant osseointegration in ovariectomized rats. *Biomaterials* 31, 3266-3273.

Listgarten, M. A. & Lai, C. H. (1999). Comparative microbiological characteristics of failing implants and periodontally diseased teeth. *J Periodontol* 70, 431-437.

Liu, C., Zhao, Q., Liu, Y., Wang, S. & Abel, E. W. (2008). Reduction of bacterial adhesion on modified DLC coatings. *Colloids Surf B Biointerfaces* 61, 182-187.

Loe, H., Theilade, E. & Jensen, S. B. (1965). Experimental Gingivitis in Man. *J Periodontol* 36, 177-187.

Maddikeri, R. R., Tosatti, S., Schuler, M., Chessari, S., Textor, M., Richards, R. G. & Harris, L. G. (2007). Reduced medical infection related bacterial strains adhesion on bioactive RGD modified titanium surfaces: A first step toward cell selective surfaces. *J Biomed Mater Res A* 84, 425-435.

Martin, J. Y., Dean, D. D., Cochran, D. L., Simpson, J., Boyan, B. D. & Schwartz, Z. (1996). Proliferation, differentiation, and protein synthesis of human osteoblast-like cells (MG63) cultured on previously used titanium surfaces. *Clin Oral Implants Res* 7, 27-37.

Merritt, K. & Chang, C. C. (1991). Factors influencing bacterial adherence to biomaterials. *J Biomater Appl* 5, 185-203.

Mombelli, A. (2002). Microbiology and antimicrobial therapy of peri-implantitis. *Periodontol 2000* 28, 177-189.

Mombelli, A., van Oosten, M. A., Schurch, E., Jr. & Land, N. P. (1987). The microbiota associated with successful or failing osseointegrated titanium implants. *Oral Microbiol Immunol* 2, 145-151.

Morrison, M. L., Buchanan, R. A., Liaw, P. K., Berry, C. J., Brigmon, R. L., Riester, L., Abernathy, H., Jin, C. & Narayan, R. J. (2006). Electrochemical and antimicrobial properties of diamondlike carbon-metal composite films. *Diamond and Related Materials* 15, 138-146.

Mosmann, T. (1983). Rapid colorimetric assay for cellular growth and survival: application to proliferation and cytotoxicity assays. *J Immunol Methods* 65, 55-63.

Niu, X. F., Liu, B. Q., Du, Z. X., Gao, Y. Y., Li, C., Li, N., Guan, Y. & Wang, H. Q. (2011). Resveratrol protects leukemic cells against cytotoxicity induced by proteasome inhibitors via induction of FOXO1 and p27Kip1. *BMC Cancer* 11, 99.

Nohr, R. S. & Macdonald, J. G. (1994). New biomaterials through surface segregation phenomenon: new quaternary ammonium compounds as antibacterial agents. *J Biomater Sci Polym Ed* 5, 607-619.

Olivares, R., Rodil, S. E. & Arzate, H. (2004). In vitro studies of the biomineralization in amorphous carbon films. *Surface & Coatings Technology* 177, 758-764.

Papaioannou, W., Quirynen, M. & Van Steenberghe, D. (1996). The influence of periodontitis on the subgingival flora around implants in partially edentulous patients. *Clin Oral Implants Res* 7, 405-409.

Patel, R. (2005). Biofilms and antimicrobial resistance. *Clin Orthop Relat Res*, 41-47.

Pereira da Silva, C. H., Vidigal, G. M., Jr., de Uzeda, M. & de Almeida Soares, G. (2005). Influence of titanium surface roughness on attachment of Streptococcus sanguis: an in vitro study. *Implant Dent* 14, 88-93.

Pontoriero, R., Tonelli, M. P., Carnevale, G., Mombelli, A., Nyman, S. R. & Lang, N. P. (1994). Experimentally induced peri-implant mucositis. A clinical study in humans. *Clin Oral Implants Res* 5, 254-259.

Quirynen, M., Bollen, C. M., Papaioannou, W., Van Eldere, J. & van Steenberghe, D. (1996). The influence of titanium abutment surface roughness on plaque accumulation and gingivitis: short-term observations. *Int J Oral Maxillofac Implants* 11, 169-178.

Rai, M., Yadav, A. & Gade, A. (2009). Silver nanoparticles as a new generation of antimicrobials. *Biotechnol Adv* 27, 76-83.

Rams, T. E. & Link, C. C., Jr. (1983). Microbiology of failing dental implants in humans: electron microscopic observations. *J Oral Implantol* 11, 93-100.

Robertson, J. (2002). Diamond-like amorphous carbon. *Materials Science & Engineering R-Reports* 37, 129-281.

Rodil, S. E., Olivares, R. & Arzate, H. (2005). In vitro cytotoxicity of amorphous carbon films. *Biomed Mater Eng* 15, 101-112.

Rodil, S. E., Olivares, R., Arzate, H. & Muhl, S. (2003). Properties of carbon films and their biocompatibility using in-vitro tests. *Diamond and Related Materials* 12, 931-937.

Rodil, S. E., Olivares, R., Arzate, H. & Muhl, S. (2006) Biocompatibility, cytotoxicity and bioactivity of amorphous carbon films. In: *Topics in Applied Physics 100; The future material for advanced technology applications*, (eds.) G. Messina & S. Santangelo, pp. 55-75. Germany: Springer-Verlag.

Sahithi, K., Swetha, M., Prabaharan, M., Moorthi, A., Saranya, N., Ramasamy, K., Srinivasan, N., Partridge, N. C. & Selvamurugan, N. (2010). Synthesis and characterization of nanoscale-hydroxyapatite-copper for antimicrobial activity towards bone tissue engineering applications. *J Biomed Nanotechnol* 6, 333-339.

Salvi, G. E., Furst, M. M., Lang, N. P. & Persson, G. R. (2008). One-year bacterial colonization patterns of Staphylococcus aureus and other bacteria at implants and adjacent teeth. *Clin Oral Implants Res* 19, 242-248.

Santavirta, S. (2003). Compatibility of the totally replaced hip. Reduction of wear by amorphous diamond coating. *Acta Orthop Scand Suppl* 74, 1-19.

Schatzle, M., Mannchen, R., Balbach, U., Hammerle, C. H., Toutenburg, H. & Jung, R. E. (2009). Stability change of chemically modified sandblasted/acid-etched titanium palatal implants. A randomized-controlled clinical trial. *Clin Oral Implants Res* 20, 489-495.

Schierholz, J. M., Lucas, L. J., Rump, A. & Pulverer, G. (1998). Efficacy of silver-coated medical devices. *J Hosp Infect* 40, 257-262.

Schmidmaier, G., Lucke, M., Wildemann, B., Haas, N. P. & Raschke, M. (2006). Prophylaxis and treatment of implant-related infections by antibiotic-coated implants: a review. *Injury* 37 Suppl 2, S105-112.

Schwartz, Z., Lohmann, C. H., Oefinger, J., Bonewald, L. F., Dean, D. D. & Boyan, B. D. (1999). Implant surface characteristics modulate differentiation behavior of cells in the osteoblastic lineage. *Adv Dent Res* 13, 38-48.

Schwarz, F., Sager, M., Kadelka, I., Ferrari, D. & Becker, J. (2010). Influence of titanium implant surface characteristics on bone regeneration in dehiscence-type defects: an experimental study in dogs. *J Clin Periodontol* 37, 466-473.

Sela, M. N., Badihi, L., Rosen, G., Steinberg, D. & Kohavi, D. (2007). Adsorption of human plasma proteins to modified titanium surfaces. *Clin Oral Implants Res* 18, 630-638.

Shi, C., Zhu, Y., Ran, X., Wang, M., Su, Y. & Cheng, T. (2006). Therapeutic potential of chitosan and its derivatives in regenerative medicine. *J Surg Res* 133, 185-192.

Shibli, J. A., Melo, L., Ferrari, D. S., Figueiredo, L. C., Faveri, M. & Feres, M. (2008). Composition of supra- and subgingival biofilm of subjects with healthy and diseased implants. *Clin Oral Implants Res* 19, 975-982.

Socransky, S. S. & Haffajee, A. D. (2005). Periodontal microbial ecology. *Periodontol 2000* 38, 135-187.

Socransky, S. S., Haffajee, A. D., Cugini, M. A., Smith, C. & Kent, R. L., Jr. (1998). Microbial complexes in subgingival plaque. *J Clin Periodontol* 25, 134-144.

Stanford, C. M. (2010). Surface modification of biomedical and dental implants and the processes of inflammation, wound healing and bone formation. *Int J Mol Sci* 11, 354-369.

Stein, G. S., Lian, J. B. & Owen, T. A. (1990). Relationship of cell growth to the regulation of tissue-specific gene expression during osteoblast differentiation. *FASEB J* 4, 3111-3123.

Tenovuo, J. (1998). Antimicrobial function of human saliva - how important is it for oral health? *Acta Odontologica Scandinavica* 56, 250-256.

Tiller, J. C., Liao, C. J., Lewis, K. & Klibanov, A. M. (2001). Designing surfaces that kill bacteria on contact. *Proc Natl Acad Sci U S A* 98, 5981-5985.

Truong, V. K., Lapovok, R., Estrin, Y. S., Rundell, S., Wang, J. Y., Fluke, C. J., Crawford, R. J. & Ivanova, E. P. (2010). The influence of nano-scale surface roughness on bacterial adhesion to ultrafine-grained titanium. *Biomaterials* 31, 3674-3683.

Tyagi, M. & Singh, H. (1997). Preparation and antibacterial evaluation of urinary balloon catheter. *Biomed Sci Instrum* 33, 240-245.

Wang, J., Huang, N., Yang, P., Leng, Y., Sun, H., Liu, Z. Y. & Chu, P. K. (2004). The effects of amorphous carbon films deposited on polyethylene terephthalate on bacterial adhesion. *Biomaterials* 25, 3163-3170.

Wilson, M. & Henderson, B. (1995). Virulence factors of Actinobacillus actinomycetemcomitans relevant to the pathogenesis of inflammatory periodontal diseases. *FEMS Microbiol Rev* 17, 365-379.

Wu, Y., Zitelli, J. P., TenHuisen, K. S., Yu, X. & Libera, M. R. (2011). Differential response of Staphylococci and osteoblasts to varying titanium surface roughness. *Biomaterials* 32, 951-960.

Xie, H., Cook, G. S., Costerton, J. W., Bruce, G., Rose, T. M. & Lamont, R. J. (2000). Intergeneric communication in dental plaque biofilms. *J Bacteriol* 182, 7067-7069.

Yamazaki, Y., Ebisu, S. & Okada, H. (1988). Partial purification of a bacterial lectinlike substance from Eikenella corrodens. *Infect Immun* 56, 191-196.

Yorganci, K., Krepel, C., Weigelt, J. A. & Edmiston, C. E. (2002). In vitro evaluation of the antibacterial activity of three different central venous catheters against gram-positive bacteria. *Eur J Clin Microbiol Infect Dis* 21, 379-384.

Yoshinari, M., Oda, Y., Kato, T. & Okuda, K. (2001). Influence of surface modifications to titanium on antibacterial activity in vitro. *Biomaterials* 22, 2043-2048.

Zhang, F., Zhang, Z., Zhu, X., Kang, E. T. & Neoh, K. G. (2008). Silk-functionalized titanium surfaces for enhancing osteoblast functions and reducing bacterial adhesion. *Biomaterials* 29, 4751-4759.

Zhao, Q., Liu, Y., Wang, C. & Wang, S. (2007). Evaluation of bacterial adhesion on Si-doped diamond-like carbon films. *Applied Surface Science* 253, 7254-7259.

Zhou, H., Xu, L., Ogino, A. & Nagatsu, M. (2008). Investigation into the antibacterial property of carbon films. *Diamond and Related Materials* 17, 1416-1419.

Zitzmann, N. U., Berglundh, T., Marinello, C. P. & Lindhe, J. (2001). Experimental peri-implant mucositis in man. *J Clin Periodontol* 28, 517-523.

8

Biological Sealing and Defense Mechanisms in Peri-Implant Mucosa of Dental Implants

Takayoshi Yamaza and Mizuho A. Kido
Department of Molecular Cell Biology and Oral Anatomy, Graduate School of Dental Science, Kyushu University, Fukuoka Japan

1. Introduction

Much attention during the early stages of basic and clinical research on dental implants has been focused on the bone (jaw)-to-titanium (implant) interface, because direct bone contact with the implant was thought to be a critical factor in implant therapeutics. However, since wide acceptance of the important concept of "osseointegration", developed by Branemark et al. (1977) in the late 1960's, biomaterial implants, usually titanium, have been shown to be able to bind directory and tightly to the bone surface at the engraftment sites, with no tissue intervention. This concept also avoids the risk of fibrous encapsulation, indicating that successful biological and clinical sealing can occur at the bone-to-implant interface (Kajiwara et al., 2005). The applications of titanium implant therapy have therefore increased for patients in medical and dental clinics.

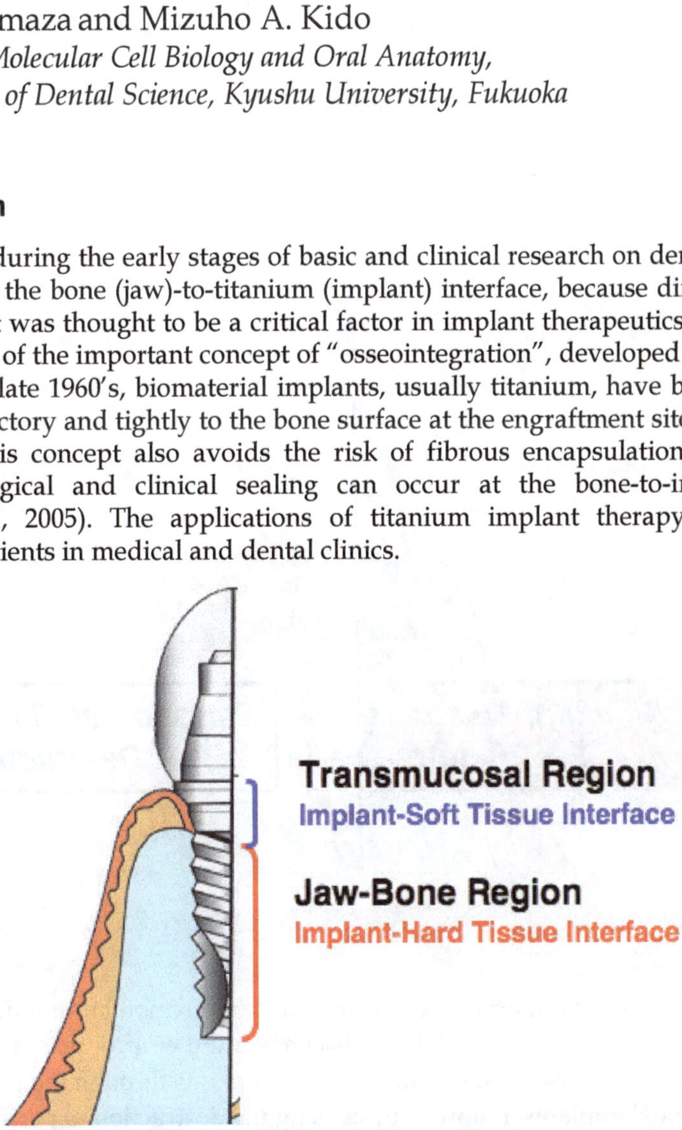

Fig. 1. Schema of biological region around dental implants. A unique part of dental implants is their pierce through oral mucosa. The dental implants are hided in jaw-bone to support the implant body. For functional and aesthetic matters, dental implants expose to the oral cavity. The surrounding tissue of dental implants is biologically divided into two regions; jaw-bone and transmucosal regions.

To date, several factors have been considered to improve the outcomes of clinical dental implants. The functional and aesthetic constraints on dental implants require their insertion through the oral mucosa/gingiva, thus inevitably establishing a transmucosal region between the oral cavity and the dental implant body (Figure 1). This environment exposes dental implants to several external stimuli from the oral cavity through the implant-soft tissue interface. Inflammation of the area surrounding the dental implant is one of most critical problems associated with the clinical failure and short- and long-term maintenance of dental implants, in a similar manner to the problems of tooth-loss caused by periodontal disease (Baillie et al., 2004; Esposito et al., 2010). Bacterial invasion of the transmucosal region leads to the progressive destruction of the peri-implant tissues and their subsequent failure (Mombelli, 1999), indicating that effective protection of the peri-implant mucosa is mandatory (Pontoriero et al., 1994; Tonetti & Schmid, 1994) (Figure 2). Regeneration of firm soft tissues surrounding dental implants, especially in the transmucosal region, is thus required for the long-term success of therapeutic dental implants (Grusovin et al., 2008; Canullo et al., 2011).

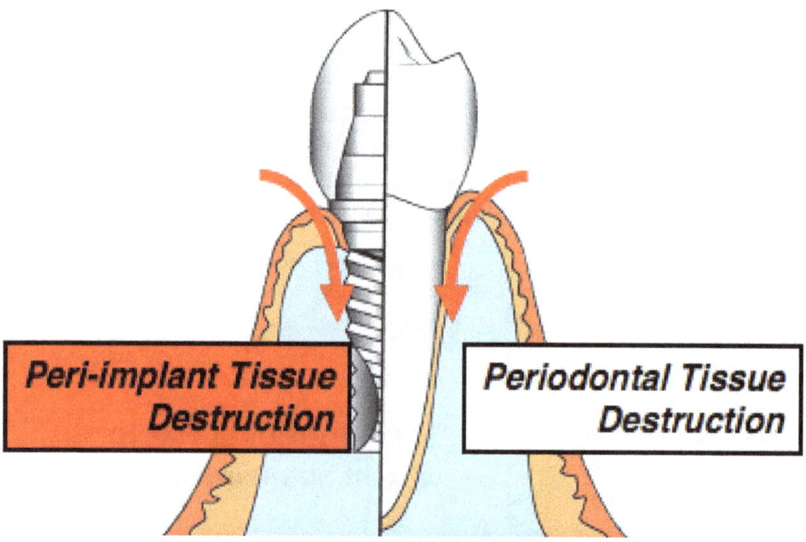

Fig. 2. Schema of a clinical importance of the transmucosal region around dental implants. A variety of oral pathogens (red arrows), likely bacteria and their products, are able to penetrate into the submucosal tissue around dental implants through the transmucosal region around dental implants, followed by causing the destruction of peri-implant tissue, similar to the destruction of periodontal tissue around tooth.

Dental implant research has focused on the interface between dental implants (titanium) and the surrounding soft tissues (Cairo et al., 2008; Grusovin et al., 2008). *In vivo* and *in vitro* investigations can help to understand the structural, functional and molecular properties of the biological seal and defense mechanisms acting at the interface between the peri-implant mucosa and dental implants (Baschong et al., 2001; Chai et al., 2010). Histological analysis of *in vivo* models, including animal and human subjects, is one of the gold standard methods for investigating the mechanisms at the implant-soft tissue interface. However data on peri-implant tissue from human subjects are scarce because of the limited collecting opportunities and ethical issues (Piattelli et al., 1993, 1997a, 1997b; Arvidson et al., 1996; Corpe et al., 1999; Baschong et al., 2001), animal models have therefore been widely used (Albrektsson et al., 1985; Buser et al., 1992; Berglundh et al., 1994; Berglundh & Lindhe, 1996; Weber et al., 1996; Abrahamsson et al., 1998, 2001, Fujii et al., 1998, 2003; Kawahara et al., 1998; Moon et al., 1999; Hermann et al., 2000, 2001). Peri-implant tissue contains both hard (bone) and soft (mucosa) tissues, which presents a challenge in terms of the histochemical examination of the intact implant-soft tissue interface.

This chapter reviews the morphological and functional features of the soft tissue surrounding dental implants, with emphasis on the epithelial interface between the implant and the peri-implant mucosa. The evidence is based on recent animal studies, especially our investigations using a unique oral implant rat model (Ikeda et al., 2000, 202; Atsuta et al., 2005a, 2005b; Yamaza et al., 2009). This *in vivo* model uses a 4-week implantation system, immediately after tooth extraction (maxillary first molar). Screw-type pure titanium implants (4 mm long, 2 mm in diameter) were inserted, and a complete peri-implant mucosa developed around the titanium body. Furthermore, this model allows the preserved implant-soft tissue interface to be examined at the ultrastructural level, including cellular features (e.g., microvilli, cytoplasmic processes, cytoplasmic organelles of epithelial cells, nerve fibers and terminals, blood vessel components, immune cells) and the epithelial attachment apparatus (basal lamina and hemidesmosomes).

2. Topological features of peri-implant mucosa

A tissue surrounding tooth, known as periodontium, is characterized by four types of tissue: periodontal ligament, cementum, alveolar bone, and gingiva (Schroeder, 1986). These components play critical roles in the support, maintenance, and repair of the tooth and the supporting tissue under both physiological and pathological conditions. The gingiva is a special oral mucosa that surrounds the tooth surface enamel, and covers the alveolar bone that supports the tooth (Schroeder & Listgarten, 1997). This mucosa is composed of connective tissue and epithelial components (Figures 3a and 4a). The gingival connective tissue component, the lamina propria, attach directly and tightly to the alveolar bone, while the gingival epithelium, which overlies the lamina propria, faces the oral cavity and the tooth surface. A tiny slit between the tooth surface and the gingival epithelium, known as oral sulcus, is present even under healthy conditions. This narrow space forms a route for outward flow from the sub-epithelial tissue, as well as an inward pathway into the connective tissue.

To achieve their therapeutic function based on recent established clinical techniques, dental implants pierce the oral mucosa and are inserted into the alveolar bone (Branemark et al., 1977). A tissue surrounding dental implant, known as peri-implant tissue, exhibits various morphological and structural similarities to the natural periodontium; it contains implant-supporting jaw bone and surrounding oral mucosa (peri-implant mucosa), but no intercalated tissue between the bone and implant surface equivalent to the periodontal ligament and cementum.

The peri-implant mucosa is specifically acquired after dental implant surgery, and resembles the natural gingiva, consisting of peri-implant connective tissue and peri-implant mucosal epithelium (Ikeda et al., 2000) (Figures 3b and 4b). The peri-implant connective tissue integrates with the surface of the jaw bone supporting the dental implant body, while the peri-implant mucosal epithelium faces the oral cavity and the implant surface. There is also an acquired fissure between the implant surface and the peri-implant mucosa, known as the peri-implant sulcus.

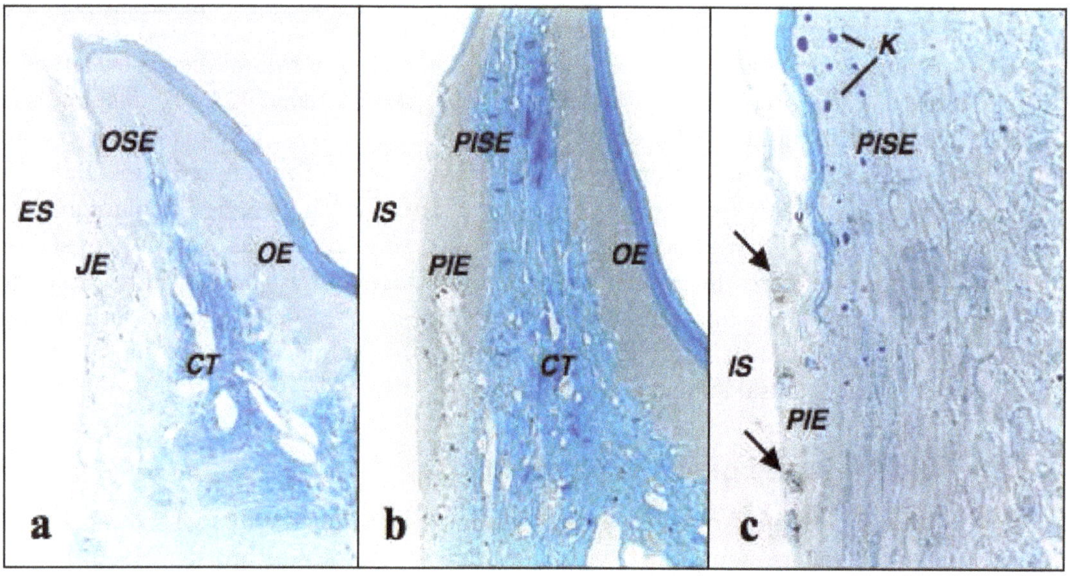

Fig. 3. Light micrographs of healthy gingiva and peri-implant mucosa in rats. (a) Healthy gingiva consists of an epithelial component and a connective tissue component (*CT*). The gingival epithelium can be divided into three parts: oral epithelium (*OE*), oral sulcular epithelium (*OSE*), and junctional epithelium (*JE*). *ES*: enamel space. (b, c) The components of peri-implant mucosa resemble those of the healthy gingiva. The peri-implant mucosa epithelium consists of oral epithelium, peri-implant sulcular epithelium (*PISE*), and peri-implant epithelium (*PIE*). The oral epithelium and peri-implant sulcular epithelium in the peri-implant mucosa, as well as the oral epithelium and oral sulcular epithelium in healthy gingiva, are keratinized, stratified squamous epithelia, while the PIE and junctional epithelium are non-keratinized epithelia with invading neutrophils (arrows). Blood vessels are developed under the PIE and junctional epithelium. *IS*: implant space. *K*: keratohyaline granules. Toluidine blue staining.

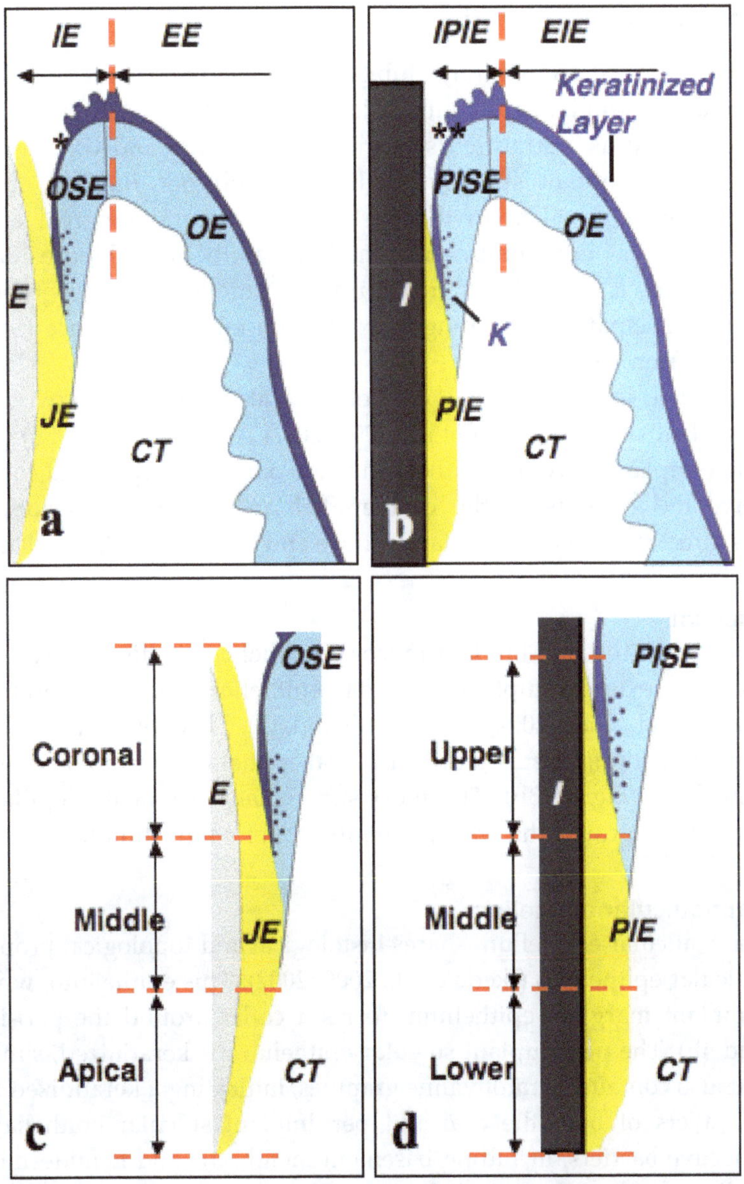

Fig. 4. Schemata of gingiva and peri-implant mucosa. (a) The gingival epithelium can be divided into oral epithelium (*OE*), oral sulcular epithelium (*OSE*), and junctional epithelium (*JE*). The external marginal epithelium (*EE*) covers the gingiva facing the oral cavity, while the inner marginal epithelium (*IE*) covers the gingiva facing the tooth. The space (asterisk) between the enamel (*E*) and inner marginal epithelium is the oral sulcus. *CT*: connective tissue. (b) Epithelia in the peri-implant mucosa consist of the oral epithelium, peri-implant sulcular epithelium (*PISE*), and peri-implant epithelium (*PIE*). The external peri-implant epithelium (*EPIE*) faces the oral cavity, while the inner peri-implant epithelium (*IPIE*) faces the implant (*I*). The peri-implant sulcus (double asterisk) comprises a narrow space between the inner peri-implant epithelium and the implant surface. (c) Natural junctional epithelium is divided into three regions: the coronal, middle and apical regions. (d) The PIE is also divided into three regions: the upper, middle and lower regions.

3. Peri-implant mucosal epithelium

The peri-implant mucosal epithelium exhibits histological and structural features similar to those of the natural gingival epithelium (Ikeda et al., 2000, 2002) (Figures 3 and 4). This epithelium is classified as a stratified squamous epithelium, and consists of three parts: oral epithelium, peri-implant sulcular epithelium, and peri-implant epithelium (PIE) (Figures 3b and 4b), equivalent to the parts of the natural gingival epithelium: oral epithelium, oral sulcular epithelium and junctional epithelium (Figures 3a and 4a). The junctional epithelium is considered to be unique among the three types of gingival epithelium, and participates in forming a fixed tooth-gingiva interface (Schroeder, 1986; Schroeder & Listgarten, 1997).

Topologically, the peri-implant mucosal epithelium is also divided into two parts in relation to the dental implant surface (Ikeda et al., 2000, 2002; Atsuta et al., 2005b) (Figures 4a and 4b). The external-implant marginal epithelium is the part of the epithelial component facing the oral cavity, and consists of the oral epithelium, and the inner-implant marginal epithelium lies directly against the implant surface and the peri-implant sulcus.

3.1 Oral epithelium

The oral epithelium of the peri-implant mucosal epithelium is directly exposed to the oral cavity, forming the external-implant marginal epithelium of the peri-implant mucosal epithelium (Ikeda et al., 2000, 2002) (Figures 3b and 4b). This epithelium is common to the natural gingival epithelium. Histologically, the oral epithelium forms a keratinized stratified squamous epithelium (Figure 3b). The most superficial layer of this epithelium contains keratin, which helps to protect the oral epithelium from foreign stimuli.

3.2 Peri-implant sulcular epithelium

The peri-implant sulcular epithelium shares histological and topological properties with the natural oral sulcular epithelium (Ikeda et al., 2000, 2002). This epithelium, which forms part of the inner-implant marginal epithelium, forms a collar around the peri-implant sulcus (Figures 3b and 4b). The peri-implant sulcular epithelium is keratinized, similar to the oral epithelium, but also contains keratohyaline granules, indicating a keratinized barrier (Figure 3c). The basal layers of both the oral and peri-implant sulcular epithelia form general epithelial-connective barriers, including basement membrane and hemidesmosomes, which join the epithelium to the sub-epithelial tissue. The peri-implant sulcus provides a direct connection to the oral cavity, and acts as a passage for foreign substances into the peri-implant tissue (Ikeda et al., 2002) (Figure 5a), in a similar manner to the oral sulcus (Schroeder & Listgarten, 1997).

3.3 PIE

The PIE, the other part of the inner-implant epithelium, demonstrates unique and specific characteristics, forming a solid transmucosal interface around the dental implant (Ikeda et al., 2000, 2002) (Figures 3 and 4). The topological and structural features of the PIE resemble those of the tooth-enamel interface epithelium, the junctional epithelium, suggesting an important function for the transmucosal region around dental implants in biological sealing and defense.

4. Biological characteristics of the PIE

4.1 Topological and ultrastructural features of the PIE and PIE cells

PIE is formed by epithelial cells derived from the oral epithelium and/or residues of the junctional epithelium after tooth extraction (Fujii et al., 1998; Atsuta et al., 2005a). The epithelial cells move and grow down along the implant surface whilst secreting laminin 5, resulting in reorganization of the intercalated epithelial tissue to form the PIE (Atsuta et al., 2005a).

PIE and PIE cells show some structural and cellular phenotypic similarities to natural junctional epithelium and junctional epithelial cells (Ikeda et al., 2000). The PIE is a non-keratinized and stratified squamous epithelium (Figures 3b, 3c), consisting of basal and supra-basal cell layers. It is located between the surface of the dental implant and the lamina propria of the peri-implant mucosa (Figure 5a, 5b). Blood vessels, especially post-capillary venules, mostly occur under the sub-PIE connective tissue, compared to other sub-peri-implant epithelial tissue (Figure 3b).

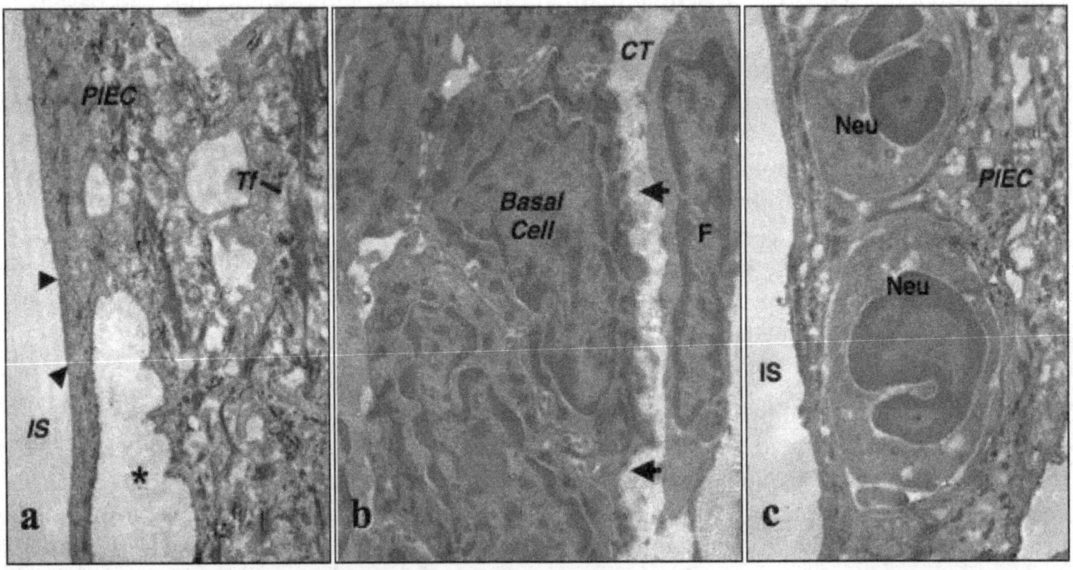

Fig. 5. Electron micrographs of the transmucosal region of the peri-implant mucosa. (a) Typical electron micrograph of the suprabasal peri-implant epithelium (*PIE*), especially the lower PIE. PIE cells (*PIEC*) are arranged parallel to the implant surface, are flattened, and contain a variety of vesicles and vacuoles. Tonofilaments (*Tf*) are localized within the PIE cells. Wide intercellular spaces (asterisk) are found between the cytoplasmic processes. Internal basement lamina (arrowheads) is laid on the innermost PIE cell. *IS*: implant space. (b) The basal part of the PIE consists of cuboidal cells (*Basal Cell*) lining the external basal lamina (arrows). *CT*: connective tissue, *F*: fibroblast. (c) Neutrophils (*Neu*) migrate into the intercellular spaces between PIE cells.

PIE cells are flattened, undifferentiated epithelial cells with few organelles, such as mitochondria and endoplasmic reticulum (Ikeda et al., 2000) (Figure 5a). The PIE cells are arranged parallel to the implant surface. They extend their cytoplasmic processes to other PIE cells, and connect via desmosomes to form wide intracellular spaces (Figure 5a). Neutrophilic granulocytes leak from the blood vessels of the sub-epithelial connective tissue and invade into the PIE (Ikeda et al., 2000; Yamaza et al., 2009) (Figure 5c). These ultrastructural characteristics support the idea that the PIE acts as a pathway not only for foreign molecules penetrating into the sub-epithelial connective tissue of the peri-implant mucosa (Ikeda et al., 2002), but also for the flow of peri-implant cervicular fluid from the sup-epithelial tissue (Eley et al., 1991). Both inward (McDougall, 1971; Romanowsky et al., 1988; Yamaza et al., 1997) and outward (Golub et al., 1976; Tanaka 1984; Tanaka and Sakano, 1987) flow are also recognized in the junctional epithelium.

The PIE cells also contain tonofilaments (Figure 5a) that associate with desmosomes and hemidesmosomes (Schroeder, 1986). Many lysosomal vesicular and vacuolar structures are located in the cytoplasm (Ikeda et al., 2000; Yamaza et al., 2009) (Figures 5a and 10c).

4.2 Ultrastructural features of transmucosal epithelial attachment around dental implants

4.2.1 Epithelial attachment around natural teeth

Epithelial attachment components in the junctional epithelium are located throughout the tooth-gingiva interface. The attachment apparatus includes hemidesmosomes and basement lamina, which in turn comprises the external basement lamina (EBL) and the internal basement lamina (IBL) (Schroeder, 1986). The EBL, which is formed between the basal cells of the junctional epithelium and the connective tissue, shows a typical basement-membrane structure. The IBL, however, is a unique and specific adhesive structure at the interface between the innermost junctional epithelial cells and the enamel surface. Both the IBL and the EBL consist of two laminal structures, known as the lamina densa and the lamina lucida. These contain the major components of the basal lamina, laminin-1 and laminin-5 (Sawada et al., 1990; Hormia et al., 1998; Mullen et al., 1999). Hemidesmosomes are arranged in the cytoplasm under the plasma membrane of the junctional epithelial cells to anchor the IBL and EBL (Schroeder, 1986).

4.2.2 Epithelial attachment around dental implants

The PIE is divided to three regions: the upper, middle and lower regions (Ikeda et al., 2000) (Figure 4c), equivalent to the three regions of the junctional epithelium: the coronal, middle, and apical regions (Tanaka, 1984) (Figure 4d). The upper region of the PIE is closest to the peri-implant sulcus, while the lower region is connected to the sub-PIE tissue. The middle region is intercalated between the upper and lower regions. The PIE expresses a unique distribution of epithelial attachment, compared to the junctional epithelium (Ikeda et al., 2000; Atsuta et al., 2005b).

Several studies have demonstrated the formation of attachment structures at the titanium-epithelium interface both *in vivo* and *in vitro* (Gould et al., 1984; Mckinney et al., 1985; Donley & Gillette, 1991). At the internal interface between the implant and the PIE, the epithelial attachment apparatus, including the basal lamina and hemidesmosomes, are limited to the lower region of the PIE (Ikeda et al., 2000; Atsuta et al., 2005b) (Figures 5a and 6c). The hemidesmosomes lie beneath the plasma membrane of the innermost PIE cells. The basal lamina of the IBL shows structural similarity with the lamina densa and lamina lucida of the natural junctional epithelium. Laminin-1 and laminin-5 are strongly expressed and distributed heterogeneously in both the lamina densa and lamina lucida of the PIE IBL-like structure similar to the IBL of the junctional epithelium (Ikeda et al, 2000: Atsuta et al., 2005b) (Figure 6c). This indicates that the lower PIE provides epithelial attachment structures similar to those in the natural junctional epithelium. However, no comparative studies have yet elucidated the distribution of hemidesmosomes at the internal interface of the PIE.

In the upper and middle regions of the innermost interface, the innermost PIE cells are close to the implant surface, but epithelial attachment structures are absent or rare (Ikeda et al., 2000; Atsuta et al., 2005b) (Figure 6b). The innermost PIE cells extend short cytoplasmic processes to the titanium surface, probably forming a loose attachment (Ikeda et al., 2000) (Figure 6b). Laminin-1 and laminin-5 are located in the innermost cells, but are not deposited on the interface (Ikeda et al., 2000; Atsuta et al., 2005b) (Figure 6b).

The external interface is formed between the basal PIE cells and the sub-epithelial connective tissue (Figure 5b). Basal lamina and hemidesmosomes are located throughout the external interface (Ikeda et al., 2000; Atsuta et al., 2005b). The basal lamina contains laminin-1 and laminin-5 and shows feature in common with the EBL of the natural junctional epithelium. Some part of the EBL of the PIE, especially in the lower region, is discontinuous, indicating epithelial migration of PIE/PIE cells (Atsuta et al., 2005b).

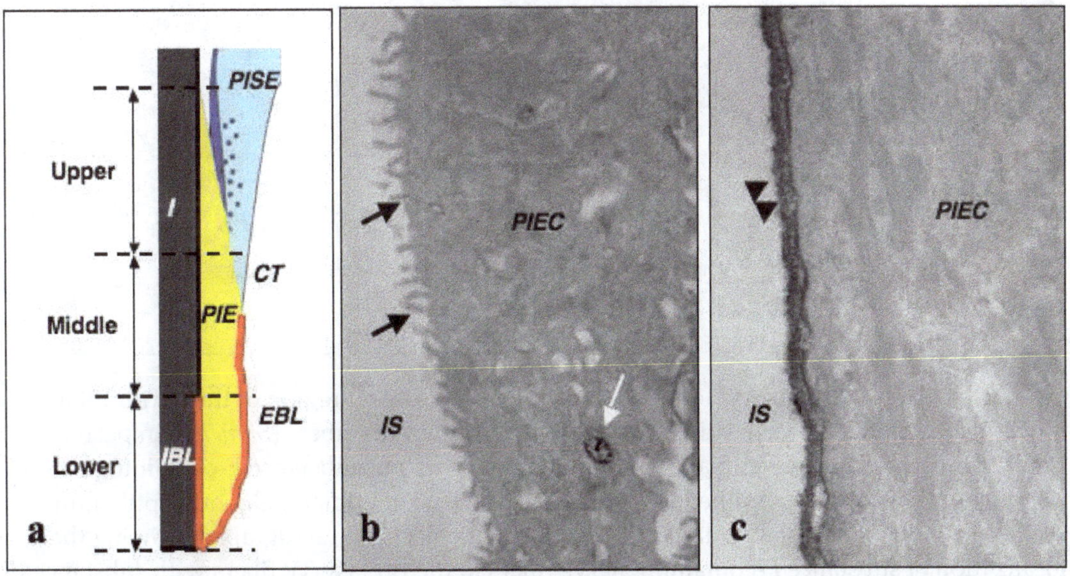

Fig. 6. Interface of the transmucosal region of the peri-implant mucosa (a) Schema of the transmucosal region of the peri-implant mucosa. The transmucosal region consists of the peri-implant epithelium (*PIE*). Only the inner interface of the lower portion of the PIE has an internal basement lamina (*IBL*), and IBL-like structure is lacking in the other portions. The external interface, the external basement lamina (*EBL*), is found through the PIE. *I*: implant, *PISE*: peri-implant sulcular epithelium. *CT*: connective tissue. (b, c) Immunoelectron micrographs showing the localization of laminin 5 at the inner interface (*IS*) of the PIE. (b) No specific epithelial attachment structures are found in the upper region of the PIE. An innermost PIE cell (*PIEC*) extends short cytoplasmic processes (arrows) to the implant surface. No laminin 5 is detected at the interface between the PIE cell and titanium, but laminin 5 is recognized in vesicles within PIE cells (white arrow). (c) In the lower region, IBL-like structure is found between the innermost PIE cell and the implant surface. Laminin 5-immunnoproducts (arrows) are deposited in the IBL structures, the lamina densa and lamina lucida.

4.3 Innervation of PIE by sensory nerve fibers

The natural junctional epithelium, as well as its sub-epithelial connective tissue, is abundantly supplied by nerve fibers derived from the trigeminal ganglion (Byers & Holland, 1977; Kondo et al, 1992; Sugaya et al., 1994). The sensory nerve fibers contain the neuropeptides, calcitonin gene-related peptide (Byers et al., 1987; Nagata et al., 1992, 1994) and substance P (Nagata et al., 1992, 1994; Tanaka et al., 1996; Kido et al., 1999), and terminate close to endothelial cells, neutrophils, and junctional epithelial cells (Kondo et al, 1992; Tanaka et al., 1996).

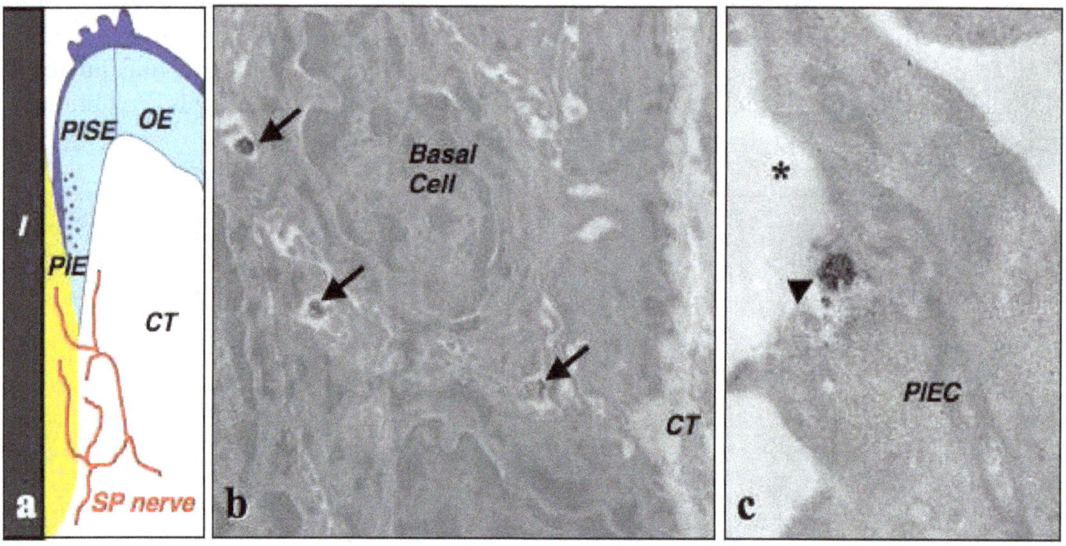

Fig. 7. Distribution of sensory nerve fibers in the transmucosal region of the peri-implant mucosa. (a) Schema of innervation by substance P-containing fibers (*SP nerve*) in peri-implant mucosa. The peri-implant epithelium (*PIE*) is rich in substance P-containing nerve fibers, compared to other epithelia. *CT*: connective tissue, *I*: implant, *OE*: oral epithelium, *PISE*: peri-implant sulcular epithelium. (b, c) Immunoelectron micrographs showing the localization of substance P-containing nerve fibers in the PIE. Nerve fibers with substance P immununoproducts (arrows) penetrate into the PIE via the intercellular spaces between basal PIE cells (*Basal Cell*) (b). The substance P-positive nerve ending (arrowhead) is closely localized to a PIE cell (*PIEC*) (c) Asterisk: intercellular space between PIE cells.

The peri-implant mucosa is also supplied with sensory nerves containing calcitonin gene-related peptide (Fujii et al., 2003) and substance P (Yamaza et al, 2009) (Figure 7a). The innervation of the PIE is denser than in other parts of the epithelium (peri-implant sulcular epithelium and oral epithelium) (Figure 7b). The free ends of the nerve fibers terminate close to PIE cells (Figure 7c), neutrophils and endothelial cells (Yamaza et al, 2009). In addition, neurokinin-1 receptors, which are receptors for substance P, are expressed on the extra- and intra-epithelial nerve fibers, endothelial cells and PIE cells (Yamaza et al, 2009) (Figures 8a, 8b, and 8d). These receptors are also localized in neutrophils invading into the intercellular spaces between PIE cells (Figure 8c). Overall, the PIE shows a similar distribution of substance P-containing sensory nerve fibers and their neurokinin-1 receptors, compared to junctional epithelium (Kondo et al, 1992; Tanaka et al., 1996; Kido et al., 1999).

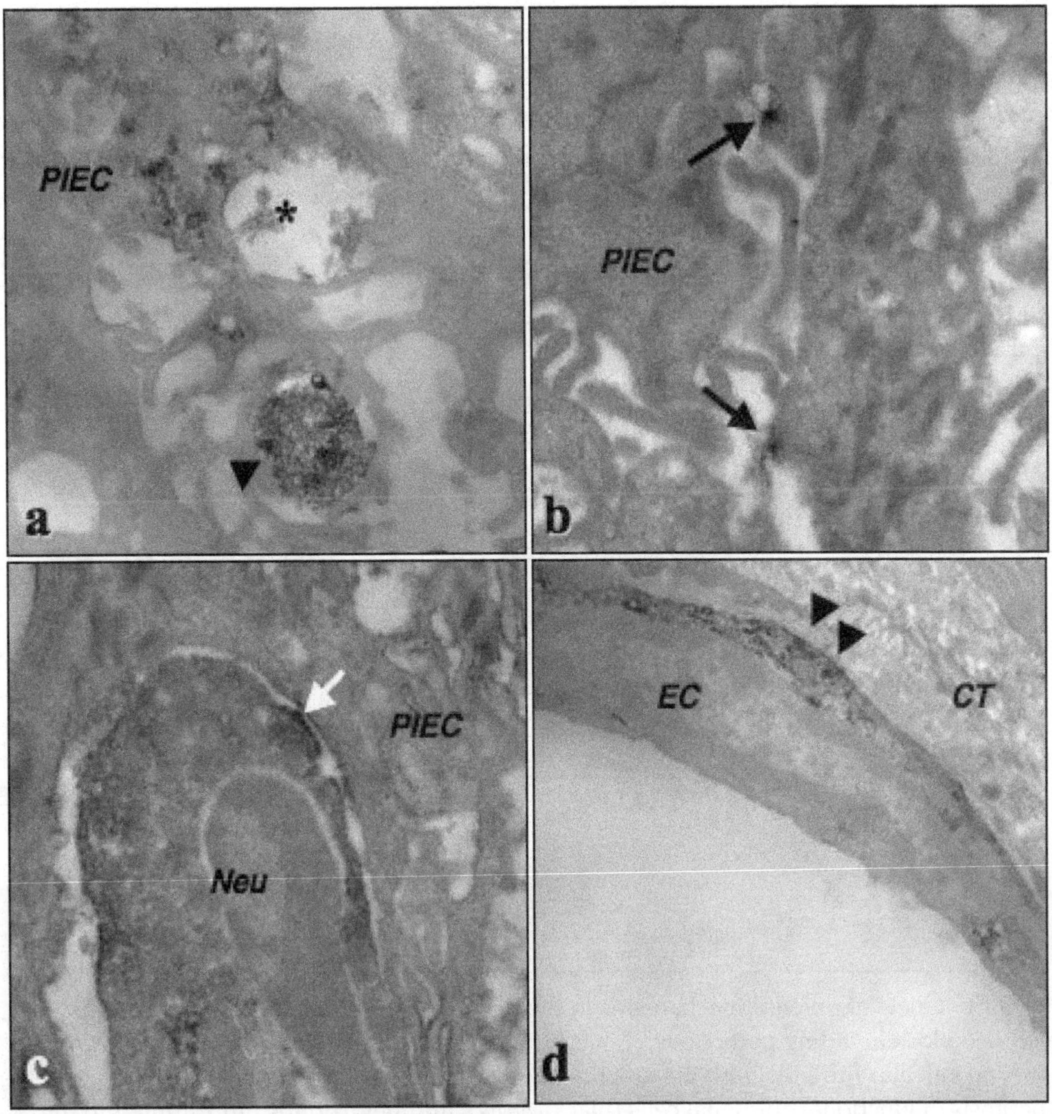

Fig. 8. Distribution of neurokinin 1 receptors in the peri-implant epithelium (*PIE*). (a) Neurokinin 1 receptor-positive products (arrowhead) are seen in a nerve ending close to a PIE cell (*PIEC*). Asterisk: intercellular space between PIE cells. (b) Neurokinin 1 receptor-positivity (arrows) can be detected on the plasma membrane of a PIE cell. (c) An invading neutrophil (*Neu*) was positive for neurokinin 1 receptors (white arrow). (d) A nerve fiber close to an endothelial cell (*EC*) was also positive for neurokinin 1 receptors (double arrowhead). *CT*: connective tissue.

5. Biological sealing and defense mechanisms in the transmucosal region around dental implants

The junctional epithelium is a critical transmucosal region for innate defense against periodontal inflammation. Various mechanisms of peripheral host defense have been demonstrated in this epithelium (Schroeder & Listgarten, 1997) (Figure 9): (1) phagocytosis and anti-bacterial activity of neutrophils infiltrating into the junctional epithelium (Yamasaki et al., 1979, Tanaka et al., 1988), (2) outward flow of gingival sulcular fluid through the junctional epithelium (McDougall, 1970; Tanaka, 1984; Tanaka and Sakano, 1987), (3) fast turnover or apoptosis of junctional epithelial cells (Schroeder, 1986, Ekuni et al., 2005), (4) continuous epithelial attachment via the IBL throughout the enamel surface (Squier, 1991; Bartold, et al., 2000), (5) endocytotic capacity of junctional epithelial cells for external pathogens (Yamasaki et al., 1979; Tanaka 1984; Tanaka & Sakano, 1987; Ayasaka et al., 1989, Yamaza et al., 1997), and (6) neurotrophic modulation in the junctional epithelium (Kondo et al., 1995; Tanaka et al., 1996; Kido et al, 1999).

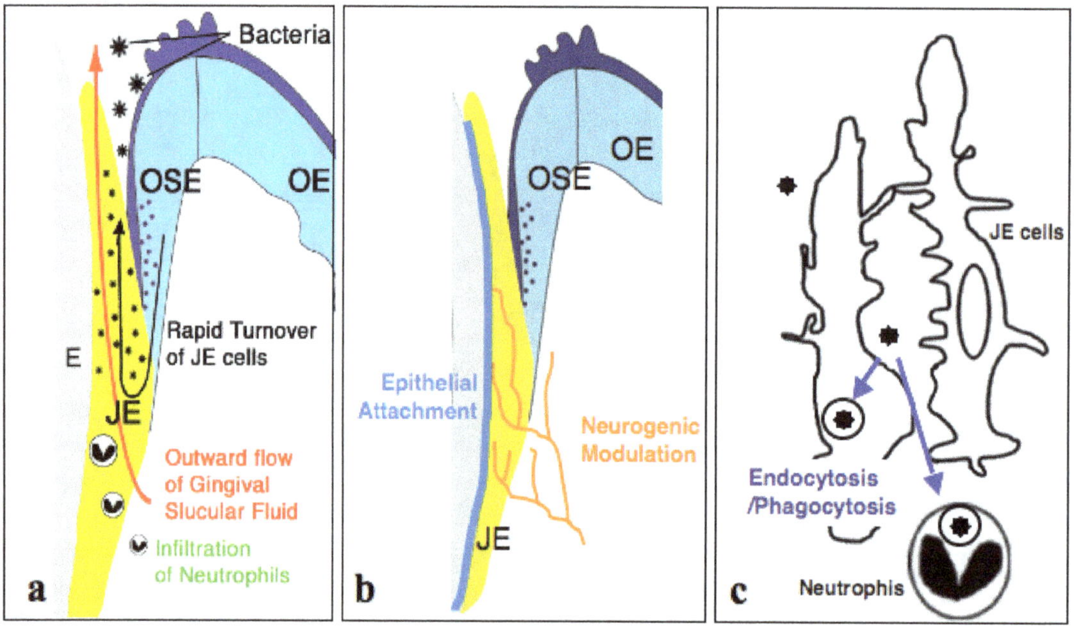

Fig. 9. Schemata of defense mechanisms in the junctional epithelium (JE) around natural teeth. To block invading pathogens, JE has defensive mechanism of (a) outward flow of gingival sulcular fluid through the junctional epithelium (red arrow), fast turnover or apoptosis of junctional epithelial cells (black arrow), and neutrophils infiltrating into the junctional epithelium, (b) continuous epithelial attachment via the internal basement lamina throughout the enamel surface (blue line, and neurotrophic modulation by sensory nerve innervation in the junctional epithelium (orange lines), and (c) endocytotic capacity of junctional epithelial cells and phagocytosis of neutrophils for external pathogens (blue arrows). E: enamel, OE: oral epithelium, OSE: oral sulcular epithelium.

The ultrastructural findings support the idea that the PIE can allow the penetration of foreign molecules into the sub-epithelial connective tissue, indicating that the PIE acts as a first line of defense in protecting against the invasion of several pathogens (Ikeda et al., 2000, 2002). Transmucosal defense around dental implants is suggested to involve the acquisition and maintenance of a similar defense system to that shown by the junctional epithelium. This review considers three aspects of the mucosal defense system around dental implants; (1) PIE-titanium barrier (2) endocytotic system in the PIE, and (3) neurogenic regulation in the PIE (Figure 13).

5.1 Epithelial attachment of PIE-titanium barrier

Laminin-1 and laminin-5 are major components of the basal lamina, and participate in the formation of a molecular network in the basal lamina (Tryggvason, 1993; Burgeson et al., 1994; Aumailley & Krieg, 1996). They also play important roles in cell differentiation, migration, and adhesion, as well being involved in determining cell phenotype and survival (Timpl, et al., 1979). Laminin 5 forms anchoring filaments in hemidesmosomes and promotes their assembly, indicating a strong binding function in the basal lamina (Green & Jones, 1996). This suggests that IBL- and hemidesmosome-like structures contribute, at least in part, to the formation of a tight attachment at the inner interface between the PIE and the dental implant (Ikeda et al., 2000; Atsuta et al., 2005b).

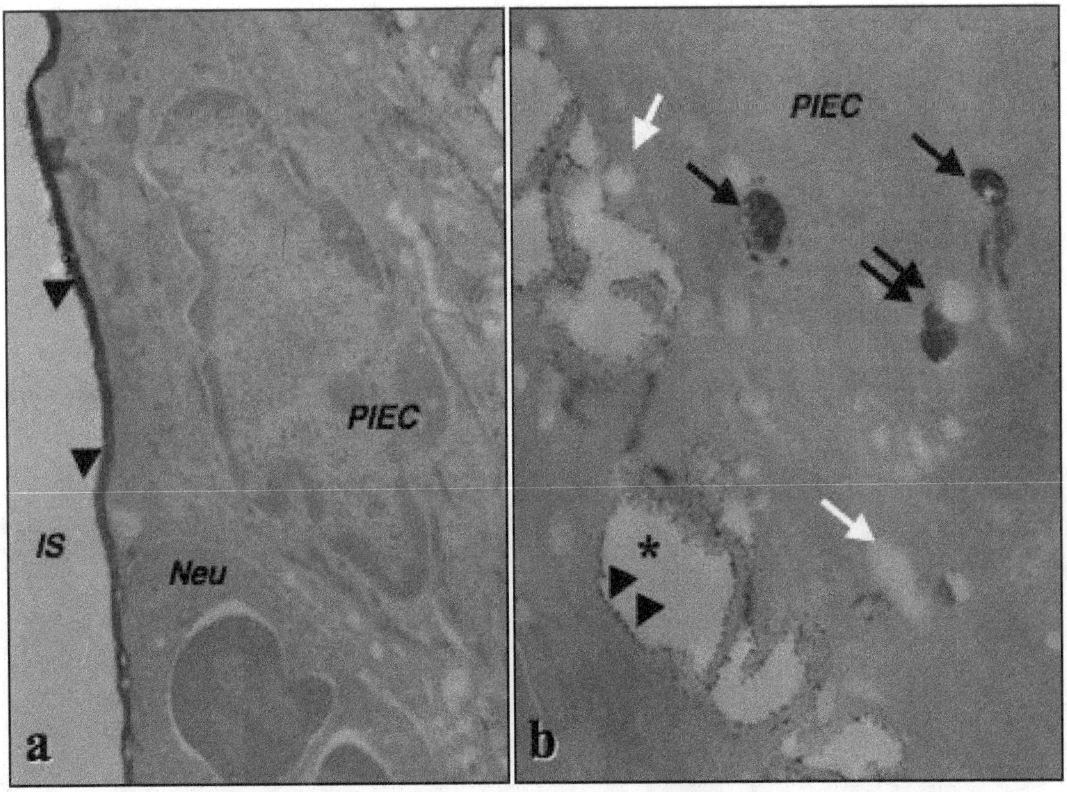

Fig. 10. Electron micrographs showing the localization of applied horseradish peroxidase in the periimplant epithelium. (a) Horseradish peroxidase-reactive products (arrowheads) were found in the internal basement lamina in the lower PIE. However, horseradish peroxidase was not found in the intercellular spaces between PIE cells (*PIEC*). *Neu*: neutrophil, *IS*: implant space. (b) Horseradish peroxidase-reactive organelles show several feature in PIE cells. Endosome-like structures in the cells contained various densities of horseradish peroxidase-reactive products (arrows). Horseradish peroxidase-negative endosomes (white arrows) were also found in PIE cells. Some endosomes were fused with other horseradish peroxidase-negative endosomes (double arrow). Horseradish peroxidase-reactive products (arrowheads) were deposited on the plasma membrane of PIE cells. Asterisk: intercellular space between PIE cells.

The application of horseradish peroxidase (HRP) as a tracer in the mucosa around dental implants or teeth shows a different distribution at each transmucosal interface (Ikeda et al., 2002) (Figures 10, 11). At the natural interface, abundant HRP is stopped at the coronal region of the junctional epithelium and IBL (Yamaza et al., 1997). In contrast, high levels of horseradish peroxidase are widely distributed from the upper to middle regions of the PIE around the dental implants (Ikeda et al., 2002) (Figures 10a, 11a). The lower region also contains HRP, but in smaller amounts (Figures 10b, 11a). The IBL of the lower PIE accumulates exogenous HRP, suggesting a functional role for the IBL in protecting against external invasion (Ikeda et al., 2002) (Figure 11). These findings indicate that the IBL in the PIE participates in local defense around dental implants (Figure 13a).

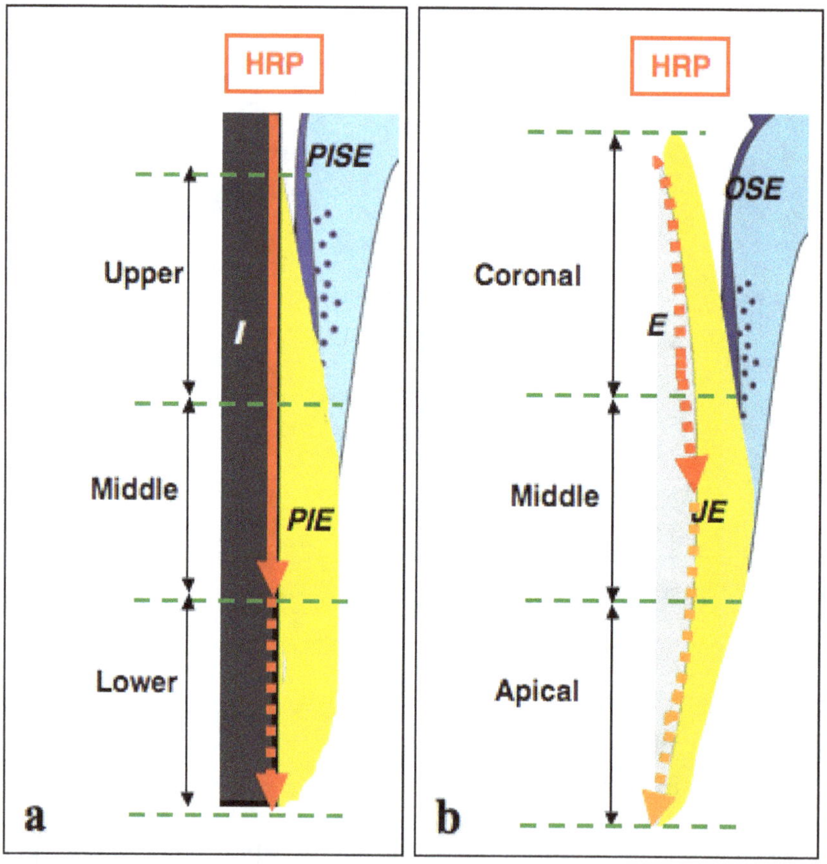

Fig. 11. Schema of the difference of barrier capability of internal basement lamina in the peri-implant epithelium (*PIE*) and junctional epithelium (*JE*). (a) In the PIE, only the lower region has a solid epithelial attachment structure, not in the middle and upper portions. Locally applied horseradish peroxidase (HRP) is easy to penetrate into the PIE thorouth the direct interface between the dental implant (*I*) and PIE (red arrow), but the lower interface showing basal lamina structure defend the penetration (red dot arrow). *PISE*: peri-implant sulcular epithelium. (b) In the natural teeth, basal lamina structure is present throughout the interface between enamel (*E*) and junctional epithelium (*JE*). Loccaly appile HRP is hard to invade along not only to the internal interface of the coronal to middle portion of JE (red dot arrow), but also to the middle to lowe interface (orange dot line).

5.2 Endocytotic system in PIE

Neutrophils generally play an important role in the front-line defense against foreign bodies, through their phagocytotic capacity. They infiltrate into the PIE (Ikeda et al., 2002), suggesting that they are resident or transient leukocytes in the PIE, as well as in the natural junctional epithelium (Yamaza et al., 1997), and function effectively to prevent peri-implant inflammation/disease by their phagocytotic capacity (Ikeda et al., 2002).

Junctional epithelial cells have the ability to endocytose foreign substances (Tanaka et al., 1984; Yamasaki et al., 1985; Ayasaka & Tanaka, 1989; Yamaza et al., 1997). These cells can also digest materials using the intracellular lysosomal system containing aspartic proteinase, cathepsin D (Ayasaka et al., 1993), and the cysteine proteinases, cathepsins B and H (Yamaza et al., 1997). Lysosomal compartments participate in intracellular degradation using lysosomal enzymes (Mellman et al., 1986). The cathepsins show high protein degradative activities (Barrett & Kirschke, 1981), especially in the case of cathepsin B and H (Nishimura et al., 1988). Periodontal pathogens can invade the gingival epithelial cells (Lamont et al., 1995; Rautemaa et al., 2004). PIE cells also contain a variety of intracellular endosome/lysosome systems, suggesting a capacity to take up and digest foreign materials in the vesicles and vacuoles (Ikeda et al., 2000, 2002). PIE cells also show the ability to endocytose HPR applied locally to the peri-implant mucosa, indicating their digestive capacity against foreign materials (Ikeda et al., 2002) (Figure 10b). These results suggest that the endocytotic system of PIE cells, as well as the presence of neutrophils, may play a role in the local defense of the transmucosal region around dental implants (Figure 13).

Cystatin C is an endogenous cysteine proteinase inhibitor (Abrahamson et al., 1986) expressed in junctional epithelial cells, and secreted extracellularly (Yamaza et al., 2005). This natural inhibitor also plays a role in the anti-bacterial activity against the periodontal microorganism, *Porphyromonas gingivalis* (Blankenvoorde et al., 1998), which releases a specific cysteine proteinase (Chen et al., 1992). Cystatin C is present in gingival cervicular fluid (Ulker et al., 2008), supporting the extracellular secretion of this inhibitor into gingival tissues, including the intercellular spaces of the junctional epithelium. Secreted cystatin C from junctional epithelial cells may participate in the inhibition of *P. gingivalis*-derived proteinase activity and suppression of *P. gingivalis* growth, suggesting that cystatin C also acts as a candidate molecule governed by the PIE cell-mediated defense system. Thus several functions of PIE cells may contribute to local defense in the transmucosal region around dental implants.

5.3 Neurogenic regulation in PIE

Substance P is a nociceptive neuropeptide responsible for transmitting pain stimuli, such as those due to chemical irritants, heat, cold or other noxious stimuli. It is expressed in sensory nerves of the peripheral nervous system and participates in the afferent transmission of pain impulses from the mucosa through sensory receptors at the nerve endings (Lundy & Linden, 2004) (Figure 12). In contrast, this transmitter is also released efferently from nerve endings on stimulation by noxious phenomena (Figure 12). Released substance P can affect the responses of the target cells through direct interaction with neurokinin-1 receptors (Scholzen et al., 1998) (Figure 12). The presence of substance P in gingival cervicular fluid supports the release of this neuropeptide from nerve terminals (Linden et al., 1997). Acting via neurokinin-1 receptors, substance P induces several cellular responses (Figure 12), In the endothelial cells, vasodilation, and modulates blood flow and plasma leakage are occurred by the substance P-nurokin 1 receptor binding (Lembeck & Holzer 1979; Nicoll et al., 1980; Otsuka & Yoshida 1993). The substance P-neurokinin-1 receptor pathway can also enhance endocytosis in neutrophils (Bar-Shavit et al., 1980; Tanabe et al., 1996). Substance P also stimulates the chemotaxis of neutrophils and macrophages, the proliferation and migration of keratinocytes and fibroblasts, degranulation of mast cells, the expression of various adhesion proteins on endothelial cells, and the release of inflammatory cytokines from immune cells (Kähler et al., 1993; Ziche et al., 1994; Scholzen et al., 1998; Koon et al., 2006; Liu et al., 2007). Furthermore, substance P-binding neurokinin-1 receptors are known to regulate the innate immune system (Tuluc et al., 2009; Douglas & Leeman, 2011), and participate in immunomodulation in immune diseases (Koon & Pothoulakis, 2006).

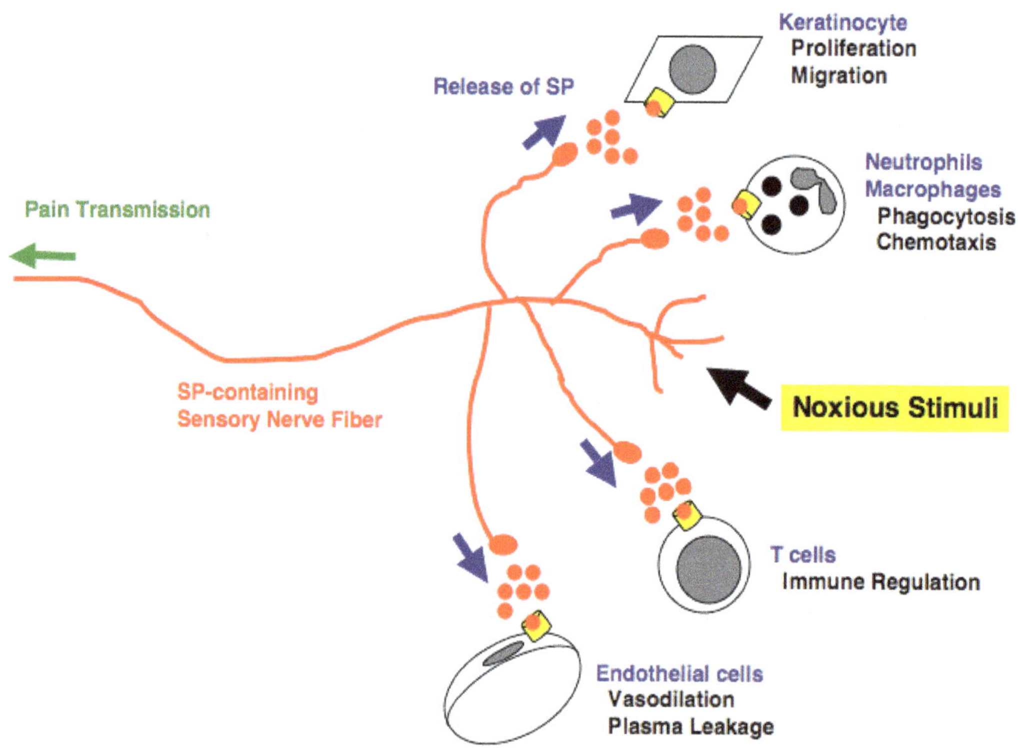

Fig. 12. Scheme of biological functions of substance P. Once the nerve ending catch noxious stimuli such as chemical irritants, heat, cold stimuli, (black arrow) to substance P-containing nerve fibers, substance P has a capable of transmitting pain stimuli (green arrow). On the other hand, substance P can be released from the free nerve endings by the noxious stimuli (blue arrows). Released substance P (red dots) are able to bind to their receptors neurokinin 1 recetors (yellow squeares) on the several types of cells, such as keratinocytes, neutrophils, macrophages, endothelial cells of blood vessels, and T cells to induce a variety of cellular functions, as shown on the scheme.

The distribution of substance P-containing sensory nerve terminals and neurokinin-1 receptors in the PIE (Yamaza et al., 2009) suggests that released substance P may bind to neurokinin-1 receptors on PIE cells, endothelial cells, and intraepithelial neutrophils, and induce a variety of innate defense mechanisms in the PIE (Figure 13). These mechanisms might include the induction of neutrophil infiltration from blood vessels into the PIE, the promotion of plasma extravasation from blood vessels beneath the PIE subjected to peri-implant sulcular fluid, and up-regulation of the endocytotic capabilities of PIE cells and neutrophils.

Substance P is also known to have anti-microbial activity (Kowalska et al., 2002; El Karim et al., 2008; Douglas & Leeman, 2011). Substance P released from nerve terminals into the intercellular spaces between the nerve endings and neurokinin receptor-bearing cells may inhibit intraepithelial growth of peri-implant bacteria in the PIE. Thus substance P-neurokinin-1 receptor function could, at least partly, govern the local defense mechanisms in this transmucosal region around dental implants, as in the natural junctional epithelium (Kido et al., 1999; Brogden et al., 2005).

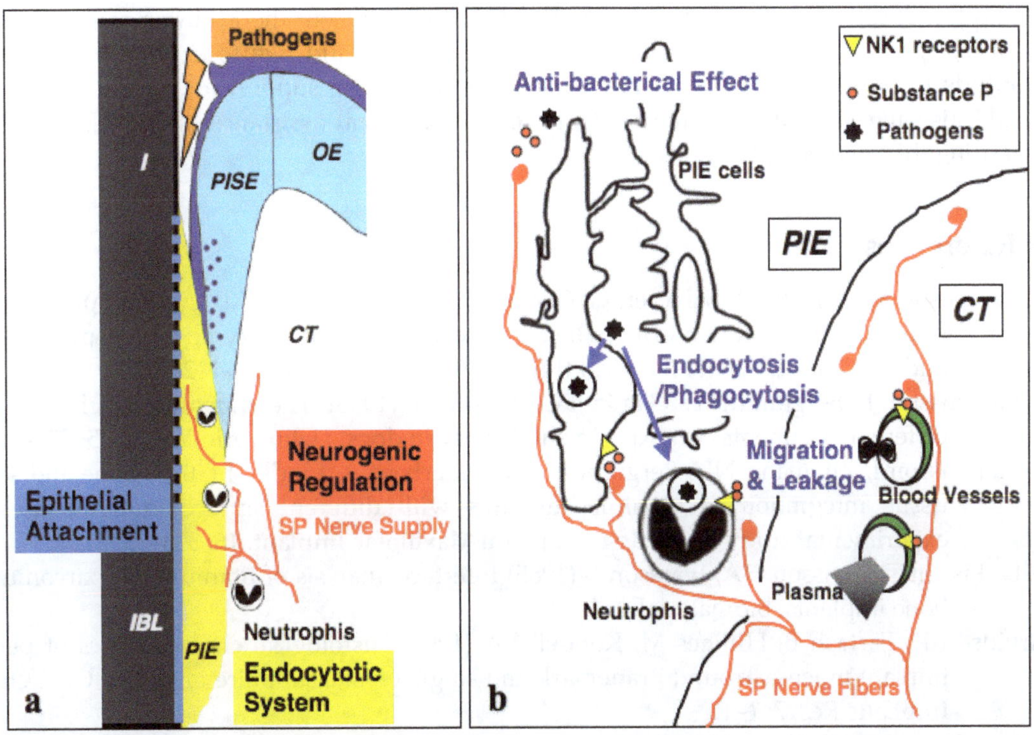

Fig. 13. Schemata of defense mechanisms in the transmucosal region around dental implants. (a) Epithelial attachment structure, internal basement lamina (*IBL*) and substance-P (SP) nerve supply in the peri-implant epithelium (*PIE*) and its subepithelial connective tissuesuggests the restoration of biological seals and defenses against several pathogens (bacteria or their products) from the oral cavity. *CT*: connective tissue, *I*: implant, *OE*: oral epithelium, *PISE*: peri-inplant sulcular epithelium. (b) Invaded pathogens stimulate the release of substance-P from the nerve endings of extra-and intra-epithelial nerve fibers. The released substance-P induces various cellular functions by binding to neurokinin-1 (NK1) receptors localized on endothelial cells, neutrophils, and peri-implant epithelial cells. This linkages result in migration of neutrophils from blood vessels into the peri-implant epithelium, and increased permeability of blood vessels to pass outwardly throughout the peri-implant epithelium. The cascades also promote the endocytosis or phagocytosis of peri-implant epithelial cells or neutrophils. The released substance P may also leads to act as a direct anti-bacterial agent.

6. Conclusion

The transmucosal region around dental implants demonstrates similar anatomical and biological features to the natural interface between the tooth enamel and the junctional epithelium. Regeneration of the PIE with its defense functions will produce a more secure implant-soft tissue interface, and thus improve the success of clinical dental implant therapy.

7. Acknowledgments

This work was supported by grants-in-aid for Scientific Research (C) (no. 21592334 to M.A.K.) and Scientific Research (C) (no. 21592333 to T.Y.) from the Ministry of Education, Culture, Sports, Science and Technology of Japan. We would like to express our sincere gratitude to Professor Emeritus Teruo Tanaka for continuing support for our research. We would also like to thank Dr. Ikiru Atsuta for his technical assistance and special advice regarding this manuscript.

8. References

Abrahamson M, Barrett AJ, Salvesen G, Grubb A (1986) Isolation of six cysteine proteinase inhibitors from human urine. Their physicochemical and enzyme kinetic properties and concentrations in biological fluids. J Biol Chem. 261:11282-11289

Abrahamsson I, Berglundh T, Glantz PO, Lindhe J (1998) The mucosal attachment at different abutments. An experimental study in dogs. J Clin Periodontol. 25: 721–727

Abrahamsson I, Zitzmann NU, Berglundh T, Wennerberg A, Lindhe J (2001) Bone and soft tissue integration to titanium implants with different surface topography: an experimental study in the dog. Int J Oral Maxillofac Implant. 16: 323–332

Albrektsson T, Hansson HA, Ivarsson B (1985) Interface analysis of titanium and zirconium bone implants. Biomaterial. 6: 97–101

Arvidson K, Fartash B, Hilliges M, Kondell PA (1996) Histological characteristics of peri-implant mucosa around Branemark and single-crystal sapphire implants. Clin. Oral Implants Res. 7: 1–10

Atsuta I, Yamaza T, Yoshinari M, Mino S, Goto T, Kido MA, Terada Y, Tanaka T (2005a). Changes in the distribution of laminin-5 during peri-implant epithelium formation after immediate titanium implantation in rats. Biomaterials 26:1751-1760

Atsuta I, Yamaza T, Yoshinari M, Goto T, Kido MA, Kagiya T, Mino S, Shimono M, Tanaka T (2005b). Ultrastructural localization of laminin-5 (gamma2 chain) in the rat peri-implant oral mucosa around a titanium-dental implant by immuno-electron microscopy Biomaterials 26:6280-6287

Aumailley M, Krieg T (1996) Laminins: a family of diverse multifunctional molecules of basement membranes. J Invest Dermatol. 106:209-214

Ayasaka N, Tanaka T (1989) A cytochemical study of horseradish peroxidase uptake in rat junctional epithelium. J Dent Res 68:1503-1507

Ayasaka N, Goto T, Tsukuba T, Kido MA, Nagata E, Kondo T, Yamamoto K, Tanaka T (1993) Immunocytochemical localization of cathepsin D in rat junctional epithelium. J Dent Res. 1993 72:502-507

Barrett AJ, Kirschke H (1981) Catepisin B, cathepisin H and cathepsin L. Methods Enzymol. 80:535-561

Bar-Shavit Z, Goldman R, Stabinsky Y, Gottlieb P, Fridkin M, Teichberg VI, Blumberg S (1980) Enhancement of phagocytosis—a new found activity of substance P residing in its N-terminal tetrapeptide sequence. Biochem Biophys Res Commun 94:1445–1451

Bartold PM, Walsh LJ, Narayanan AS (2000). Molecular and cell biology of the gingiva Periodontol 2000 24:28-55

Baschong W, Suetterlin R, Hefti A, Schiel H (2001) Confocal laser scanning microscopy and scanning electron microscopy of tissue Ti-implant interfaces. Micro. 32: 33–41

Berglundh T, Lindhe J, Jonsson K, Ericsson I (1994) The topography of the vascular systems in the periodontal and peri-implant tissues in the dog. J Clin Periodontol. 21: 189–193

Blankenvoorde MF, van't Hof W, Walgreen-Weterings E, van Steenbergen TJ, Brand HS, Veerman EC, Nieuw Amerongen AV (1998) Cystatin and cystatin-derived peptides have antibacterial activity against the pathogen Porphyromonas gingivalis. Biol Chem. 379:1371-1375

Brånemark PI, Hansson BO, Adell R, Breine U, Lindström J, Hallén O, Ohman A (1977) Osseointegrated implants in the treatment of the edentulous jaw. Experience from a 10-year period.Scand J Plast Reconstr Surg. 16:1-132

Brogden KA, Guthmiller JM, Salzet M, Zasloff M (2005) The nervous system and innate immunity: the neuropeptide connection. Nat Immunol. 6:558-564

Burgeson RE, Chiquet M, Deutzmann R, Ekblom P, Engel J, Kleinman H, Martin GR, Meneguzzi G, Paulsson M, Sanes J, Timpl R, Tryggvason K, Yamada Y, Yurchenco PD (1994) A new nomenclature for the laminins. Matrix Biol. 3:209-211

Buser D, Weber HP, Donath K, Fiorellini JP, Paquette DW, Williams RC (1992) Soft tissue reactions to non-submerged unloaded titanium implants in beagle dogs. J Periodontol. 63: 225–235

Byers MR, Holland GR (1977) Trigeminal nerve endings in gingiva, junctional epithelium and periodontal ligament of rat molars as demonstrated by autoradiography. Anat Rec 188:509-523

Byers MR, Mecifi KB, Kimberly CL (1987) Numerous nerves with calcitonin gene-related peptide-like immunoreactivity innervate junctional epithelium of rats. Brain Res 419:311-314

Cairo F, Pagliaro U, Nieri M. Soft tissue management at implant sites (2008) J Clin Periodontol 35:163-167

Canullo L, Pellegrini G, Allievi C, Trombelli L, Annibali S, Dellavia C (2011) Soft tissues around long-term platform switching implant restorations: a histological human evaluation. Preliminary results. J Clin Periodontol. 38:86-94.

Chai W, Moharamzadeh K, Vannoort R (2010) A review of histomorphometric analysis techniques for assessing implant-soft tissue interface. Biotech Histochem. *In press.*

Chen Z, Potempa J, Polanowski A, Wikstrom M, Travis J (1992) Purification and characterization of a 50-kDa cysteine proteinase (gingipain) from Porphyromonas gingivalis J Biol Chem. 267:18896-18901

Corpe RS, Steflik DE, Young TR, Wilson MR, Jaramillo CA, Hipps M, Sisk A, Parr GR (1999) Retrieval analyses of implanted biomaterials: light microscopic and scanning electron microscopic analyses of implants retrieved from humans. J Oral Implantol. 25: 161–178

Donley TG, Gillette WB (1991) Titanium endosseous implant-soft tissue interface: a literature review. J Periodontol. 62:153-160

Douglas SD, Leeman SE (2011) Neurokinin-1 receptor: functional significance in the immune system in reference to selected infections and inflammation. Ann N Y Acad Sci. 1217:83-95

Ekuni D, Tomofuji T, Yamanaka R, Tachibana K, Yamamoto T, Watanabe T (2005) Initial apical migration of junctional epithelium in rats following application of lipopolysaccharide and proteases. J Periodontol. 76:43-48

Eley BM, Cox SW, Watson RM (1991) Protease activities in peri-implant sulcus fluid from patients with permucosal osseointegrated dental implants. Correlation with clinical parameters. Clin Oral Implants Res 2:62-70

El Karim IA, Linden GJ, Orr DF, Lundy FT (2008) Antimicrobial activity of neuropeptides against a range of micro-organisms from skin, oral, respiratory and gastrointestinal tract sites. J Neuroimmunol. 200:11-16

Fujii N, Kusakari H, Maeda T (1998) A histological study on tissue responses to titanium implantation in rat maxilla: the process of epithelial regeneration and bone reaction. J Periodontol. 69:485-495

Fujii N, Ohnishi H, Shirakura M, Nomura S, Ohshima H, Maeda T (2003) Regeneration of nerve fibres in the peri-implant epithelium incident to implantation in the rat maxilla as demonstrated by immunocytochemistry for protein gene product 9.5 (PGP9.5) and calcitonin gene-related peptide (CGRP). Clin Oral Implants Res. 14:240-247

Golub LM, Kennett S, McEwan H, Curran JB, Ramamurthy NS (1976) Collagenolytic activity of crevicular fluid from pericoronal gingival flaps. J Dent Res 55:177-181

Gould TR, Westbury L, Brunette DM (1984) Ultrastructural study of the attachment of human gingiva to titanium in vivo. J Prosthet Dent. 52:418-420

Green KJ, Jones JC (1996) Desmosomes and hemdesmosomes: structure and functon of molecular components. FASEB J. 10:871-881

Grusovin MG, Coulthard P, Worthington HV, Esposito M (2008) Maintaining and recovering soft tissue health around dental implants: a Cochrane systematic review of randomised controlled clinical trials. Eur J Oral Implantol. 1:11-22

Hermann J, Buser D, Schenk R, Higginbottom F, Cochran D (2000) Biologic width around titanium implants. A physiologically formed and stable dimension over time. Clin Oral Implants Res. 11: 1–11

Hermann JS, Buser D, Schenk RK, Schoolfield JD, Cochran DL (2001) Biologic Width around one- and two-piece titanium implants. Clin Oral Implants Res. 12: 559–571

Hormia M, Sahlberg C, Thesleff I, Airenne T (1998) The epithelium-tooth interface--a basal lamina rich in laminin-5 and lacking other known laminin isoforms. J Dent Res. 77:1479-1485.

Ikeda H, Yamaza T, Yoshinari M, Ohsaki Y, Ayukawa Y, Kido MA, Inoue T, Shimono M, Koyano K, Tanaka T (2000) Ultrastructural and immunoelectron microscopic studies of the peri-implant epithelium-implant (Ti-6Al-4V) interface of rat maxilla. J Periodontol 71:961–973

Ikeda H, Shiraiwa M, Yamaza T, Yoshinari M, Kido MA, Ayukawa Y, Inoue T, Koyano K, Tanaka T (2002) Difference in the penetration of horseradish peroxidase tracer as a foreign substance into the peri-implant epithelium or junctional epithelium of rat gingivae. Clin Oral Implant Res 13:243–251

Kähler CM, Sitte BA, Reinisch N, Wiedermann CJ (1993) Stimulation of the chemotactic migration of human fibroblasts by substance P. Eur J Pharmacol. 249:281-286

Kajiwara H, Yamaza T, Yoshinari M, Goto T, Iyama S, Atsuta I, Kido MA, Tanaka T (2005) The bisphosphonate pamidronate on the surface of titanium stimulates bone formation around tibial implants in rats. Biomaterials. 6:581-587

Kawahara H, Kawahara D, Mimura Y, Takashima Y, Ong JL (1998) Morphologic studies on the biologic seal of titanium dental implants. Report II. In vivo study on the defending mechanism of epithelial adhesions/attachment against invasive factors. Int J Oral Maxillofac Implant. 13: 465–473

Kido MA, Yamaza T, Goto T, Tanaka T (1999) Immunocytochemical localization of substance P neurokinin 1 receptors in rat gingival epithelium. Cell Tissue Res 297:213–222

Kondo T, Ayasaka N, Nagata E, Tanaka T (1992) A light and electron microscopic anterograde WGA-HRP tracing study on the sensory innervation of junctional and sulcular epithelium in the rat molar. J Dent Res 71:60-65

Kondo T, Kido MA, Kiyoshima T, Yamaza T, Tanaka T (1995) An immunohistochemical and monastral blue-vascular labelling study on the involvement of capsaicin-sensitive sensory innervation of the junctional epithelium in neurogenic plasma extravasation in the rat gingiva. Arch Oral Biol 40:931-940

Koon HW, Pothoulakis C (2006) Immunomodulatory properties of substance P: the gastrointestinal system as a model. Ann N Y Acad Sci. 1088:23-40

Koon HW, Zhao D, Zhan Y, Rhee SH, Moyer MP, Pothoulakis C (2006) Substance P stimulates cyclooxygenase-2 and prostaglandin E2 expression through JAK-STAT activation in human colonic epithelial cells. J Immunol. 176:5050-5059

Kowalska K, Carr DB, Lipkowski AW (2002) Direct antimicrobial properties of substance P. Life Sci. 71:747–750

Lamont RJ, Chan A, Belton CM, Izutsu KT, Vasel D, Weinberg A (1995) Porphyromonas gingivalis invasion of gingival epithelial cells. Infect Immun. 63:3878-3885.

Lembeck F, Holzer P (1979) Substance P as a neurogenic mediator of antidromic vasodilation and neurogenic plasma extravasation. Naunyn Schmiedebergs Arch Pharmacol 310:175–183

Linden GJ, McKinnell J, Shaw C, Lundy FT (1997) Substance P and neurokinin A in gingival crevicular fluid in periodontal health and disease. J Clin Periodontol. 24:799-803

Liu JY, Hu JH, Zhu QG, Li FQ, Wang J, Sun HJ (2007) Effect of matrine on the expression of substance P receptor and inflammatory cytokines production in human skin keratinocytes and fibroblasts. Int Immunopharmacol. 7:816-823

Lundy FT, Linden GJ (2004) Neuropeptides and neurogenic mechanisms in oral and periodontal inflammation. Crit Rev Oral Biol Med. 15:82–98

Mellman I, Fuchs R, Helenius A (1986) Acidification of the endocytotic and exocytotic pathway. Annu Rev Biochem. 55:663-700

McDougall WA (1970) Pathways of penetration and effects of horseradish peroxidase in rat molar gingiva. Arch Oral Biol :621-633

McDougall WA (1971) Penetration pathways of a topically applied foreign protein into rat gingiva. J Periodontal Res 6:89-99

McKinney RV Jr, Steflik DE, Koth DL (1985) Evidence for a junctional epithelial attachment to ceramic dental implants. A transmission electron microscopic study. J Periodontol. 56:579-591

Mombelli A (1999) In vivo model of biological responces to implant microbiological models. Adv Dent Res. 13:67-72

Moon IS, Berglundh T, Abrahamsson I, Linder E, Lindhe J (1999) The barrier between the keratinized mucosa and the dental implant. An experimental study in the dog. J Clin Periodontol. 26: 658–663

Mullen LM, Richards DW, Quaranta V (1999) Evidence that laminin-5 is a component of the tooth surface internal basal lamina, supporting epithelial cell adhesion. J Periodontal Res. 34:16-24

Nagata E, Kondo T, Ayasaka N, Nakata M, Tanaka T (1992) Immunohistochemical study of nerve fibres with substance P- or calcitonin gene-related peptide-like immunoreactivity in the junctional epithelium of developing rats. Arch Oral Biol. 37:655-662

Nagata E, Kondo T, Kiyoshima T, Nakata M, Tanaka T (1994) Immunohistochemical evidence for the presence of nerve fibres with substance P- or calcitonin gene-related peptide-like immunoreactivity in the proliferating epithelium in the developing teeth of rats. Arch Oral Biol. 39:197-203

Nicoll RA, Schenker C, Leeman SE (1980) Substance P as a transmitter candidate. Annu Rev Neurosci 3:227-268

Nishimura Y, Amano J, Sato H, Tsuji H, Kato K (1988) Biosynthesis of lysosomal cathepsins B and H in cultured rat hepatocytes. Arch Biochem Biophys. 262:159-170

Otsuka M, Yoshida K (1993) Neurotransmitter function of mammalian tachykinins. Am J Physiol 73:229–308

Piattelli A, Paolantonio M, Corigliano M, Scarano A (1997a) Immediate loading of titanium plasma-sprayed screw-shaped implants in man: a clinical and histological report of two cases. J Periodontol. 68: 591–597

Piattelli A, Sacarano A, Piattelli M, Bertolai R, Panzoni E (1997b) Histologic aspects of the bone and soft tissues surrounding three titanium non-submerged plasma-sprayed implants retrieved at autopsy: a case report. J Periodontol. 68: 694–700

Piattelli A, Trisi P, Romasco N, Emanuelli M (1993) Histologic analysis of a screw implant retrieved from man: influence of early loading and primary stability. J Oral Implantol. 19: 303–306

Pontoriero R, Tonelli MP, Carnevale G, Mombelli A, Nyman SR, Lang NP (1994) Experimentally induced peri-implant mucositis. A clinical study in humans. Clin Oral Implants Res. 5:254-259.

Rautemaa R, Järvensivu A, Kari K, Wahlgren J, DeCarlo A, Richardson M, Sorsa T (2004) Intracellular localization of Porphyromonas gingivalis thiol proteinase in periodontal tissues of chronic periodontitis patients. Oral Dis. 5:298-305.

Romanowski AW, Squier CA, Lesch CA (1988) Permeability of rodent junctional epithelium to exogenous protein. J Periodontal Res 23:81-86

Sawada T, Yamamoto T, Yanagisawa T, Takuma S, Hasegawa H, Watanabe K (1990) Electron-immunocytochemistry of laminin and type-IV collagen in the junctional epithelium of rat molar gingiva. J Periodontal Res. 25:372-376

Scholzen T, Armstrong CA, Bunnett NW, Luger TA, Olerud JE, Ansel JC (1998) Neuropeptides in the skin: interactions between the neuroendocrine and the skin immune systems. Exp Dermatol. 7:81–96

Schroeder HE (1986) Gingiva. In: Oksche A, Vollrath L (eds) Handbook of microscopic anatomy, vol. 5, The periodontium, pp. 233–323. Springer-Verlag, Berlin, Germany

Schroeder HE, Listgarten MA (1997) The gingival tissues: the architecture of periodontal protection. Periodontology 2000 13:91–120

Squier CA (1991) The permeability of oral mucosa. Crit Rev Oral Biol Med 2:13-32.

Sugaya A, Chudler EH, Byers MR (1994) Uptake of exogenous fluorescent Di-I by intact junctional epithelium of adult rats allows retrograde labeling of trigeminal sensory neurons. Brain Res. 653:330-334

Tanabe T, Otani H, Bao L, Mikami Y, Yasukawa T, Ninomiya T, Ogawa R, Inagaki C (1996) Intracellular signaling pathway of substance P-induced superoxide production in human neutrophils. Eur J Pharmacol 299:187–195

Tanaka T (1984) Transport pathway and uptake of microperoxidase in the junctional epithelium of healthy rat gingiva. J Periodontal Res 19:26–39

Tanaka T, Ayasaka N, Sakano A (1988) An in vivo study of degradation of azurophil granules in the neutrophilsduring phagocytosis of cationized ferritin in the gingival sulcus. Acta Histochem Cytochem 21:15-24

Tanaka T, Kido MA, Ibuki T, Yamaza T, Kondo T, Nagata E (1996) Immunocytochemical study of nerve fibers containing substance P in the junctional epithelium of rat. J Periodont Res 31:187–194

Tanaka T, Sakano A (1987) Ultrastructural localization and passage of cationized-ferritin and microperoxidase as tracers in the outward flow of rat gingival crevicular fluid. J Periodontal Res 22:482-490

Timpl R, Rohde H, Robey PG, Rennard SI, Foidart JM, Martin GR (1979) Laminin - a glycoprotein from basement membranes. J Biol Chem 254: 9933–9977

Tonetti MS, Schmid J (1994) Pathogenesis of implant failures. Periodontol 2000. 4:127-138

Tryggvason K (1993) The laminin family. Curr Opin Cell Biol. 5:877-882

Tuluc F, Lai JP, Kilpartrick LE, Evance DL, Douglas SD (2009) Neurokinin 1 receptor isoforms and the control of innate immunity. Trends Immunol. 30:271-276

Ulker AE, Tulunoglu O, Ozmeric N, Can M, Demirtas S (2008) The evaluation of cystatin C, IL-1beta, and TNF-alpha levels in total saliva and gingival crevicular fluid from 11- to 16-year-old children. J Periodontol. 79:854-860

Weber HP, Buser D, Donath K, Fiorellni JP, Doppalapudi V, Paquette DW, Williams RC (1996) Comparison of healed tissues adjacent to submerged and non-submerged unloaded titanium dental implants. A histometric study in beagle dogs. Clin Oral Implants Res. 7: 11–19

Yamasaki A, Nikai H, Niitani K, Ijuhin N (1979) Ultrastructure of the junctional epithelium of germfree rat gingiva. J Periodontol. 50:641-648

Yamasaki A, Nikai H, Ijuhin N, Takata T, Ito H (1985). Cytochemical identification of lysosomal system of the rat junctional epithelium. J Periodontal Res 20:591-601

Yamaza T, Kido MA, Kiyoshima T, Nishimura Y, Himeno M, Tanaka T (1997) A fluid-phase endocytotic capacity and intracellular degeneration of a foreign protein (horseradish peroxidase) by lysosomal cysteine proteinases in the rat junctional epithelium. J Periodont Res 32:651–660

Yamaza T, Mino S, Atsuta I, Danjo A, Kagiya T, Nishijima K, Zang JQ, Kido MA, Tanaka T (2005) Localization of theendogenous cystein proteinase inhibitor, cystatin C,and the cystein proteinase, cathepsin B, to the junctional epithelium in rat gingiva. Acta Histochem Cytochem 38:121-129

Yamaza T, Kido MA, Wang B, Danjo A, Shimohira D, Murata N, Yoshinari M, Tanaka T (2009) Distribution of substance P and neurokinin-1 receptors in the peri-implant epithelium around titanium dental implants in rats. Cell Tissue Res 335:407-415

Ziche M, Morbidelli L, Masini E, Amerini S, Granger HJ, Maggi CA, Geppetti P, Ledda F (1994) Nitric oxide mediates angiogenesis in vivo and endothelial cell growth and migration in vitro promoted by substance P. J Clin Invest. 94:2036-2044

9

Implant Insertion Methods and Periimplant Tissues – Experimental Study

Smiljana Matić, Novak Stamatović, Zoran Tatić
and Aleksandra Petković-Ćurčin
Military Medical Academy
Serbia

1. Introduction

The replacement of missing teeth with dental implants has become predictable treatment modality over the past several decades. The function of dental implants depends on the process of osseointegration, defined by Brånemark (Brånemark, 1985, as cited in Abrahamsson & Cardaropoli, 2006) as „direct structural and functional connection between living ordered bone and the surface of load carrying implant". The process through which osseointegration is achieved depends on several factors, such as biocompatibility of the metal used as well as the design and surface characteristics of the implant, the condition of the implant socket, the surgical technique used and the loading conditions applied (Abrahamsson & Cardaropoli, 2006).

Endosteal implants are available in various designs, forms and materials. The earliest implant designs were one-component devices, i.e. implant body and implant abutment were connected in a single unit. Those implants could only be inserted in one-stage surgical method and are collectively referred to as "one-stage" or non-submerged implant systems. When inserted, implants penetrate through the oral mucosa into the oral cavity thus risking the possible contamination and/or early loading that could result in implant failure.

Within the past five decades numerous types of implant designs have evolved. Almost all of them have a common characteristic: they consist of two parts - the implant body and the implant abutment or transmucosal part. The first part (implant body) is placed into the bone socket and covered with mucoperiosteal flap. The second part (implant abutment) is connected to the implant after a period of healing in the secondary surgical procedure. These designs are recommended for so called "two-stage" or submerge surgical approach, and the components of the soft tissue cover, epithelial and subepithelial tissue, act as a barrier between the internal (bone tissue) and external (oral cavity) environment.

The studies on both surgical methods have been well documented (Adell et al., 1990, as cited in Heydenrijk et al., 2002; Lindquist et al., 1996; Ericsson et al., 1996; Buser et al., 1996; Levy et al., 1996; Brägger et al., 1998; Abrahamsson et al., 1999; Hermann et al., 2001; Lindquist et al., Heydenrijk et al., 2002).

On the basis of early research in dogs, Brånemark and his coworkers introduced submerged implant placement believing it was one of the key prerequisites for osseointegration (Weber & Cochran, 1998). Namely, implants were placed under cover of the oral mucosa for a healing period of 3-6 months and after that period a second surgical procedure was performed i.e. the implant exposure and transmucosal components (implant abutments) were placed on the implants. Implants that accidentally became exposed to the oral cavity through wound dehiscence exhibited less favorable periimplant healing than the implants that had been submerged under oral mucosa. This concept, which requires a second stage procedure, is still followed today. An opportunity exists at the second stage surgery to correct soft tissue defects, poor soft tissue relationships, poor implant placement and bone defects (Fig. 1).

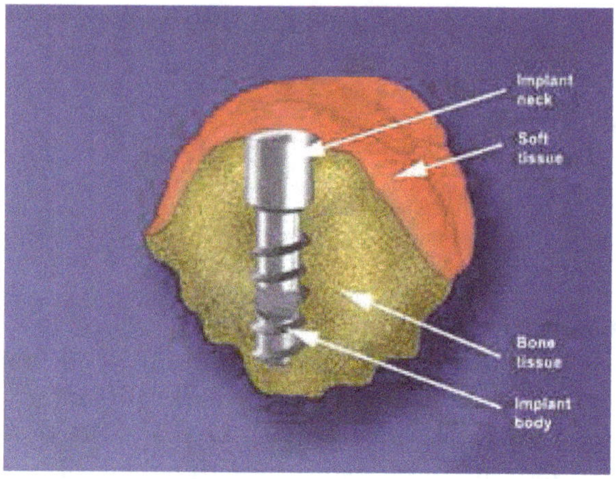

Fig. 1. Two-stage implant insertion method

However, Schroeder and al. (Schroeder, 1981, as cited in Weber & Cochran, 1998) demonstrated in the late 1970s that non-submerged or one-stage surgical method allows successful outcome of implant insertion, i.e. successful osseointegration. After the insertion the implant penetrates through the gingival tissue into the oral cavity and it is covered with the healing cap which does not interfere with the opposing or adjacent teeth. The fact that only one surgical intervention is necessary allows for soft tissue healing to the transmucosal portion of the implant by primary intention from the moment of implant insertion. This simplified method which eliminates the need for a re-entry (second surgery) is more attractive to both patients and clinicians (Fig. 2).

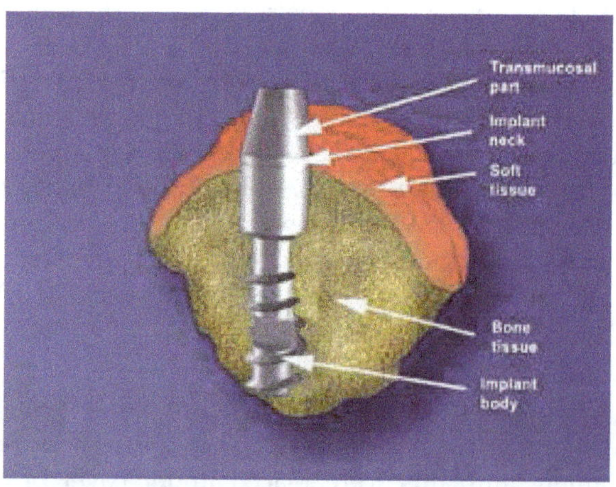

Fig. 2. One-stage implant insertion method

For a long time it was considered that implant failure was a result of soft tissue ingrowth in the coronal aspect of bony implant bed, inflammatory infiltrate, granulation tissue, bone resorption and implant mobility that was caused by the implant communication to the oral cavity.
It is now recognized that the requirement to submerge the implant during healing is not obligatory, and even has the advantages over submerged approach including: 1) the lack of secondary surgical intervention to connect the implant body and transgingival component; 2) a more mature soft tissue healing due to avoiding the second stage surgery; 3) the lack of an interface/microgap between the implant and the abutment at or below the alveolar crest level; 4) healed periimplant mucosa is not disturbed with second stage procedure for abutment placement or abutment exchanges; 5) during the osseointegration period the implants are accessible for clinical monitoring; 6) cost and time benefit advantage (Heydenrijk et al., 2002). However, one-stage implantation is not preferred treatment modality in the cases of: 1) prevention of undesirable implant loading during the osseointegration period when implants are inserted in low-density bone; 2) alveolar ridge augmentation procedures or guided bone regeneration with simultaneous implant placement when the wound has to be closed perfectly to prevent the infection of bone or membrane exposure; 3) integrated implant abutment interference with opposing jaw (in the case of one-piece implant design).
A review of literature reveals that there is no agreement as to which of these two surgical methods has achieved better outcome.

2. Experimental research

Numerous reports have compared the submerged and non-submerged implant types in animal models (Ericsson et al., 1996; Weber et al., 1996; Abrahamsson et al., 1996, 1999; Levy et al., 1996; Fiorellini et al., 1999; Moon et al., 1999; Hermann et al., 2000; Berglundh et al., 2007). The amount of scientific work was focused on the achieving and maintaining a healthy relationship of dental implants to the surrounding hard and soft tissues over extended periods. To evaluate osseointegration of dental implants by animal studies many methods have been established: radiographic evaluation of bone healing, pathohistological, immunohistochemical and histomorphometric analyses. Radiographic evaluations provide the results of periimplant bone changes, i.e. the differences of periimplant bone levels. Histomorphometric analysis is the measurement of direct bone-to-implant contact without connective tissue interposition, but all these analyses include no information about functional and structural bone architecture, bone maturity or inflammatory signs. Also, because the implants are transmucosal devices and periimplant tissues are expected to act as a barrier, pathohistological evaluations of soft tissues around dental implants were performed in order to examine the morphologic characteristics of epithelial and subepithelial tissue.

2.1 Studies on periimplant soft tissue

The role of gingival epithelium in forming a biologic seal is of great importance in implant dentistry. This seal must be effective enough to prevent the ingress of bacterial plaque, toxins, oral debris and other substances taken into the oral cavity. The initial breakdown of soft tissue was first seen around implant abutments as gingival inflammatory reaction that was followed by osteoclastic activity of underlying hard tissue and chronic resorption of the supporting bone.

James and Kelln were the first to begin a systemic study to investigate gingival attachment to the implant (James & Kelln, 1974). Although they investigated oral implants made of Vitalium (stainless steel) they concluded that an adhesion exists at the interface between the junctional epithelial cells and the penetrating implant surfaces.

Current concepts of the biologic formation of mucosal attachment are based on scientific investigations using a combination of light and electron microscopy. Periimplant epithelial tissue most closely resembles that of the natural dentition. The oral epithelium lines the lateral surface of the gingival sulcus as sulcular epithelium. Its apical part is lined with the coronal cells of the junctional epithelium which provides an epithelial union between the implant and the surrounding gingival tissue. The junctional epithelium adheres to the implant surface through a basal lamina and hemidesmosomes thus preventing external agents from moving into the internal environment of the jaw. Long-term implant maintenance depends significantly on the achievement and preservation of this attachment.

In our experimental study nine dogs (German shepherds), mean age: 4,5 years, mean weight: 32 kg were used. In the first experimental phase third and forth lower premolars were extracted bilaterally. After a healing period of eight weeks in the second phase the implants were inserted. Using split mouth design 36 c.p. (commercially pure) titanium implants were inserted using one-stage surgical method on the right mandibular side and two-stage method on the left side respectively. Three months after the implantation the animals were sacrificed and the third experimental phase - pathohistological analysis was performed.

Analyses were performed on 90 specimens from the two soft tissue regions (epithelial and subepithelial ttissue) thus comprising 180 specimens. Semi-quantitative analysis was performed for each site (evaluation of basal membrane degradation, inflammatory cell infiltration, tissue necrosis, number of blood vessels, appearance of blood vessel walls) and graded. Quantitative analyses of pathohistological findings were performed according to the established grading indices for each evaluated region. Outcomes of two surgical methods were compared using non-parametric Wilcoxon-Mann-Whitney rank-sum test for two small independent samples.

The analysis of epithelial tissue: According to the results on the basis of descriptive statistics better results were achieved by one-stage surgical method, but there were no statistically significant differences between the two applied surgical methods. Pathohistological analyses of 9 specimens inserted in one-stage approach revealed preserved basal membranes in 7 sections, massive inflammatory cell infiltrates in 2 specimens, complete tissue necrosis in 2 and partial in 3 sections (Fig. 3).

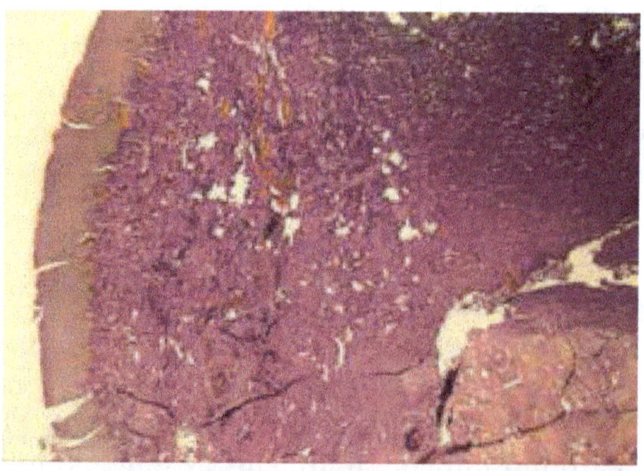

Fig. 3. Preserved epithelial tissue with basal membrane. Presence of inflammatory cells with initial necrotic lesions in subepithelial connective tissue (HE X 40).

Regarding the findings of two-stage implants, the absence of epithelial tissue, marked inflammatory infiltrate and complete necrosis were observed in 6 specimens. Basal membrane structure was preserved in only 3 sections (Fig. 4).

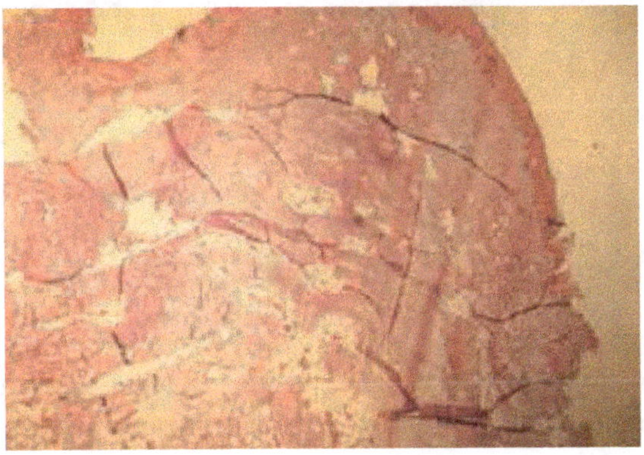

Fig. 4. Partial necrosis of gingival epithelial tissue, degradation of basal membrane, partial inflammatory cell infiltrate and initial necrosis (HE X 40)

The analysis of subepithelial tissue: According to the results on the basis of descriptive statistics, better results were achieved by one-stage surgical method regarding the number of blood vessels and vascular volume, while regarding blood vessel walls and inflammatory cell infiltrate, two methods achieved identical results. No statistically significant difference was found between the two methods. Pathohistological analyses of the implants inserted in one-stage method revealed marked neovascularization, dilated blood vessels with thick walls and inflammatory infiltrate in 3 specimens (Fig. 5).

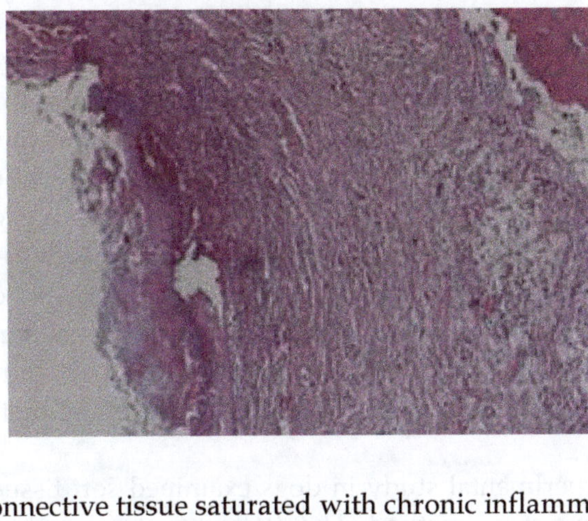

Fig. 5. Subepithelial connective tissue saturated with chronic inflammatory cells and increased vascular proliferation and dilatation (HE X 40)

Increased number of blood vessels was found in 6 specimens and marked inflammation in 4 sections of the implants inserted in two-stage method (Fig. 6).

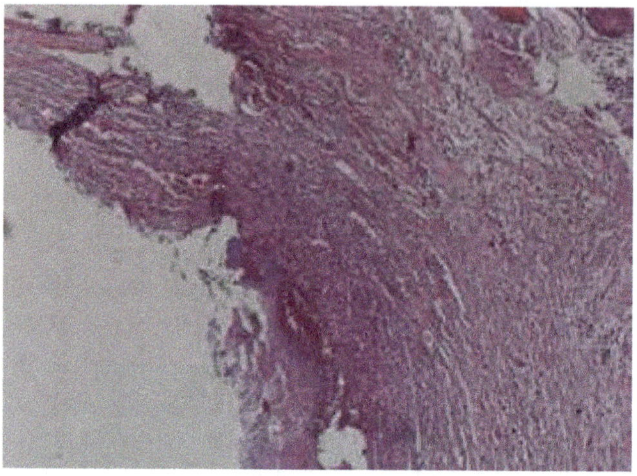

Fig. 6. Presence of partially necrotic epithelial tissue and torn subepithelial connective tissue with necrotic lesions, marked inflammatory cell infiltrate and increased vascular proliferation (HE X 40)

Dynamic changes that occur during soft tissue healing process are related to the periimplant sulcus depth, connective tissue-implant contact and the length of periimplant epithelial attachment (Buser at al., 1990; Cochran et al., 1997).

In a beagle dog study of crystal sapphire implants that were placed in one-stage procedure Fartash et al. (Fartash et al., 1990) observed discrete inflammatory infiltrate in periimplant soft tissue, while Chavrier et al. (Chavrier et al., 1994, as cited in Weber & Cochran, 1998) observed inflammatory cells in approximately half the biopsies in their study on experimental dogs. Buser et al. (Buser at al., 1990) detected the presence of periimplant epithelial attachment in one-stage implants in experimental dogs, while Abrahmsson et al. (Abrahamsson et al., 1996, 1999) in their similar experimental studies reported that surgical method had not influence on the formation and structure of periimplant soft tissue. Weber et al. comparing non-submerged and submerged implants in beagle dogs, found significant differences between implant types. In every case where the implant was initially submerged, the epithelium was found apical to the interface (microgap) between the implant and transgingival abutment. Attachment level for non-submerged implants was located more coronally compared to submerged implants. Comparing one- and two-stage implants statistically, the authors concluded that there was a significant difference in position and epithelium extension between the two methods (Weber et al., 1996).

In their review article Weber and Cochran (Weber & Cochran, 1998) described in details the significance of soft tissue response to submerged and non-submerged osseointegrated implants. Periimplant epithelium was described as junctional epithelium, in many ways analogous to the natural tooth and no difference between the methods of insertion was observed.

Moon et al. in their experimental study in dogs examined soft tissue attachment to dental implants inserted in one-stage method. The attachment was comprised of two portions: marginal junctional epithelium and connective tissue. Epithelium was observed in all examined specimens. The authors consider the connective tissue that is in direct contact with the implant surface and located apically of junctional epithelium significantly more

important. The portion of connective tissue which is next to implant surface is characterized by its absence of blood vessels and abundance of fibroblasts. The authors assume that the fibroblast rich region is „responsible" for establishment and maintenance of proper seal between oral environment and periimplant bone (Moon et al. 1999).
Herman et al. (Hermann et al., 2000) in their research on one- and two-stage implantation concluded that implant abutment/interface had an impact on gingival position and periimplant sulcus depth. Placing the microgap (the connection of the abutment and the implant body) below the bone level significantly increased the forming of infrabony periimplant pockets. If the microgap was placed 0,5 -1,0 mm below the bone level, bone resorption was increased. Microbial contamination of the microgap associated with micromovement of the implant can cause the bone resorption and chronic inflammation of the adjacent tissues. That is the reason it is not recommendable to place two-stage implants with microgap positioned apically in order to avoid negative effects on periimplant tissues. This problem has not been reported for transmucosally placed one-stage implants.
Regarding the morphogenesis of periimplant mucosal attachment, Berglundh et al. (Berglundh et al. 2007) observed epithelial proliferation and the first signs of a barrier (junctional) epithelium two weeks after implantation. Tissue maturation and collagen fiber organization was evident 6 to 12 weeks of healing.
Epithelial and subepithelial periimplant tissues were not analyzed in details in most investigations. In the experimental study in dogs Ponguarison et al. (Ponguarison et al., 2007) investigated inflammation associated with implants with different surface types inserted in one-stage method. The junctional epithelium and oral epithelium were examined for assessment of the inflammatory infiltrate. The areas of infiltrate were categorized into three grades according to the density of inflammatory cells. Pathohistological findings revealed that the periimplant tissues surrounding all types of abutment surfaces tested, exhibit some degree of inflammation. Subepithelial areas had the greatest density of infiltration (3+ grade). Implants with machined surface with circumferential groove had the largest area of inflammatory infiltrate, but there were no statistically significant differences in number of infiltrating cell types between the four investigated transmucosal surfaces, suggesting that the surface of the implant has little if any influence on the nature of the surrounding inflammation, which is in agreement with the results of numerous authors who studied the influence of implant surface on periimplant soft tissue attachment or the initiation and progression of inflammation (Abrahamsson et al., 2002; Klinge & Meyle, 2006).

2.2 Studies on periimplant bone tissue

Bone is an active biologic tissue that undergoes resorption and remodeling periods in response to various factors. Attention must be paid to maintain bone in a healthy state during the surgical procedure of implant insertion so as not to damage the cell viability and nutrient blood supply to the bone. The use of slow-speed rotary cutting instruments with internally and/or externally applied irrigation provides less amount of cell damage during surgery. Following the osteotomy, the bone must heal around the endosteal implant surface.
The concept of osseointegration arose from the studies of osseous wound healing that had started in the 1950s by Bränemark. Titanium chambers containing a transillumination system were inserted into the fibulae of rabbits to observe cellular changes during endostael

wound healing. At the completion of the study, retrieval of the titanium chamber required the fracture of bone tissue that has integrated with the chamber surface. Bränemark's team found that implants made of commercially pure (c.p.) titanium, careful bone preparation and immobilization of the implant during the initial healing phase were necessary to effect a rigid fixation of the implant to the surrounding bone tissue (LeGeros & Craig, 1993).

Surgical placement of endosteal implants elicits an osteogenic response largely driven by local factors. The initial healing response is independent of direct mechanical control because bone heals optimally in the absence of functional loading. The vascularly dependent ostegenic process can be easily disrupted by micromotion at a healing bone-implant interface. This is one of the main reasons why some surgeons advocate two-stage implant placement. Following a maturation phase of about 1 week newly formed osteoid is primarily mineralized when osteoblasts deposit about 70% of the mineral found in mature vital bone. Adequate resistance to loading in humans is achieved in about 18 weeks, but there are no quantitative data (Misch, 1999).

Two theories for the mechanism responsible for osteogenesis at implant interface exist in the literature. According to Davies et al. (Davies et al., 1991, as cited in Steflik et al., 1999) there is no fibrillar material directly at the implant-bone interface. Bone derived cells deposit calcified accretions to condition the implant surface prior bone formation, thus no collagen fibers directly interface with the implant. The second theory, based on the studies and investigations of Steflik, Albrektsson and Linde (Steflik et al., 1998; Albrektsson et al., 1981; Linder et al., 1983, as cited in Steflik et al., 1999) suggests that an unmineralized collagen fiber matrix is deposited at the implant interface and is subsequently mineralized.

The aforementioned experimental study of the authors on implant insertion in canine mandibles included pathohistological analyses of three bone regions surrounding implants: bone-to-implant contact region, bone-implant interface and bone tissue adjacent to the implant (0,03-0,04 mm) aiming specifically to provide information on bone structure, bone maturity and inflammatory reaction.

Analyses were performed on 90 specimens from each of the three bone tissue regions thus comprising 270 specimens. Semi-quantitative analysis was performed for each site (evaluation of the amount of connective - collagen tissue fibers, osteoblastic activity, number of blood vessels, inflammatory cell infiltration, bone tissue necrosis, appearance of blood vessel walls and blood vessel volume) and graded. Quantitative analyses of pathohistological findings were performed according to the established grading indices for each evaluated region. Outcomes of two surgical methods were compared using non-parametric Wilcoxon-Mann-Whitney rank-sum test for two small independent samples.

The analysis of bone-to-implant contact region: With regard to the results obtained on the basis of descriptive statistics, better results were achieved by two-stage method regarding the amount of collagen tissue fibers and this difference was statistically significant while regarding the osteoblastic activity and bone necrosis the results were identical. Pathohistological analysis of the implants inserted in one-stage method revealed increased amount of connective-collagen tissue fibers in 5 specimens. Necrosis was also observed in the same samples. In remainder moderate osteoblastic activity was found (Fig. 7).

The pathohistological findings of bone tissue in contact with the implants inserted in two-stage method revealed increased amount of connective-collagen tissue fibers in all specimens. No osteoblastic activity was observed. Partial bone tissue necrosis was found in 8 specimens and in 1 necrosis was complete (Fig. 8).

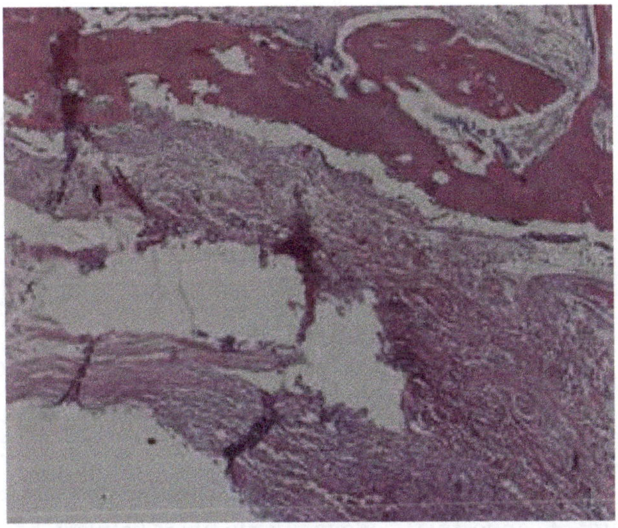

Fig. 7. Increased amount of connective tissue with marked chronic inflammatory cell infiltration, partial necrosis and marked vascular proliferation. Presence of compact bone tissue regions with osteoblastic activity can be detected (HEX40).

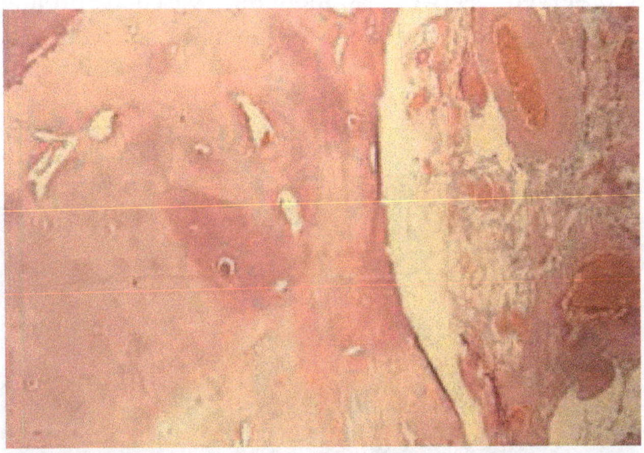

Fig. 8. On the left: compact lamellar bone. On the right: increased amount of connective - collagen tissue, with numerous dilated blood vessels, marked inflammatory cell infiltrate and partial necrotic lesions (HE X 40).

The analysis of the bone-implant interface: According to the results on the basis of descriptive statistics the results were identical regarding median values of osteoblastic activity, blood vessels, inflammatory cell infiltrate and bone tissue necrosis. Better results were achieved by two-stage method regarding the amount of collagen tissue, but there were no statistically significant differences between the methods. The pathohstological analysis of bone-implant interface of the implants inserted in one-stage method revealed increased amount of connective-collagen tissue fibers in all specimens, moderate increase of the number of osteoblasts (osteoblastic activity) was observed in 2 specimens Marked neovascularization was found in 2 and moderate in 1 specimen. Inflammation was absent in all specimens, while necrosis was found in only 1 specimen (Fig. 9).

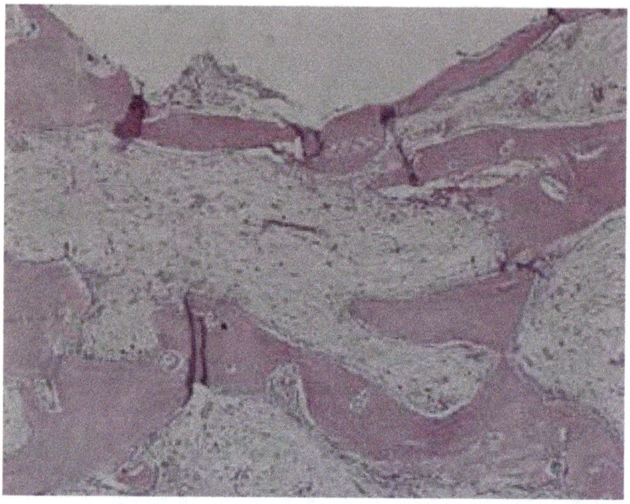

Fig. 9. Marked amount of connective - collagen tissue fibers between bone lamellae with vascular proliferation and marked osteoblastic reaction (HE X 40)

The pathohistological analysis of the implants inserted in two-stage method revealed marked increase of connective tissue fibers in 5 specimens, in 1 specimen moderate increase of osteoblasts was observed, as well as moderate vascular proliferation and marked neovascularization. Inflammation and bone tissue necrosis were also found in only 1 specimen (Fig. 10).

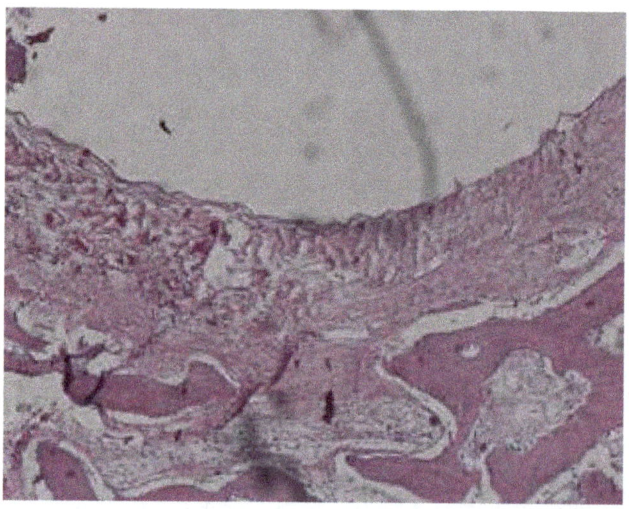

Fig. 10. Loose subepithelial connective tissue. Trabecular bone lattice with collagen tissue proliferation, marked neovascularization, poor osteoblastic activity, moderate inflammatory cell infiltrate and partial bone tissue necrosis (HEX40).

The analysis of bone tissue adjacent to the implant: According to the results on the basis of descriptive statistics the results were identical regarding the median values of amount of collagen tissue, osteoblastic reaction and bone tissue necrosis while better results were achieved regarding the number of osteocytes by two-stage surgical procedure. The latter result was also statistically significant.

Pathohistological analysis of the implants inserted in one-stage method revealed moderate increase of connective-collagen tissue fibers in only 1 specimen where also no osteoblasts and osteocytes could be observed; moderate increase of osteoblasts and osteocytes was found in 3 samples; the number of osteocytes was increased in 4 specimens. Necrotic bone tissue was not found in any of analyzed specimens. In 1 specimen bone structure was completely preserved with no connective tissue fibers, but with no osteoblasts and osteocytes as well (Fig. 11).

Pathohistological analysis of the implants inserted in two-stage method revealed moderate increase of connective tissue fibers in only 1 specimen. No osteoblastic activity could be observed in all specimens. Moderate increase of osteocytes was observed in 3 specimens and marked increase in 6 remained specimens. Necrotic bone tissue was not found in any of analyzed specimens (Fig. 12).

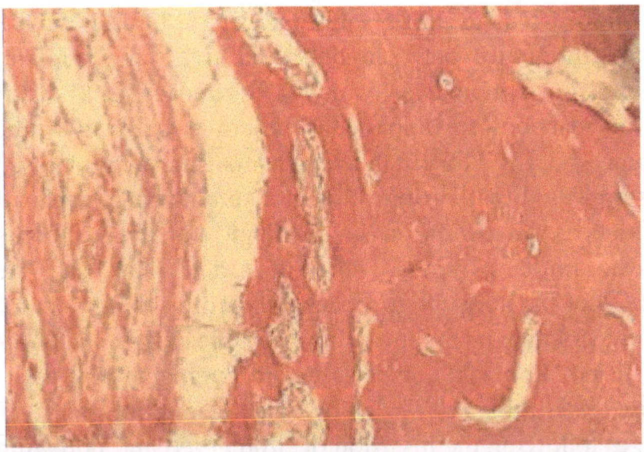

Fig. 11. On the left: loose subepithelial connective tissue, underneath scattered interconnected bone trabeculae with osteoblastic reaction, collagen tissue proliferation between trabeculae. On the right: preserved lamellar bone tissue with osteocytes in lacunae (HEX10).

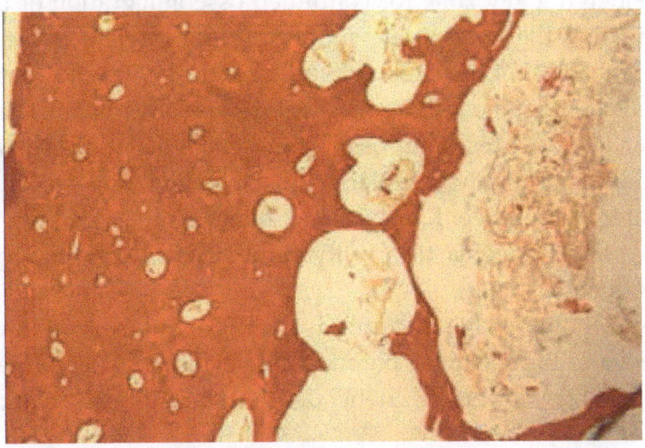

Fig. 12. Mature lamellar bone, underneath interconnected bone trabeculae and intertrabecular collagen tissue proliferation (HE X10).

Experimental study conducted by Ericsson et al. on Labrador dogs analyzed certain characteristics of periimplant tissues following one- and two-stage surgical installation of Bränemark implants. The results demonstrated that titanium implants can obtain proper bone anchorage (osseointegration) despite being exposed to oral cavity during the initial 3-month healing phase (Ericsson et al., 1996).

Implant surface characteristics have been the focus of research in implantology since 1960s. The interrelationship of surgical methods and implant surface was investigated by Levy et al. who analyzed bone-to-implant contact around porous coated root form implants placed in the canine model in one- and two-stage surgical method. After six weeks of healing, the absolute bone-to-implant contact was greater for submerged implants, although significantly on the buccal aspects only (Levy et al., 1996). Similar results were reported by Sagara et al. (Sagara et al.,1993, as cited in Levy et al., 1996) who analyzed bone-to-implant contact of submerged and non-submerged implants placed in dogs after a healing period of 12 weeks. In contrast, Gotfredsen et al. (Gotfredsen et al., 1991, as cited in Levy et al., 1996) found no significant difference between one- and two-stage implant methods in their experimental research on 6 monkeys. Namely, Gotfredsen et al. performed histological evaluations of tissue reactions to unloaded submerged implants without reopening and unloaded non-submerged ITI TPS (titanium plasma spray) implants. After 22 weeks of healing the results indicated that both groups had similar bone levels at the end of healing period and no differences were found in the histological analysis of bone-to-implant contact regions between the implant types. They concluded that osseointegration could be established regardless of the surgical approach. According to Levy et al. (Levy et al., 1996) this difference in protocol may be the important variable in that the long healing period may have provided sufficient time for bone healing to overcome any early inhibitory factors affecting non-submerged implants. Fiorellini et al. (Fiorellini et al., 1999) evaluated the radiographic changes following the insertion of submerged and non-submerged implants in beagle dogs and concluded that there were no differences between the implants on the overall amount and rate of periimplant bone loss, although distinctive patterns of bone resorption existed between the implant types.

The region of bone adjacent to the implant has been investigated in not so many studies. This region is considered a key zone for continued osseointegration of the implant. One of the studies investigating the bone tissue supporting the implant is the one conducted by Meenaghan (Meenaghan, 1974, as cited in Steflik et al., 1999) who first described a triple layer of osseous cells in the remodeling process close to blade implant. He suggested that an outer dense cellular layer existed comprised of mesenchymal-like cells interfaced with the implant. A middle layer of highly vascularized osteogenic tissue existed to a third layer of osteoblasts associated with osteoid matrix and bone. Similar findings were reported by Steflik et al. who observed osteoblastic activity in the zone adjacent to implant. (Steflik et al., 1994, as cited in Steflik et al., 1999).

Investigating crestal bone changes around titanium submerged and non-submerged implants in canine mandibles histomorphometrically, Hermann et al. (Hermann et al., 2000) concluded that bone changes were not dependent on the surgical technique (one- and two-stage insertion).

Koch et al. (Koch et al., 2010) investigated the osseointegration of the implants of different materials inserted in one- and two-stage surgical procedure in dogs. Healing modalities did not influence the rate of bone-to-implant contact between the implants, among which were the implants of c.p. titanium.

2.3 Future research

Oral implants have developed rapidly. New technical and technological improvement upon diagnostic tools and medical equipment have considerably reduced the risk of operative complications. Basic studies within physical and biologic sciences have resulted in development of various surgical implant systems where special attention has been paid to surface topography and technology as well as to the processes of wound healing along biomaterial interfaces.

Currently direct bone-to-implant contact is considered the optimal healing outcome around endosteal implants. The character of tissues around the implants and the quality of tissue attachment to the implant surface influence the biomechanical response of this integration.

The interfacial interactions between recipient tissues and implanted material are limited to the surface layer of the implant and a few nanometers into the living tissue. The surface property has been recognized as important factor for successful osseointegration because it can promote early and secure bone formation around dental implants. Titanium is by far the material of choice for dental implants and various surface treatments have been proposed to enhance the osseointegration: blasting of the surface, acid or fluoride etching or anodizing. In recent years chemically modified surfaces have been proven to enhance bone-to-implant contact. These modifications increase the hydrophilic property of titanium surfaces and accelerate and enhance the initial adsorption of extracellular matrix proteins (Rupp et al., 2004; Buser et al., 2004, as cited in Jimbo et al., 2011). In their experimental study on Japanese White rabbits Jimbo et al. (Jimbo et al., 2011) investigated bone apposition during the early phases of osseointegration of anodized porous titanium implants modified with hydrogen fluoride solution and ultraviolet irradiated. Histomorphometric analyses revealed that photo-induced hydrophilic surface enhanced bone apposition thus shortening the healing period. In addition, photo-reactive implant surface provide photo-induced sterilization as well as a decontamination of infected implant parts (eg. transmucosal abutments) by simple irradiation.

Recently, much attention has been given to implant surface treatment with biologically active substances. These include purified proteins and synthetic peptides that mediate the binding of osteoblast cell adhesion receptors. When dental implants inserted into the bone a sequence of cellular and molecular events are involved. Undifferentiated mesenchymal cells proliferate and migrate into the implant socket from adjacent marrow, endosteum and periosteum. These cells differentiate into osteoblasts or osteoclasts under the influence of locally acting growth factors, leading to bone maturation and mineralization. Bone morphogenetic proteins (BMPs) are members of the TGF-β (transforming growth factor) - β super family, a group of cytokines with the expression in various tissues. They have numerous functions, among which is to induce the osteoblasts to differentiate and form bone tissue (Asahina et al., 1996; Yamaguchi et al., 1996).

In their study on the influence of recombinant human BMP-2 (rhBMP-2) on bone-implant osseointegration, Lan et al. (Lan et al., 2007) investigated whether osseointegration can be enhanced by the use of rhBMP-2. Titanium implants were coated by rhBMP-2 with polylactic acid as a carrier. The results showed that osseointegration was improved in quality as well as in quantity, however further studies are necessary to evaluate the optimal dose range of rhBMP-2 and research new carriers.

Most studies evaluating growth, differentiation and matrix factor as potential agents in support alveolar bone augmentation have focused on rhBMP-2, but it is not the only member of BMP family of proteins approved for clinical use. Susin et al. (Susin et al., 2010) have used rhBMP-7 (also known as recombinant human osteogenic protein - rhOP-1) coated onto the titanium porous-oxide surface implants to attain vertical alveolar ridge augmentation and implant osseointegration. Two different doses of BMP-7 were compared. No statistically significant differences were observed. Both doses produced clinically relevant bone formation. The authors concluded that rhBMP-7 coated onto titanium implants exhibits a convincing potential to stimulate local bone formation. Lee et al. (Lee et al., 2010) also investigated osseointegration of implants coated with rhBMP-2 and concluded that significant bone formation was achieved. Huh et al. (Huh et al., 2010) investigated the effects of anodized implants coated with Escherichia coli-derived rhBMP-2 (ErhBMP-2) on alveolar ridge augmentation in beagle dogs. The results suggest that ErhBMP-2 can induce vertical bone augmentation when placed in the vertical defects of alveolar bone that has been healed after tooth extraction thus improving the stability of implants and excluding the need for additional bone transplantation.

Functioning arrangement of connective tissue around endosteal implants that would act as a periodontal ligament does not exist, but the efforts are made in order to make an implant resemble a natural tooth. One direction of investigations is to regenerate periodontal ligament from periodontal cells (for example in immediate implantation) and the other direction is from mesenchymal stem cells or periodontal progenitor cells.

Early experimental studies on new formation of periodontal ligament have started in 1980s.Those studies indicated that only cells residing in PDL (periodontal ligament) were capable of forming new cementum with inserting collagen fibers on exposed root surfaces. Periodontal ligament is lost with the natural tooth loss, it cannot be restored after implant placement. Buser et al. (Buser et al., 1990) analyzed the wound healing around titanium implants in the presence of retained root tips. The experiment was performed on 5 monkeys. After a period of 12 months pathohistologic examination revealed that in regions the implants were placed close to retained roots, a periodontal ligament had formed around large portions of the implant. In polarized light it was apparent that the collagen fibers were oriented perpendicularly to the implant surface and were inserted in the cementum on the implant surface as well as in the opposing bone.

The discovery of a periodontal ligament around titanium implants opens new perspectives in implantology. Parlar et al. (Parlar et al., 2005) performed unique experiment on mongrel dogs to explore the formation of periodontal tissues around titanium implants using maxillary canine roots. They created chambers within the roots and prepared slits in the cavity walls to connect the chamber to the periodontal space. Implants were placed into the center of each chamber. Following 4 months of healing pathohistological analysis was performed. Fibrous encapsulation was observed around most implants, but cellular cementum was deposited on 2 implants, most likely formed through cementoconductivity rather than by differentiation of periodontal ligament cells upon contact with the implant surface. Partial generation of periodontal ligament on endosteal dental implants in dogs was also observed by approximating a tooth–to-implant contact using orthodontics (Jahangari et al., 2005).

In a pilot experimental study Craig et al. (Craig et al., 2006) reported on the effect of autogenous periodontal cell grafts on the implant-connective tissue interface with and without enamel matrix derivative (EMD). After 8 weeks histomorphometric and microscopic analyses revealed that EMD and the type of cell population present in the implant wound-healing environment may alter the implant-connective tissue interface.

Technically implant carrying periodontal ligament (PDL) may be inserted in the extraction socket of the missing tooth. One of the recent investigations regarding a tissue-engineered periodontal ligament around dental implants was performed by Gault et al. (Gault et al., 2010). They developed so called "ligaplant" which is the combination of PDL cells with the implant biomaterial. Following implant placement a new PDL-like tissue is produced. The authors claim that ligaplants have the capacity to induce the formation of new bone tissue. Investigations were performed in animal and human models. Hydroxyapatite (HAP)-coated titanium implants were combined with canine-derived PDL cells and inserted into the jaws of respective cell donors. The dogs were sacrificed after 20 weeks and pathohistological analyses were performed on 11 implants. The results indicated that the formation of PDL-like tissue can be attained *in vivo,* if a suitable implant surface and sufficient amounts of PDL cells are provided. A PDL-like tissue was formed with perpendicular fibers between the implant and alveolar bone. However, formation of this tissue is a slow process.

Dental and non-dental derived stem cells have the periodontal regeneration capability. As Liu et al. suggested in their study on miniature pigs, autologous periodontal ligament stem cells (PDLSC) are capable of forming bone, cementum and PDL if they are transplanted onto to HA/TCP (hydroxyapatite/tricalciumphosphate) carrier into surgically created periodontal defects (Liu, 2008, as cited in Batistella et al., 2010). PDLSC used with HA/TCP as a carrier showed the capacity to differentiate into cementoblasts and to form cementum/PDL-like structures (Batistella et al., 2010). These cells (PDLSC) also have the capacity to form collagen fibers similar to Sharpey's fibers and suggest the potential to regenerate PDL attachment.

Non-dental derived stem cells have also been the source of periodontal regeneration cells. Marei et al. (Marei et al., 2005) investigated the formation of periodontal structure around titanium implants utilizing bone marrow mesenchymal stem cells (MSCs). In their pilot experimental study on goats they placed immediate implants after canine teeth extractions bilaterally. Experimental side received a porous hollow root-form poly DL-Lactide co-Glycolide scaffold with autogenous bone-marrow-derived mesenchymal stem cells. The results showed that periodontal-like tissue with newly formed bone was observed. The authors concluded that undifferentiated MSCs were capable of differentiating to provide three critical tissues required for periodontal tissue regeneration: cementum, bone and periodontal ligament. Adipose-derived stem cells were used in a work of Tobita combined with platelet-rich plasma (PRP) and implanted into the periodontal tissue defects in rats. Partial alveolar bone regeneration and a periodontal ligament-like structure were observed 8 weeks after implantation (Tobita et al., 2008, as cited in Batistella et al., 2010).

However the precautions must be taken, since using stem cells may have some risks. Carcinoma-associated fibroblasts (CAF) play important role in the growth of epithelial solid tumors. Although the cell type of origin of CAFs has not been conclusively established it has been shown that they may be marrow derived. When cultured in conditioned medium MSCs) derived from cancer cell lines for prolonged periods, assume CAF properties. These activated MSCs have increased expression of CAF markers and in addition, support growth of breast cancer cells *in vitro* as well as *in vivo* in xenograft model (Mishra et al., 2009).

3. Conclusion

Over the past few decades, an improved understanding of the various parameters that influence osseointegration has resulted in high predictability and clinical success of dental implants. One- and two-stage implant insertion give acceptable results regarding certain important characteristics of investigated soft and bone periimplant tissues (epithelial basal membrane structure, inflammatory reaction, tissue degradation and/or necrosis, osteoblastic activity, collagen tissue proliferation, neovascularization). Most of the experimental study designs area based on a limited number of investigated samples, so there are no significant differences between the two methods.

Numerous other phenomena that occur after the functional loading of implants are common for all implant systems, irrespective of the method of their surgical placement. Moreover, it seems that surgical methods are of lesser importance for the long term implant maintenance compared with implant design characteristics, especially those related to their surface. Ultimately, with the increasing knowledge about tissue engineering, when tooth loss does occur, regeneration of the entire tooth may be advantageous in comparison with replacement by implants.

4. Acknowledgement

The authors would like to thank Prof. Vujadin Tatić, Ph.D. for his assistance in histology preparations and Mr. Dušan Stanković for his valuable contribution to the statistical analysis and technical assistance in manuscript preparation.

5. References

Abrahamsson, I., Berglundh, T., Wennstrom, J. & Lindhe, J. (1996). The peri-implant hard and soft tissues at different implant systems. Comparative study in the dog. *Clin. Oral Impl. Res,* Vol. 7, No 3 , (September 1996), 212-219, ISSN 0905-7161

Abrahamsson, I., Berglundh, T., Moon, IS. & Lindhe, J. (1999). Periimplant tissues at submerged and non-submerged titanium implants. *J Periodontol,* Vol. 26, No 9, (September 1999), 600-607, ISSN 0303-6979

Abrahamsson, I., Zitzmann, NU., Berglundh, T., Linder, E., Wennerberg, A. & Lindhe, J. (2002). The mucosal attachment to titanium implants with different surface characteristics: an experimental study in dogs. *J Clin Periodontol,* Vol. 29, No. 5, (May 2002), 448-455, ISSN 0303-6979

Abrahamsson , I. & Cardarpoli G. (2007). Peri-implant hard and soft tissue integration to dental implants made of titanium and gold. *Clin. Oral Impl. Res,* Vol. 18, No 3, (June 2007), 269-274, ISSN 0905-7161

Asahina, I., Sampath, TK. & Hauschka, PV. (1996). Human osteogenic protein-1 induces chondroblastic, osteoblastic and/or adipocytic differentiation of clonal murine target cells. *Exp Cell Res,* Vol. 222, No. 1, (January 1996), 38-47, ISSN 0014-4827

Batistella, E., Mele, S. & Rimondini, L. (2010). Dental tissue engineering: a new approach to dental tissue reconstruction. In: *Biomimetics Learning from Nature,* Editor Amitava Mukherjee, InTech, (March 2010), ISBN 978-953-307-025-4, Wienna, Austria

Berglundh, T., Abrahamsson, I., Welander, M., Lang, N. & Lindhe, J. (2007). Morphogenesis of the peri-implant mucosa: an experimental study in dogs. *Clin.Oral Impl. Res,* Vol. 18, No. 1, (February 2007), 1-8, ISSN 0905-7161

Bräger, U., Häfeli, U., Huber, B., Hämmerle, CHF. & Lang, N. (1998). Evaluation of postsurgical crestal bone levels adjacent to non-submerged dental implants. *Clin.Oral Impl. Res,* Vol. 9, No. 4, (August 1998), 218-224, ISSN 0905-7161

Buser, D., Warrer, K. & Karring, T. (1990). Formation of a Periodontal Ligament around Titanium Implants. *J Periodontol,* Vol. 61, No. 9 (September 1990), 597-601, ISSN 0022-3492

Buser, D., Mericke-Stern, R., Dula, K. & Lang, N. (1996). Clinical Experience with One-stage, Non-submerged Dental Implants. *Adv Dent Res,* Vol. 13, No. 1, (June 1999), 153-161, ISSN 0895-9374

Cochran, DL., Hermann, JS., Schenk, RK., Higginbottom, FL. & Buser, D. (1997). Biologic width around titanium implants. A histometric analysis of the implanto-gingival junction around unloaded and loaded nonsubmerged implants in the canine mandible. *J Periodontol,* Vol. 68, No 2, (February 1997), 186-198, ISSN 0022-3492

Craig, RG., Kamer, AR., Kallur, SP., Inoue, M. & Tarnow, DP. (2006). Effects of Periodontal Cell Grafts and Enamel Matrix Proteins on the Implan-Connective Tissue Interface: A Pilot Study in the Minipig. *J Oral Implant,* Vol. 32, No. 5, 228-236, ISSN 1048-1842

Ericsson, I., Nilner, K., Klinige, B. & Glantz, P-O. (1996). Radiographical and histological characteristics of submerged and nonsubmerged titanium implants. An experimental study in the Labrador dog. *Clin. Oral Impl. Res,* Vol. 7, No 1, (March 1996), 20-26, ISSN 0905-7161

Fartash, B., Arvidson, K. & Harmann, DJ. (1990). Histology in tissues surrounding single crystal sapphire endosseous dental implants. *Clin. Oral Impl. Res,* Vol. 1, No. 1, (December 1990), 13-21, ISSN 0905-7161

Fiorellini, JP., Buser, D., Paquette, DW., Williams, RC., Haghighi, D. & Weber, HP. (1999). A Radiographic Evaluation of Bone Healing around Submerged and Non-Submerged Dental Implants in Beagle Dogs. *J Periodontol,* Vol. 70, No. 3 (March 1999), 248-254, ISSN 0022-3492

Gault, P., Black, R., Romette, J-L., Fuente, F., Schroeder, K., Thilou, F. et al. (2010). Tissue - engineered ligament: implant constructs for tooth replacement. *J Clin Periodontol,* Vol. 37, No. 8, (August 2010), 750-758, ISSN 0303-6979

Hermann, JS, Buser, D., Schenk, RK., Higginbottom, FL., & Cohran, DL. (2000). Biologic width around titanium implants. A physiologically formed and stable dimension over time. *Clin. Oral Impl. Res,* Vol. 11, No. 1, (February 2000), 1-11, ISSN 0905-7161

Hermann, JS., Buser, D., Schenk, RK. & Cochran, DL. (2000). Crestal bone changes around titanium implants. A histometric evaluation of unloaded submerged and nonsubmerged implants in the canine mandible. *J Periodontol,* Vol. 71, No.9, (September 2000), 1412-1424, ISSN 0022-3492

Hermann, JS., Buser, D., Schenk, RK., Schoolfield, JD. & Cochran, DL. (2001). Biologic Width around one- and two-piece titanium implants. A histometric evaluation of unloaded nonsubmerged and submerged implants in canine mandible. *Clin. Oral Impl. Res,* Vol. 12, No. 6, (December 2001), 559-571, ISSN 0905-7161

Heydenrijk, K.,Raghoebar, GM., Meijer, HJ., van der Reijden, WA., van Winkelhoff., AJ. & Stegenga, B. (2002). Two-stage IMZ implants and ITI implants inserted in a single stage procedure. A prospective comparative study. *Clin. Oral Impl. Res,* Vol. 13, No. 4, (August 2002), 371-380, ISSN 0905-7161

Huh, JB., Park, CK., Kim, SE., Shim, KM., Choi, KH., Kim, SJ. et al. (2010). Alveolar ridge augmentation using anodized implants coated with *Escherichia coli* - derived recombinant human bone morphogenetic protein 2. *Oral Surg Oral Med Oral Pathol Oral Radiol Endod,* in press, doi: 10.1016/ij.tripleo.2010.09.063

Jahangiri, L., Hessamfar, R. & Ricci, JL. (2005). Partial generation of periodontal ligament on endosseous dental implants in dogs. *Clin. Oral Impl. Res,* Vol. 16, No. 4 , (August 2005), 394-401, ISSN 0905-7161

James, RA. & Kelln, E. (1974). A histopathological report on the nature of the epithelium and underlining connective tissue which surrounds implant posts. *J Biomed Mat Res,* Vol. 8, No. 4, 385-390, ISSN 1097-4636

Jimbo, R., Ono, R., Hirakawa, Y., Odatsu, T., Tanaka, T. & Sawase, T. (2011). Accelerated Photo-Induced Hydrophilicity Promotes Osseointegration: An Animal Study. *Clin Implant Dent and Rel Res,* Vol. 13, No. 1, (March 2011), 79-85, ISSN 1523-0899

Klinge, B. & Meyle, J. (2006). Soft tissue integration of implants. Consensus report of Working Group 2. *Clin. Oral Impl. Res,* Vol. 17 (Suppl.), No S2, (October 2006), 93-96, ISSN 0905-7161

Koch, FP., Weng, D., Kramer, S., Biesterfeld, S., Jahn-Eimermacher A. & Wagner, W. (2010). Osseointegration of one-piece zirconia implants compared with a titanium implant of identical design: a histomorphometric study in the dog. *Clin. Oral Impl. Res,* Vol. 21, No. 4, (April 2010), 350-356, ISSN 0905-7161

Lan, J, Wang, ZF., Shi., Xia, HB. & Cheng, XR. (2007). The influence of recombinant human BMP-2 on bone-implant osseointegration: biomechanical testing and histomorphometric analysis. *Int. J. Oral Maxillofac. Surg.* Vol. 36, No.4, (April 2007), 345-349, ISSN 0901-5027

Lee, J., Decker, JF., Polimeni, G., Cortella, CA., Rohrer, MD., Wozney, JM et al. (2010). Evaluation of implants coated with rhBMP-2 using two different coating strategies:

a critical-size supraalveolar peri-implant defect study in dogs. *J Clin Periodont,* Vol. 37, No. 6, (June 2010), 582-590, ISSN 0303-6979

Levy, D., Deporter, DA., Piliar, RM., Watson, PA. & Valiquette, N. (1996). Initial healing in the dog of submerged versus non-submerged porous-coated endosseous dental implants. *Clin. Oral Impl. Res,* Vol. 7, No 2, (June 1996), 101 - 110, ISSN 0905-7161

LeGeros, RG. & Craig, RG. (1993). Strategies to Affect Bone Remodeling: Osteointegration. *J Bone Min Res,* Vol. 8, No S2, (December 1993), S583-S596, ISSN 0884-0431

Linquist, LW., Carlsson, GE. & Jemt, T. (1996). A prospective 15-year follow-up study of mandibular fixed prostheses supported by osseointegrated implants. Clinical results and marginal bone loss. *Clin. Oral Impl. Res,* Vol. 7, No. 4, (December 1996), 329-336, ISSN 0905-7161

Marei, KM., Saad, MM., El-Ashwah, AM., El-Backly, RM & Al-Khodary, MA. (2009). Experimental Formation of Periodontal Structure Around Titanium Implants Utilizing Bone Marrow Mesenchymal Stem Cells: A Pilot Study. *J Oral Implant,* Vol. 35, No. 3, 106-129, ISSN 1048-1842

Micsh, CE. (1999). Contemporary Implant Dentistry, Second Edition, Mosby Inc., ISBN 0-8151-7059-9, St. Louis, USA

Mishra, PJ., Mishra PJ. & Glod, JW. (2009). Mesenchymal Stem Cells: Flip Side of the Coin. *Cancer Res,* Vol.69, No. 4, (Febraury 2009), 1255-1257, ISSN 0008- 5472

Moon, I-S., Berglundh, T., Abrahamsson, I. & Linder J. (1999). The barrier between the keratinized mucosa and the dental implant. An experimental study in the dog. *J Clin Periodontol,* Vol. 26, No. 10, (October 1999), 658-663, ISSN 0303-6979

Parlar, A., Bosshardt, DD., Ünsal, B., Çetiner,D., Haytaç, C. & Lang, NP. (2005). New formation of periodontal tissues around titanium implans in a novel dentin chamber model. *Clin. Oral Impl. Res,* Vol. 16. No. 3, (June 2005), 259-367, ISSN 0905-7161

Ponguarison, NJ., Gemmell, E., Tan, AES., Henry, PJ., Marshall, RI. & Seymour, GJ. (2007). Inflammation associated with different surface types. *Clin. Oral Impl. Res,* Vol. 18, No. 1, (February 2007), 114-125, ISSN 0905-7161

Steflik, DE., Corpe, RS., Young, TR., Sisk, AI. & Parr, GR. (1999), The Biologic Tissue Responses to Uncoated and Coated Implanted Biomaterials. *Adv Dent Res,* Vol. 13, No. 1, (June 1999), 27-33, ISSN 0895-9374

Susin, C., Qahash, M., Polimeni, G., Lu, PH., Prasad, HS., Rohrer, MD. et al. (2010). Alveolar ridge augmentation using implants coated with recombinant human bone morphogenetic protein-7 (rhBMP-7/rhOP-1): histological observations. *J Clin Periodont,* Vol. 37, No. 6, (June 2010), 574-581, ISSN 0303-6979

Weber, HP., Buser, D., Donath, K., Fiorellini, JP., Doppalapudi, V., Paquette, DW. & Williams, RC. (1996). Comparison of healed tissues adjacent to submerged and non-submerged titanium implants. A histometric study in beagle dogs. *Clin. Oral Impl. Res,* Vol. 17, No 1, (March 1996), 11-19, ISSN 0905-7161

Weber, HP. & Cochran DL. (1998). The soft tissue response to osseointegrated dental implants. *J Prosthet Dent.* Vol. 79, No. 1, (January 1998), 79-89, ISSN 0022-3913

Yamaguchi, A., Ishizuya, T., Kintou, N., Wada, Y., Katagari, T., Wozney, JM. et al. (1996). Effects of BMP-2, BMP-4 and BMP-6 on osteoblastic differentiation of bone marrow-derived stromal cell lines, ST2 and MC3T3-G2/PA6. *Biochem Biophys Res Commun*, Vol. 220, No. 2, (March 1996), 336-371, ISSN 0006-291X

10

Biomechanics of Cantilevered Implant-Supported Prosthesis (Biomechanics in Implant Prosthodontics)

José H. Rubo and Vinicius Cappo Bianco
Department of Prosthodontics, Bauru School of Dentistry,
University of São Paulo, Bauru, SP;
Brazil

1. Introduction

The peculiar characteristic of an implant-supported prosthesis is the fact that its fixation is given by the connection of an alloplastic material (the implant) to a living tissue (the bone). This fixation has been defined as rigid and clinically asymptomatic and must be maintained during functional loading (Albrektsson & Zarb, 1993). Under load, bone tissue will undergo a remodeling process, which ultimately influences the long-term function of a dental implant system (Meijer et al., 1993). Bone remodelling is a complex process that involves a sequence of chemical- and mechanical-mediated biologic events known as mechanotransduction (Duncan & Turner, 1995).

Because the occlusal load will be transferred to the implants and subsequently to the bone, it is believed that the biomechanics of the implant-supported prosthesis play an important role in the longevity of the bone around dental implants (Skalak, 1985). It is commonly found in the literature that, for cantilevered implant supported mandibular prosthesis, stresses tend to be concentrated at the cortical bone on the disto-lingual aspect of the implant closest to the load (Meijer et al., 1993; Murphy et al., 1995; Rubo & Souza, 2008; Sertgoz & Guvener, 1996; Weinberg & Kruger, 1995). Many researchers have focused on the steps of force transfer to gain insight into the biomechanical effect of force directions, force magnitudes, prosthesis type, prosthesis material, implant design, number and distribution of supporting implants, bone density, and the mechanical properties of the bone-implant interface (Sahin & Cehreli, 2002). The resultant stresses should be kept below the failure stress limit of the materials involved (Frost, 1994; Skalak, 1985; Wiskott & Belser, 1999).

Failures in dental implant prostheses have been correlated with biomechanical complications. Overloading factors may negatively influence implant longevity (Kim et al., 2005). According to Isidor (2006), although it has been stated that occlusal forces may be associated with the loss of oral implants, a causative relationship has never been convincingly demonstrated. The related mechanisms of these displacements are still not completely understood and studies about the influences of the several biomechanical factors are inconclusive (Rangert et al., 1989). Implant failure caused by overload has been classified as a dogma and as such should be abandoned (Carlsson, 2009). There are contradictory studies regarding bone loss in overload conditions. From those studies it can be inferred that

bone loss around implants could happen with large occlusal interferences or in the coexistence of small interferences associated with inflammation (Oh et al., 2002).
According to Brunski, (1991), three tasks need to be accomplished in implant biomechanical studies: 1) identify and quantify the biomechanical variables that can affect bone biology; 2) measure the effects of these variables quantitatively and with precision; and 3) to distinguish the effects resultant of one variable from the effects resultant of other variable. Failure prevention demands testing and stress analysis of the implants and tissues in vitro as well in vivo.
The first attempt to solve the biomechanical problem was presented by Skalak (1983), who created a mathematical model to determine force components in implants. Skalak's model considered bone and prosthesis as being infinitely rigid, while implants were considered elastic. Although this model had some limitations, part of the results are still valid and have called the attention of researchers to the biomechanical problems of implant prosthesis.
However, stress transmission to the bone must be studied taking into account bone biology aspects. During function, bone around implants is subjected to repetitive loading. Like other rigid materials, bone is subjected to fatigue. Repetitive load may result in micro fractures that, if left to build up, can lead to structural failure. The effect of tension on bone tissue has been object of discussion. The concept that bone architecture is determined by induction of tension/deformation remounts to the 19th century (Chamay & Tschantz, 1972; Duncan & Turner, 1995; Rieger et al., 1990). Today it is believed that changes in bone structure are the result of a system where local mechanic signals induce bone cell activity. Frost (1994) proposed a theory according to which there is a minimal bone tension level, the "minimal effective strain" (MES), above which adaptative response would take place, while below it bone would remain stable (Duncan & Turner, 1995).
How much load implants can withstand without jeopardizing the surrounding bone is the question that remains unanswered (Brunski, 1991, 1992; Clelland et al., 1991; Murphy et al., 1995; Sertgoz & Guvener, 1996). Although Frost's theory establishes a minimal effective strain for each loading condition, certainly there is not a single answer to the question, since individual particularities are determinants in this quantification. There is a general agreement that a well-planned and executed prosthesis is essential to avoid excessive forces on bone and implant components. Implant dentistry would greatly profit if it were provided the means to predict how bone and implant components would behave considering each patient's unique jaw anatomy, quality of bone, amount of occlusal force exerted on the prosthesis, etc.
To shed light on this issue, the influence of factors such as the curvature of the mandible, the density of cancellous bone, the length of implants and abutments, the length of cantilever, the number of implants, and the framework stiffness have been objects of study (Bidez & Misch, 1992; Meijer et al., 1993; Pierrisnard et al., 2003; van Oosterwick 1998).

2. FEA studies

The creation of a computerized model of an implant-supported fixed prosthesis allows an analysis of the possible variation in stress distribution that is likely to occur with diverse prosthetic designs and occlusal load variables. A good understanding of how each component of the implant prosthesis behaves under load could facilitate optimal prosthesis design and fabrication. This could decrease the likelihood of mechanical failures as well as improve implant prosthesis longevity.

Finite-element analysis (FEA), with all its inherent limitations (Brunski, 1988; Murphy et al., 1995), is a valuable instrument in pursuing that goal. When associated with clinical findings and accumulation of reliable data on implant loading, bone-implant contact area and other factors, FEA models could help us understand the problems encountered in daily practice (Brunski, 1991). For the reasons above mentioned, FEA studies results have to be seen with a critical eye, and the values should not be taken as absolute but rather be used to compare the possible magnitudes of stress that bone and implant components undergo during function (Meijer et al., 1993; Murphy et al., 1995; Weinberg & Kruger, 1995).
To study some of the variables that affect the biomechanics of implant prosthodontics, a computerized 3-dimensional (3-D) finite-element model of the anterior segment of a human mandible provided with an implant-supported bridge was created. The basic model consisted of a curved beam with radius 15.0 mm and dimensions 69.0 mm long, 14.0 mm high, and 6.0 mm wide. This beam was covered with a 1.0-mm-thick layer on the buccal, occlusal, and lingual surfaces and a 3.0-mm layer at the base to simulate cortical bone. The final external dimensions were therefore 71.0 3 18.0 3 8.0 mm, respectively. Five 10.0-mm cylinders 3.75 mm in diameter were placed at the center of the beam, their centers 7.0 mm apart from each other. The cylinders were provided with 3.0-mm-high extensions to simulate the abutments. A second beam (71.0 3 4.0 36.0 mm) was added in connection to the abutments to simulate a framework (Figure 1).
The model was fixed at both ends for the sake of the stress analysis. All materials, bone included, were assumed to be linearly elastic and isotropic. An FEA program (I-DEAS Structural Dynamics Research, Milford, Ohio) installed in a desktop computer was used to analyze the many possible variations in prosthetic design and occlusal load.

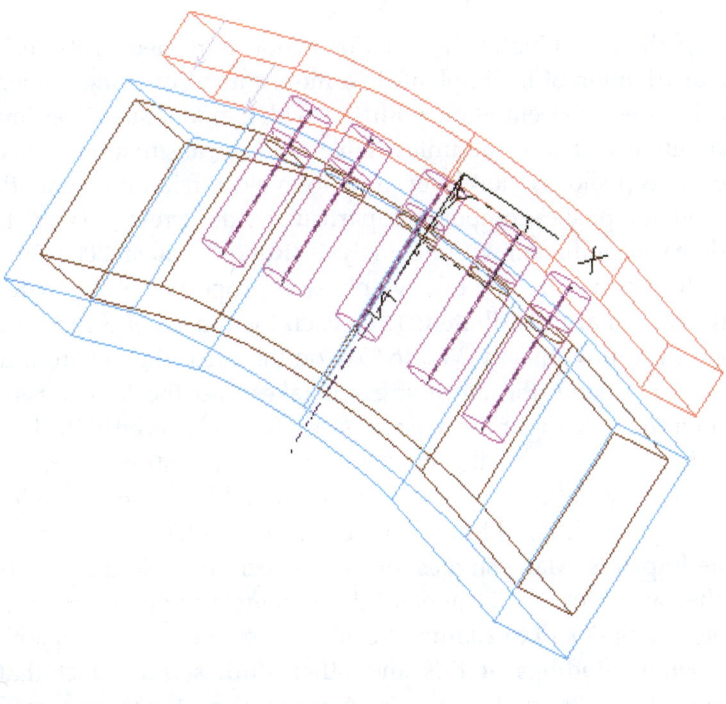

Fig. 1. 3-D model with its internal layers

The model was fed with elastic properties of the materials as derived from the literature. Elastic modulus for cortical bone was assumed to be 13.7 GPa, while for cancellous bone it was assumed to be 1.5 GPa based on a density of 25%. A 100-N vertical load was applied at 15.0 mm distally to the terminal abutment to simulate the occlusal force. Images with the fringes of stress were obtained for each of the components of the model, and maximum Von Mises stresses (σEmax) at each site were analyzed for comparison.
Seven clinical variables were chosen to be evaluated and are summarized in Table 1 for easy reference. Each variable was introduced alternately on the basic model, all other conditions being equal. Cantilever length was defined as the position where load was applied relative to the center of the terminal abutment. Quality of cancellous bone was expressed in terms of its modulus of elasticity (E) as derived from the literature. Abutment and implant lengths were based on the Brånemark system (Nobel Biocare AB, Goteborg, Sweden). Framework alloy was selected according to the modulus of elasticity of AgPd (E = 95 GPa) and CoCr (E = 218 GPa) alloys.

1) curvature of mandible	*r = 15 mm	r = 10mm	r = 18mm	
2) cantilever length	*15 mm	10mm	20mm	
3) cancellous bone quality	*E = 1.5Gpa	E = 4.0GPa	E = 7.9GPa	
4) abutment length	*3.0mm	5.5mm	7.0mm	
5) implant length	*10mm	13mm	15mm	
6) framework alloy	*E = 95GPa	E = 218GPa		
7) number of implants	*a)5	b)4	c)4	d)3

E – elastic modulus **r** – radius * - Features of the basic model

Table 1. Clinical variables selected for analysis.

The curvature of the mandible in the anterior region is related to its shape and ultimately influences the distribution of the implants in a more curved or straight line. Apparently there is an increase in stress concentration with the wider model since the implants tend to be located in a straight line creating an unfavorable mechanical situation. For conditions like that it is advisable to keep shorter cantilever arms to avoid torsion moments that could increase stress in bone and also pushes components, particularly the screws, to risk of fracture.
From the studies we conducted with FE analysis (Rubo & Souza, 2008, 2010) (Figures 2 to 7) it was possible to observe that the relative physical properties of the materials substantially affect the way stresses are distributed: 1. At each increment of 5 mm in cantilever length, stress increased by approximately 30% to 37% on the cortical bone around implants. 2. The stiffer the cancellous bone, the more stress it takes and the less stress the cortical bone appears to undergo. 3. A slight decrease in stress was observed with longer implants and abutments. 4. The use of a CoCr alloy contributes to a better stress distribution.
The conventional design of an implant supported fixed bridge on the edentulous mandible results in bilaterally cantilevered framework extensions, which under load create torque and moment on the implants. Many suggestions have been made in the literature regarding the extension of the cantilever, but in general the various authors agree that according to the quality of bone, a range of 10 to 20 mm of cantilever extension is acceptable. Perhaps one of the most compelling findings of this and other studies is the fact that the increase in cantilever length has a remarkable impact upon the stress concentration around the implants. The longer the cantilever arm, the more stress was observed.

Fortunately, this is one of the implant-supported prosthesis features most easily controlled by the dentist. The applications of the shortened dental arch concept and the express recommendation to the dental technician to keep the length of the cantilever arm to a minimum are procedures that cannot be neglected. Previous studies have demonstrated that the increase in cantilever length is directly proportional to the increase in stress concentration around the implants. Kunavisarut et al. (2002) observed that the presence of a cantilever arm significantly increased the stress in the prosthesis, implant, and surrounding bone. Besides, when no proper fit is achieved, the stress is magnified by the cantilever.

The effect of increasing the cantilever arm in this study was remarkable. Stress in the abutment/implant almost doubled when the force was moved from 10 to 20 mm along the cantilever. When analyzing the effect on the framework, a different pattern is observed. The stress increases from 10 to 15 mm but then decreases at the 15 to 20 mm change. According to Benzing et al. (1995) the load application in a framework for implant prosthesis produces deformation energy in the system that causes flexion. If a great amount of deformation energy is consumed by the framework, reduction of the transmitted energy happens, decreasing the stress in this structure.

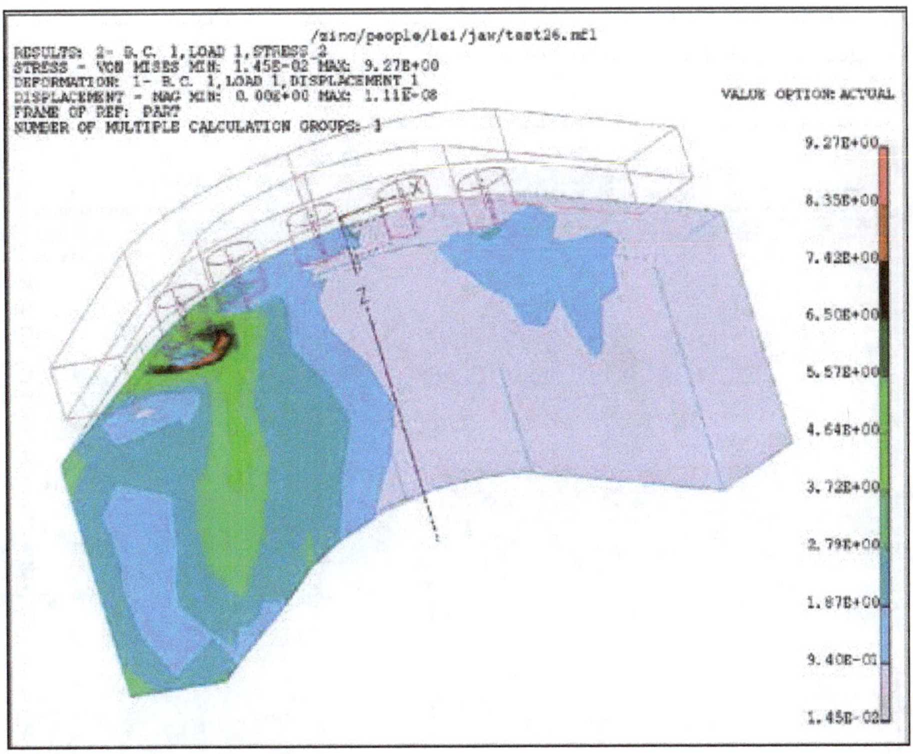

Fig. 2. Fringes of stress in cortical bone (MPa).

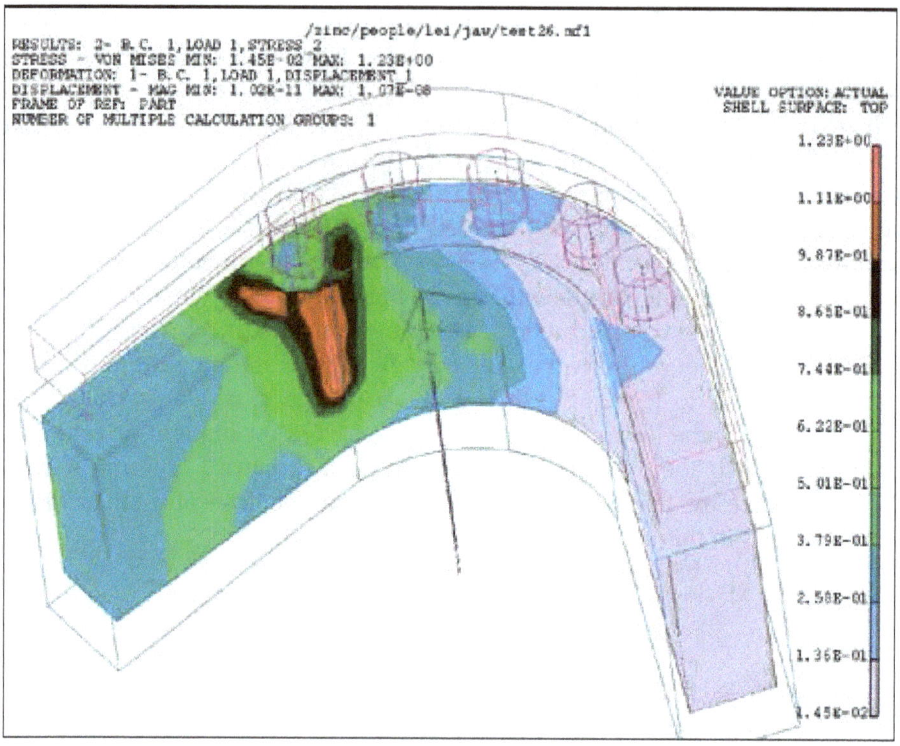

Fig. 3. Fringes of stress in cancellous bone (MPa)

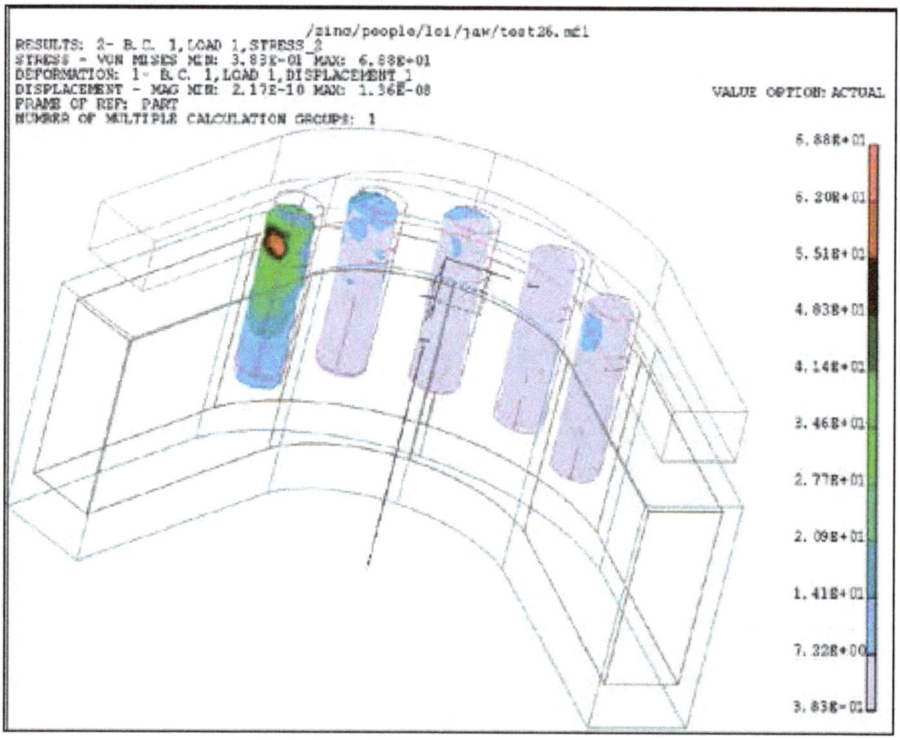

Fig. 4. Stresses on implants/abutments (lingual view).

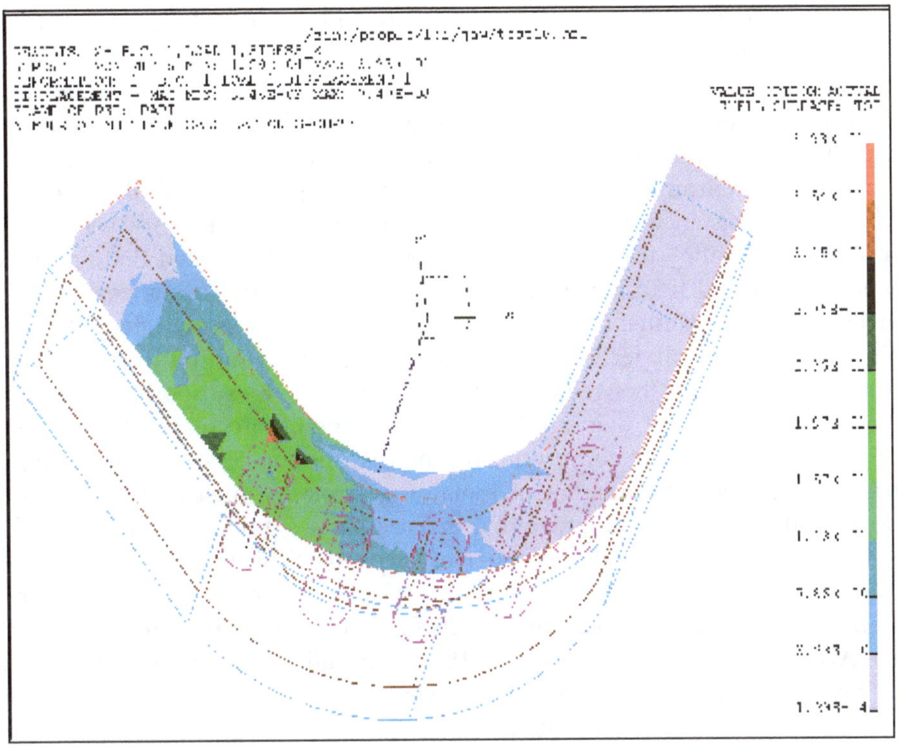

Fig. 5. Stresses on the framework (bottom view).

Structural strength is dependent on the elastic modulus, shape, and length of the prosthesis, which may affect the load distribution among the implants. The lower the elastic modulus, the greater the force applied to the abutment/implant closest to the load. Therefore, if an imaginary rubbery framework was used, nearly the totality of the load would be concentrated at the implant/abutment closest to the point of load application (Skalak, 1983). Likewise, an infinitely rigid framework would distribute the load equally among the implants. Brunski, (1992) compared two implant prosthesis frameworks of considerably different elastic moduli, one made out of acrylic resin and one made out of AgPd alloy, confirming the theory that most of the load concentrates on the terminal implant closest to the load. This finding opposes the original theory proposed by Skalak (1993) who underestimated the load on the implant closest to the load and super estimated the load on the implants on the opposite side, exactly because disregarded the mechanical properties of the structures.

The use of a CoCr alloy allowed a better stress distribution. There was an increase of the stress on the terminal abutment opposite to the load of the order of 135%, with a decrease of the stress in the remaining positions. This finding is corroborated by others in the literature (Benzing et al., 1995; Hulterstrom & Nilsson, 1994; Sertgoz & Guvener, 1996; Skalak, 1985), who found that a stiffer framework provides a more even distribution of forces among the abutments, decreasing the stress within the retaining screws, as a result of the reduced bending of the framework. Left aside the difficulties in the use of CoCr alloys, like casting shrinkage (around 2.3%) and melting point differences relative to gold cylinders, its use has been clinically tested with no complications that could be regarded to the alloy itself (Hulterstrom & Nilsson, 1994).

The analysis of the stress in the framework with different cantilever length revealed an interesting fact relative to the AgPd alloy: the increase in cantilever length is not followed by a proportional increase in stress levels of the framework. The stress in the framework increases when the cantilever changes from 10 to 15 mm, but this effect does not repeat at the 15 to 20 mm change. In fact, there is a decrease in the stress levels, denoting that, with longer cantilevers, the framework begins to bend, yielding to the load. Benzing et al. (1995) observed that the resistance to the deformation of a golden framework was two-thirds of that of a nonprecious alloy framework. Therefore, it can be suggested that, in cases of long cantilevers, there would be a benefit in the use of a more rigid framework. Nevertheless, excessive long cantilevers must be avoided even with frameworks of high elastic modulus.

When the osseointegration technique was introduced the standard procedure was the placement of six implants between the mental foramina to support a fixed prosthesis. Because of space limitations, this number was subsequently decreased to five and then to four implants without greatly compromising the distribution of stress. However, when an implant is lost, not only the number of remaining implants must be considered, but also their distribution in order to guarantee that the stresses are going to be properly dissipated (Figures 4, 6 and 7). Reducing the number of implants from five to four and then three implants resulted in an increase of stresses on the abutment nearest to the point of load application (6.88MPa with 5 implants, 71.2MPa with 4 implants and 7.72MPa with 3 implants). Also, the position of the implant that eventually is lost, for example the terminal implant, results in an even longer cantilever arm what could cause unpredictable consequences to the bone and components.

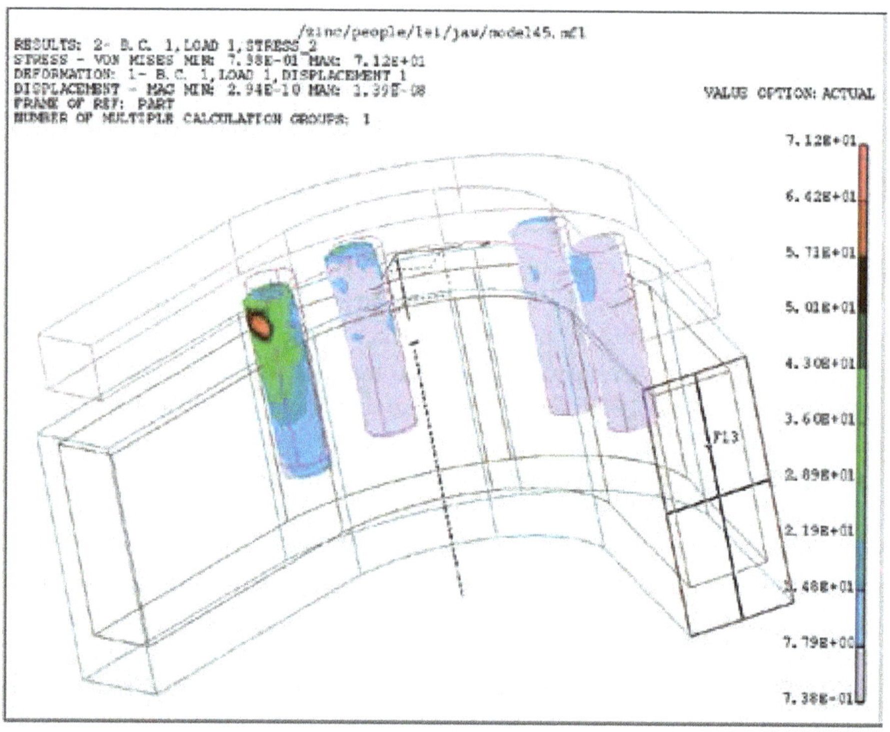

Fig. 6. Stresses on implants/abutments with four implants.

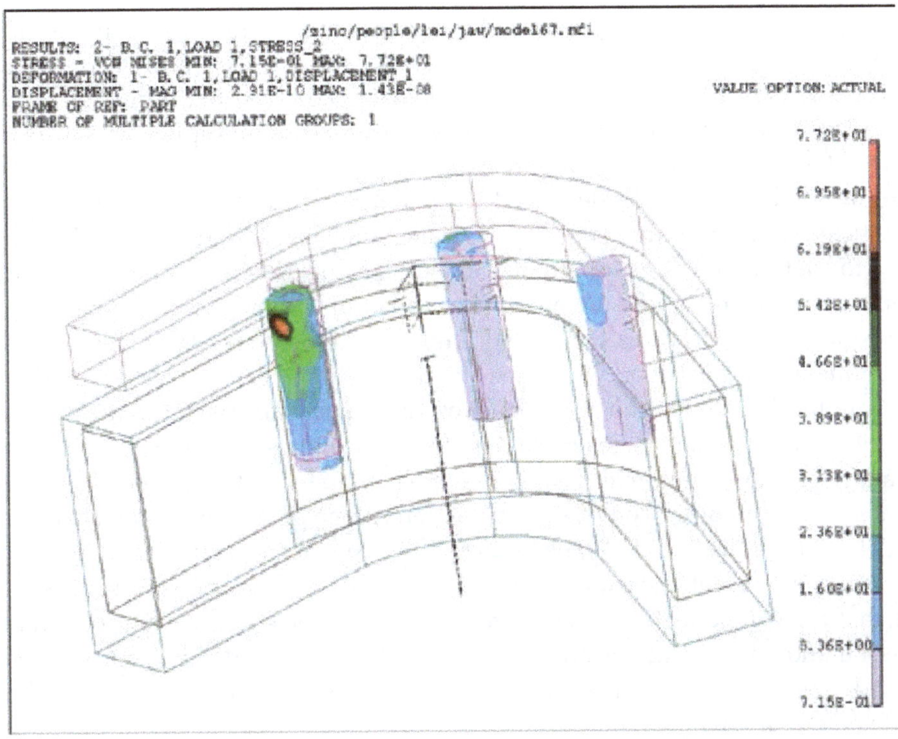

Fig. 7. Stresses on implants/abutments with three implants.

3. Strain gauge analysis

The relevance of osseointegration in today's prosthodontic practice is well recognized. Failure rates are low and easily surmounted by the improvements in function, esthetics, and quality of life. Nevertheless, failures do occur and are considered to be related to a range of biologic and mechanical factors. Among the most commonly reported failures are: resorption of the peri-implant bone crest, peri-implantitis, loss of osseointegration, screw loosening and fracture, and fracture of the prosthesis, prosthetic components, and even the implant itself (Jemt 1991; Kallus & Bessing, 1994; Worthington, 1987; Zarb & Schimitt, 1990). Many times the cause of failure is attributed to a non passive framework, which leads to implant overload (Adell et al., 1981; Carlson B, Carlsson, 1994; Patterson et al., 1995; Sahin & Cehreli, 2001; Zarb & Schimitt, 1990; Zitzmann & Marinello, 2002).

Framework passivity has become a concern in implant prosthodontics and all efforts have been made to pursue it. Restorative dentists have the task of obtaining a passive fit without any accepted clinical parameters for horizontal, vertical, or angular discrepancies. Thus, the goal is to create a fit as accurate as it is clinically possible to avoid strains in the components. Therefore, the way passivity of fit is understood leads to the belief that no stresses or strains must exist at all. But that may not be true, since when torque is applied to bring the joints together a tensile force appears on the screw, which is then elongated. This leads to the development of a compressive axial force between the cylinder and abutment, which maintains the union between the components (Isa & Hobkirk, 1995; Duyck & Naert 2002; Geng et al., 2001).

Compressive forces deform the components to a measurable level. If the compressive force is homogeneous along the periphery of the abutment-cylinder interface or, in other words, if the cylinder fits properly to the abutment, deformation of the abutment should also be homogeneous and measurable. Usually, machined components are preferred to cast ones because casting may produce a rough surface, making it even more difficult to achieve a proper fit. Machined cylinders need to be overcast to create multiple element frameworks, which is another complicating factor in itself.

Hitherto, no method has been described to establish a reliable parameter for passive fit. Photoelasticity, finite element analysis, and strain gauge measurements have been proposed as tools to determine stresses/strains in implant prostheses. With the purpose of determining a measurable parameter to what constitutes a passive fit framework, a study (Moretti-Neto et al., 2009) was conducted aiming at the evaluation of the deformation to which abutments are submitted when free-standing cylinders are screwed onto them. Strain gauges were used to define the mean level of abutment deformation that can be expected with no interference of factors, such as laboratory procedures, in passive fit. The magnitude of the values found was minimal. The highest mean value of deformation was -625.35 με for abutment screw tightening. Conversion to the percentage of deformation yields the value of 0.062% deformation. It should also be observed that low levels of abutment deformation do not necessarily represent a desirable condition. In fact, deformation levels close to 0 may indicate that the components are completely apart and consequently, not transmitting any force to one another. In this instance, the prosthetic screw and the framework would be overloaded, and the framework adaptation would be forced by the torque applied to the screws (Duyck et al., 2001).

The results of this study corroborate the findings of Isa & Hobkirk (1995) who demonstrated that screw tightening generated compression and tension stresses on the abutments, even when using a framework with a misfit as small as 10 μm. Considering a system formed by a screwed joint, only compression forces should affect the abutments in an ideal condition of passive fit. However, tension forces were observed on the machined cylinders. These results may have occurred because the prosthesis does not establish a homogeneous and uniform contact with the surfaces of the abutments and may have presented adequate fit only at one side (Duyck et al., 2001; Clelland et al., 1993).

Horizontal and angular internal misfits, whose detection is difficult, may also contribute to the instability of the screws and generate tension forces on the implant components (Sahin & Cehreli, 2001; Millington & Leung, 1995; Helldén & Dérand, 1998; Tan et al., 1993). Such distortions, which are difficult to detect, may be responsible for the variability of the results observed in this and other studies. The method employed for evaluating passive fit of prosthetic cylinders to the abutments as a function of abutment deformation could be regarded as useful, since it revealed that despite the small magnitude of the outcomes, some amount of deformation is always present and is measurable, varying from 173.29 με (Pd-Ag machined cylinders) to 200.47 με (Co-Cr cast cylinders).

There is still a difficulty to overcome to apply these parameters to the clinical situation: It is technically difficult to connect strain gauges to patients' mouths to take measurements, which would give more reliable results. Therefore, the proposed method must be regarded as a source of information for what can be expected in an ideal condition. Variations on the amount of abutment deformation and the presence of tension forces should be related to poor quality fit of frameworks.

The clinical relevance of this study relies on the importance of understanding the mechanisms of force transmission from the framework/prosthetic cylinders to the

abutments, from these to the implants, and consequently, to the surrounding bone. In this study, the abutments were rigidly fixed to a metallic master cast simulating the bone. Since bone is the living tissue that ultimately responds to the stresses in the system, a model that takes into account the mechanical properties of bone needs to be developed to quantify bone stress after implant prosthesis connection.
Therefore, studies have been conducted on simulated bone models. Polyurethane was found to present elastic modulus similar to human bone (Miyashiro et al., 2011; Moretti-Neto et al., 2011) and was chosen to verify the tension levels that are developed around implants during function (Figure 8) When prosthetic restorations were connected to the abutments, the tension levels on the bone located at the cervical area of the implant were very low, around 58 με to 100 με for single crowns and reaching 350 με to 400 με for multiple element restorations. What can be regarded as relevant in these studies is that the tension levels fall within physiologic limits, as proposed by Frost's minimal effective strain theory, between 50-200 με to 1500-2500 με. Such tension levels would not be capable of causing bone resorption around implants (Rubo, 2010).

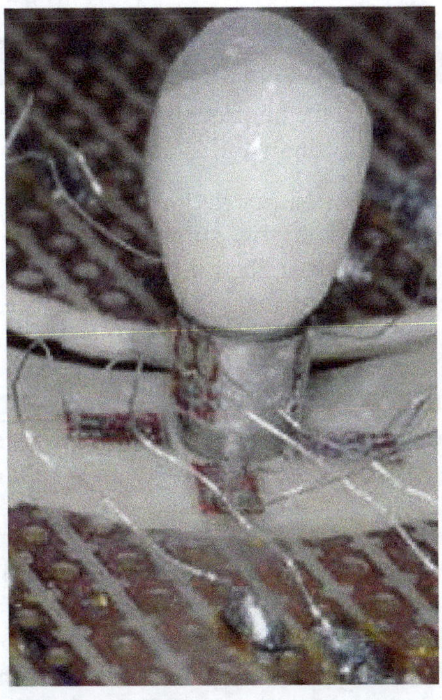

Fig. 8. A bone simulated model was used to quantify the tension around the cervical area of the implant when the restoration is connected.

The influence of cantilever length, abutment's height and framework alloy was also studied by means of strain gauge analysis (Jacques et al., 2009; Suedam et al., 2009) (Figure 9). Frameworks for implant-supported prostheses have been evolved from soldering a gold alloy framework to gold cylinders, to gold alloy frameworks cast directly onto the cylinders, to Ag-Pd alloy frameworks (Cox & Zarb, 1985; Jemt, 1991). The clinical results showed that the latter option gives consistently good results with respect to accuracy of fit, load bearing capacity, reduced cost and design versatility (Rangert et al., 1989). However, the use of an alloy with higher modulus of elasticity, such as Co-Cr, would allow for a more evenly distributed load among implants with a less bulky framework, which would be an advantage if intraoral space is limited (Hulterstrom & Nilsson, 1994; Chao et al., 1988). For these reasons, the Ag-Pd alloy framework was chosen for comparison purposes.

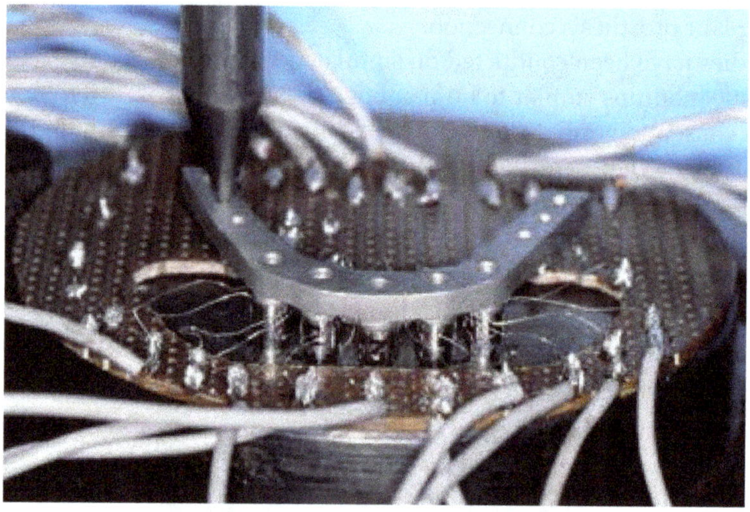

Fig. 9. A framework was screwed to the abutments with strain gages on the proximal aspects; 100N load applied at 5mm, 10mm and 20mm distal to terminal implant.

Cantilevered ends of fixed implant-supported prostheses increase the load on the first implant nearest the cantilever arm. In this study it could be noticed that the abutment closest to the point of load application on the cantilever extension registered deformation by compression, but higher levels of deformation by tension were observed in intermediary abutments. These results are according to data from other experiments (Benzing et al., 1995; Chao et al., 1988; Rubo & Souza, 2008; Skalak 1983; Suedam et al., 2009) reporting that in cantilevered prostheses, the most distal implants represent the fulcrum and, therefore, are subjected to compression forces while intermediary abutments suffer tension. For the alloy with lower elastic modulus, as the distance between the point of load application and the distal abutment increases, energy is consumed in framework deflection and low deformation levels are observed in abutments.

The results of this study showed that the pattern of deformation generated by the application of the static force varied according to the position of the strain gauges in the abutment's aspects, according to the implant position relative to the load application, to the abutment's height and also to the type of alloy used for the framework. The increase of the abutment's height promoted an increase of the deformation by compression in the strain gauges located in the abutment adjacent to the cantilever. This could be explained by the increase of the lever arm that takes place with the increase of the abutment's height leading to the deformation in the abutment adjacent to the point of load application.

The strains generated in the abutments did not present a uniform pattern among the abutment's aspects and not even in different abutments. However, deformations by compression are present in a larger intensity in the strain gauges located in abutment no. 1 closest to the point of load application in all specimens, evidencing that the abutment's proximity to the load influences the results. This brings about the importance of evaluating the implant adjacent to the lever arm, concerning its bony support, for planning the extension of the cantilever.

In Figs 10 and 11, a tendency line was added to help visualize the effect of the difference in elastic modulus of the alloy in the pattern of deformation of the framework. It clearly shows that the stiffer CoCr alloy framework is less affected by the load, resulting in compression on both ends and tension in the middle. On the other hand, the PdAg alloy framework showed a tendency to a more complex deformation pattern, resultant of its lower elastic modulus compared with the CoCr alloy framework.

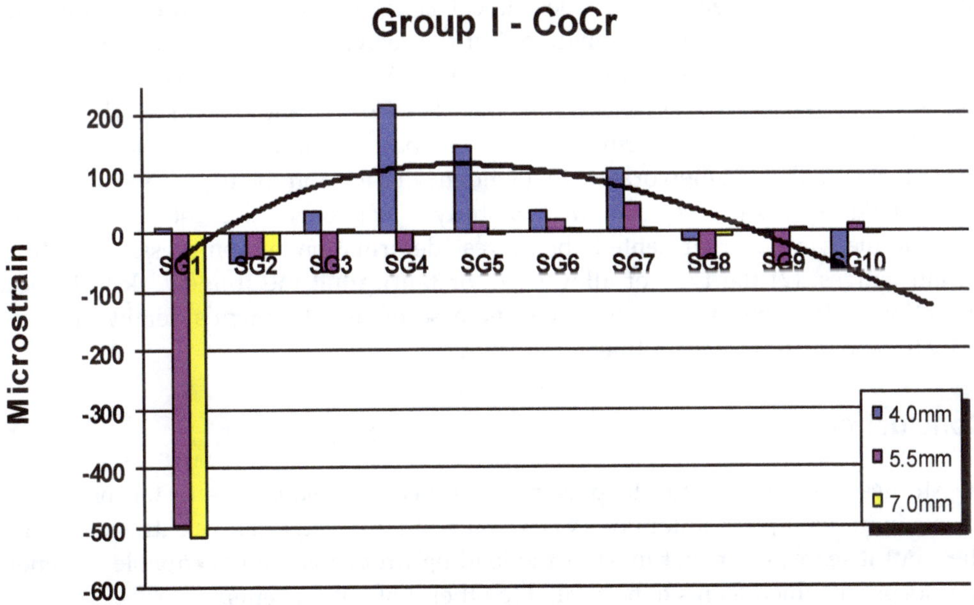

Fig. 10. Graphic of the deformation means captured by the abutment's strain gauges for CoCr frameworks.

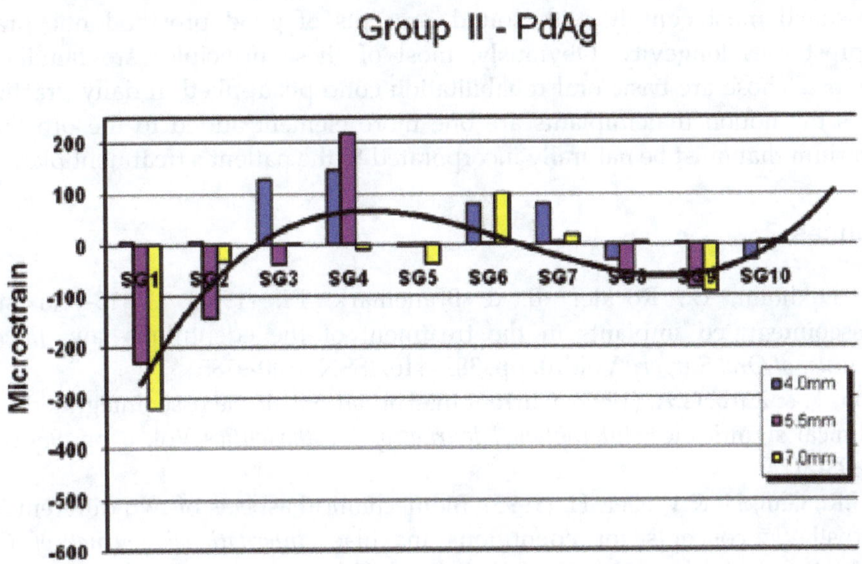

Fig. 11. Graphic of the deformation means captured by the abutment's strain gauges for PdAg frameworks.

On the other hand, the alloy with high modulus of elasticity undergoes few or no deflection with the increase of the cantilever, resulting in more abutment deformation. In both situations, the screws can be overloaded what underscores the need to keep a reduced cantilever arm, as this has been demonstrated to be the major cause of mechanical problems (Shackleton, 1992). The results observed with both alloys are inconclusive as to what material performs better.

Clearly, there is a difference in the mechanical behavior of the two frameworks and the resultant pattern of abutment deformation, but the relevance of this finding would only be determined by clinical comparative studies. (1) Abutment deformation was always higher with longer cantilever extensions; (2) The Co-Cr alloy framework resulted in higher levels of abutment deformation; (3) The pattern of abutment deformation was different for both alloy frameworks with a tendency to tension forces to appear closer to the load when Pd-Ag alloy was used. In this study it was concluded that (1) the abutment adjacent to the cantilever presented the largest deformation by compression captured by the strain gauges, (2) the type of alloy used for fabricating the framework influenced the deformation of the abutments and (3) the increase of the abutment's height increased the deformation on the terminal abutment.

4. Conclusion

Many studies have been made to present solutions or explanations to the biomechanical problems in implant prosthodontics. A large bulk of knowledge can be extracted from those studies, but it seams clear that most of the loading problems are not capable of generating bone resorption, which seems to be related to other biological events.

However, overload may be responsible for many events of screw loosening and fractures, resulting in the need for more frequent maintenance. Solving these problems may be time consuming and creates additional costs.

The professional must comply with sound concepts of good prosthodontic practice to improve prostheses longevity. Obviously, most of these principles are familiar to the prosthodontist. Those are basic oral rehabilitation concepts applied in daily practice, what underscores the notion that implants are one more element added to the prosthodontist armamentarium that must be naturally incorporated to the patient's treatment plan.

5. References

Adell, R., Lekholm, U., Rockler, B. & Brånemark, PI. (1981). A 15-year study of osseointegrated implants in the treatment of the edentulous jaw. *International Journal of Oral Surgery* Vol. 10, pp. 387–416, ISSN 0300-9785

Albrektsson, T. & Zarb, G.A. (1993). Current interpretations of the osseointegrated response: clinical significance. *International Journal of Prosthodontics* Vol. 6 pp. 95–105, ISSN 0893-2174

Benzing, U.R., Gall, H. & Weber, H. (1995). Biomechanical aspects of two different implant-prosthetic concepts for edentulous maxillae. *International Journal of Oral and Maxillofacial Implants* Vol. 10 pp. 188–198, ISSN 0882-2786

Bidez, M.W. & Misch, C.E. (1992). Force transfer in Implant Dentistry: basic concepts and principles. *Journal of Oral Implantology* Vol. 18 pp. 264–274, ISSN 0160-6972

Brunski, J.B. (1988). Biomaterial and biomechanics in dental implant design. *International Journal of Oral and Maxillofacial Implants* Vol. pp. 3:85–97, ISSN 0882-2786

Brunski, J.B. (1992). Biomechanical factors affecting the bone-dental implant interface. *Clinical Materials* Vol. 10 pp. 153–201, ISSN 0267-6605

Brunski, J.B. (1991). Influence of biomechanical factors at the bone-biomaterial interface, In: *The Bone Biomaterial Interface*, 1st ed., Davies, J.E. pp. 391-404, University of Toronto Press, ISBN 10 0802059414, Toronto.

Carlson, B. & Carlsson, G.E. (1994). Prosthodontic complications in osseointegrated dental implant treatment. *International Journal of Oral and Maxillofacial Implants* Vol. 9 pp. 90–94, ISSN 0882-2786

Carlsson, G.E. (2009). Critical review of some dogmas in prosthodontics. *Journal of Prosthodontic Research* Vol. 53 pp. 3-10.

Chamay, A. & Tschantz, P. (1972). Mechanical influences in bone remodelling. Experimental research on Wolff`s Law. *Journal of Biomechanics* Vol. 5 pp. 173-180, ISSN 0021-9290

Chao, Y., Davis, D.M., Zarb, G.A. & Judes, H. (1988). A study into the use of chromium-cobalt alloy for constructing the framework for osseointegrated prostheses. *Clinical Materials* Vol. 3 pp. 309–315, ISSN 0267-6605

Clelland, N.L., Gilat, A., McGlumphy, E.A. & Brantley, W.A. (1993). A photoelastic and strain gauge analysis of angled abutments for an implant system. *International Journal of Oral and Maxillofacial Implants* Vol. 8 pp. 541–548, ISSN 0882-2786

Clelland, N.L., Ismail, Y.H., Zaki, H.S. & Pipko, D. (1991). Three-dimensional finite element stress analysis in and around the Screw-Vent implant. *International Journal of Oral and Maxillofacial Implants* Vol. 6 pp. 391–398, ISSN 0882-2786

Cox, J. & Zarb, G.A. (1985). Alternative prosthodontic superstructure designs. *Swedish Dental Journal* Vol. 28 (Suppl.) pp. 71–75, ISSN 0348-6672

Duncan, R.L. & Turner, C.H. (1995). Mechanotransduction and the functional response of bone to mechanical strain. *Calcified Tissue International* Vol. 57 pp. 344-358, ISSN 0171-967X

Duyck, J. & Naert, I. (2002). Influence of prosthesis fit and effect of a luting system on the prosthetic connection preload: an in vitro study. *International Journal of Prosthodontics* Vol. 15 pp. 389–396, ISSN 0893-2174

Duyck, J., Van Oosterwyck, H., Vander Sloten, J., De Cooman, M., Puers, R. & Naert, I. (2001). Pre-load on oral implants after screw tightening fixed full prostheses: An in vivo study. *Journal of Oral Rehabilitation* Vol. 28 pp. 226–233, ISSN 0305-182X

Frost, H.M. (1994). Wolff's law and bone's structural adaptations to mechanical usage: an overview for clinicians. *Angle Orthodontics* Vol. 64 pp. 175-188, ISSN 0003-3219

Geng, J.P., Tan, K.B. & Liu, G.R. (2001). Application of finite element analysis in Implant Dentistry: A review of the literature. *Journal of Prosthetic Dentistry* Vol. 85 pp. 585–598, ISSN 0022-3913

Helldén, L.B & Dérand, T. (1998). Description and evaluation of a simplified method to achieve passive fit between cast titanium frameworks and implants. *International Journal of Oral and Maxillofacial Implants* Vol. 13 pp. 190–196, ISSN 0882-2786

Hulterstrom, M. & Nilsson, U. (1994). Cobalt- chromium as a framework material in implantsupported fixed prostheses: a 3-year follow-up. *International Journal of Oral and Maxillofacial Implants* Vol. 9 pp. 449–454, ISSN 0882-2786

Isa, Z.M. & Hobkirk, J.A. (1995). The effects of superstructure fit and loading on individual implant units: Part I. The effects of tightening the gold screws and placement of a superstructure with varying degrees of fit. *European Journal of Prosthodontics and Restorative Dentistry* Vol. 3 pp. 247–253, ISSN 0965-7452

Isidor, F. (2006). Influence of forces on peri-implant bone. *Clinical Oral Implants Research* Vol. 17 pp. 8–18, ISSN 0905-7161

Jacques, L.B., Moura, M.S., Suedam. V., Souza, E.A.C. & Rubo, J.H. (2009). Effect of cantilever length and framework alloy on the stress distribution of mandibular-cantilevered implant-supported prostheses. *Clinical Oral Implants Research* Vol. 20 pp. 737–741, ISSN 0905-7161

Jemt, T. (1991). Failures and complications in 391 consecutively inserted fixed prostheses supported by Brånemark implants in edentulous jaws: A study of treatment from the time of prosthesis placement to the first annual check up. *International Journal of Oral and Maxillofacial Implants* Vol. 6 pp. 270–276, ISSN 0882-2786

Kallus, T. & Bessing, C. 1994). Loose gold screws frequently occur in full arch fixed prostheses supported by osseointegrated implants after 5 years. *International Journal of Oral and Maxillofacial Implants* Vol. 9 pp. 169–178, ISSN 0882-2786

Kim, Y., Oh, T.J., Misch, C.E. & Wang, H.L. (2005). Occlusal considerations in implant therapy: clinical guidelines with biomechanical rationale. *Clinical Oral Implants Research* Vol. 16 pp. 26–35, ISSN 0905-7161

Kunavisarut, C., Lang, L.A., Stoner, B.R. & Felton D.A. (2002). Finite element analysis on dental implant-supported prostheses without passive fit. *Journal of Prosthodontics* Vol. 11 pp. 30–40, ISSN 1059-941X

Meijer, H.J.A., Starmans, F.J.M., Bosman, F. & Steen, W.H.A. (1993). A comparison of finite element models of an edentulous mandible provided with implants. *Journal of Oral Rehabilitation* Vol. 20 pp. 147–157, ISSN 0305-182X

Millington, N.D. & Leung, T. (1995). Inaccurate fit of implant superstructures. Part 1: Stresses generated on the superstructure relative to the size of fit discrepancy. *International Journal of Prosthodontics* Vol. 8 pp. 511–516, ISSN 0893-2174

Miyashiro, M., Suedam, V., Moretti-Neto, R.T., Ferreira, P.M. & Rubo, J.H. (2011). Validation of an experimental polyurethane model for biomechanical studies on implant-supported prosthesis - tension tests. *Journal of Applied Oral Science* Vol. 19 No. 3 pp. 134-138, ISSN 1678-7765

Moretti-Neto, R.T., Hiramatsu, D.A., Suedam, V., Conti, P.C.R. & Rubo, J.H. (2011). Validation of an experimental polyurethane model for biomechanical studies on implant-supported prosthesis - compression tests. *Journal of Applied Oral Science* Vol. 19 No. 1 pp. 47-51, ISSN 1678-7765

Moretti-Neto, R.T., Moura, M.S., Souza, E.A.C. & Rubo, J.H. (2009). Implant abutment deformation during prosthetic cylinder screw tightening: an in vitro study. *International Journal of Prosthodontics* Vol. 22 pp. 391-395, ISSN 0893-2174

Murphy, W.M., Williams, K.R. & Gregory, M.C. (1995). Stress in bone adjacent to dental implants. *Journal of Oral Rehabilitation.* Vol. 22 pp. 897–903, ISSN 0305-182X

Oh, T.J., Yoon, J., Mish, C.E. & Wang, H.L. (2002). The causes of early implant bone loss: myth or science? *Journal of Periodontology* Vol. 3 pp. 322-33, ISSN 0022-3492

Patterson, E.A., Burguete, R.L., Thoi, M.H. & Johns, R.B. (1995). Distribution of load in an oral prosthesis system: An in vitro study. *International Journal of Oral and*

Maxillofacial Implants Vol. 10 pp. 552–560, ISSN 0882-2786

Pierrisnard, L., Renouard, F., Renault, P. & Barquins, M. (2003). Influence of implant length and bicortical anchorage on stress distribution. *Clinical Implant Dentistry and Related Research* Vol. 5 pp. 254–262, ISSN 1523-0899

Rangert, D.F., Jemt, T. & Jorneus, L. (1989). Forces and moments on Branemark implants. *International Journal of Oral and Maxillofacial Implants* Vol. 4 No.3 pp. 241–247, ISSN 0882-2786

Rangert, B., Jemt, T. & Jorneus, L. (1989). Forces and moments on Branemark implants. *International Journal of Oral and Maxillofacial Implants* Vol. 4 pp. 241–247, ISSN 0882-2786

Rieger, M.R., Mayberry, M. & Brose, M.O. (1990). Finite element analysis of six endosseous implants. *Journal of Prosthetic Dentistry* Vol. 63 pp. 671-676, ISSN 0022-3913

Rubo, J.H. & Souza, E.A.C. (2008). Finite element analysis of stress in bone around dental implants. *Journal of Oral Implantology* Vol. 9 pp. 407- 418, ISSN 0160-6972

Rubo, J.H. & Souza, E.A.C. (2010). Finite element analysis of stress on dental implant prosthesis. *Clinical Implant Dentistry and Related Research* Vol. 12 pp. 105-113, ISSN 1523-0899

Rubo, J.H. (2010). Biomechanical studies in implant prosthodontics. *Implantnews* Vol. 7 pp. 139-44, ISSN 1678-6661

Sahin, S., Çehreli, M.C. & Yalçin, E. (2002). The influence of functional forces on the biomechanics of implant-supported prostheses - a review. *Journal of Dentistry* Vol. 30 pp. 271–282, ISSN 0300-5712

Sahin, .S & Çehreli, M.C. (2001). The significance of passive framework fit in implant prosthodontics: Current status. *Implant Dentistry* Vol. 10 pp. 85–90, ISSN 1056-6163

Sertgoz, A. & Guvener, S. (1996). Finite element analysis of the effect of cantilever and implant length on stress distribution in an implant-supported fixed prosthesis. *Journal of Prosthetic Dentistry* Vol. 76 pp. 165- 169, ISSN 0022-3913

Shackleton, J., Carr, L., Slabbert, J.C.G., Lownie, J.F. & Becker, P.J. (1992). Prosthodontic complications and problems of fixture-supported prostheses. *Journal of Dental Research* Vol. 71 No. 4 pp. 1113, ISSN 0022-0345

Skalak, R. (1985). Aspects of biomechanical considerations. In: *Tissue integrated prostheses – Osseointegration in clinical dentistry*, 1st ed. Branemark, P-I., Zarb, G.A. & Albrektsson, T. pp. 117-128 Quintessence, ISBN 0-86715-123-3, Chicago, IL.

Skalak, R. (1983). Biomechanical considerations in osseointegrated prostheses. *Journal of Prosthetic Dentistry*, Vol. 49, No. 6 pp. 843-848, ISSN 0022-3913

Suedam, V., Capello Souza, E.A., Moura, M.S., Jacques, L.B. & Rubo, J.H. (2009). Effect of abutment's height and framework alloy on the load distribution of mandibular cantilevered implantsupported prosthesis. *Clinical Oral Implants Research* Vol. 20 pp. 196–200, ISSN 0905-7161

Tan, K.B., Rubenstein, J.E., Nicholls, J.I. & Yuodelis, R.A. (1993). Three-dimensional analysis of the casting accuracy of one-piece, osseointegrated implant-retained prostheses. *International Journal of Prosthodontics* Vol. 6 pp. 346–363, ISSN 0893-2174

van Oosterwick, H., Duyck, J., Vander Sloten, J., Van der Perre, G., De Cooman, M., Lievens, S., et al. (1998). The influence of bone mechanical properties and implant fixation upon bone loading around oral implants. *Clinical Oral Implants Research* Vol. 9 pp. 407–418, ISSN 0905-7161

Weinberg, L.A., Kruger, B. (1995). A comparison of implant/prosthesis loading with four clinical variables. *International Journal of Prosthodontics* Vol. 8 pp. 421–433, ISSN 0893-2174

Wiskott, H.W.A. & Belser, U.C. (1999). Lack of integration of smooth titanium surfaces: a working hypothesis based on strains generated in the surrounding bone. *Clinical Oral Implants Research* Vol. 10 pp. 429–444, ISSN 0905-7161

Worthington, P., Bolender, C.L. & Taylor, T.D. (1987). The Swedish system of osseointegrated implants: Problems and complications encountered during a 4-year trial period. *International Journal of Oral and Maxillofacial Implants* Vol. 2 pp. 77–84, ISSN 0882-2786

Zarb, G.A. & Schimitt, A. (1990). The longitudinal clinical effectiveness of osseointegrated dental implants: The Toronto study. Part II: The prosthetic results. *Journal of Prosthetic Dentistry* Vol. 64 pp. 53–61, ISSN 0022-3913

Zitzmann, N.U. & Marinello, C.P. (2002). A review of clinical and technical considerations for fixed and removable implant prostheses in edentulous mandible. *International Journal of Prosthodontics* Vol. 15 pp. 65–72, ISSN 0893-2174

11

New Bone Formation in the Maxillary Sinus with/without Bone Graft

Dong-Seok Sohn
Catholic University of Daegu
Daegu
Republic of Korea

1. Introduction

Pneumatization of maxillary sinus causes insufficient vertical bone volume on posterior maxilla. So the restoration of edentulous posterior maxilla with dental implants is challenging due to a deficient posterior alveolar ridge, unfavorable bone quality and increased pneumatization of the maxillary sinus.[1] For maxillary sinus augmentation, the crestal approach and the lateral window approach have been used. In this chapter, sinus augmentation using crestal and lateral window approach with/without bone graft is described.

2. Indications and contraindications for sinus augmentation

Even sinus augmentation procedure is considered as highly predictable augmentation procedure, presurical evaluation on maxillary sinus and patient's medical and dental history should carefully be evaluated.

The following are indications for sinus augmentation.

- No history of sinus pathosis
- Insufficient residual bone height (less than 10mm of bone height)
- Severely atrophic maxilla
- Poor bone quality and quantity in the posterior maxilla

Sinus augmentation is not indicated when patient has history as below

- Recent radiation therapy in maxilla
- Uncontrolled systemic diseases such as Diabetes Mellitus
- Acute / chronic maxillary sinusitis (Fig. 1)
- Heavy smoker
- Alcohol abuse
- Psychosis
- Severe allergic rhinitis
- Tumor or large cyst in the maxillary sinus (Fig. 2)
- Oroantral fistula (Fig. 3)

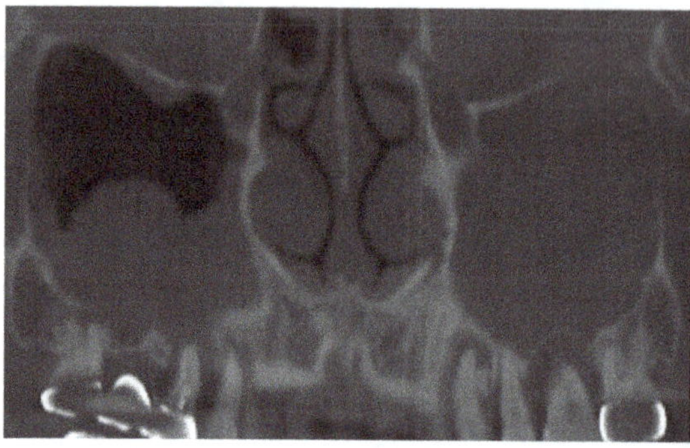
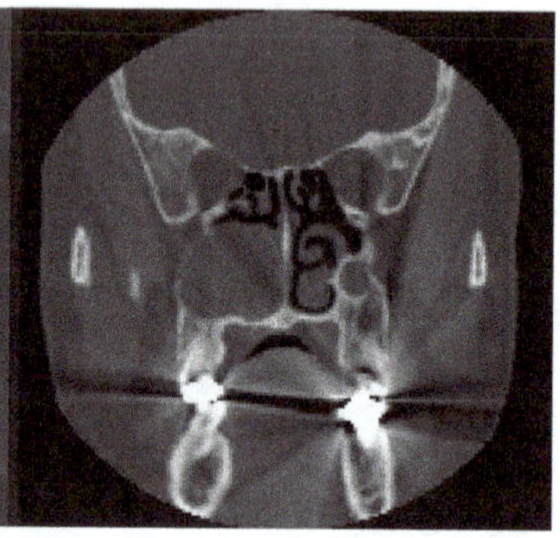

Fig. 1. (Left) demonstrates odontogenic sinusitis in the both sinus. Fig. 2. (right) shows mucocele in the right sinus. Sinus pathosis should be eliminated before sinus augmentation.

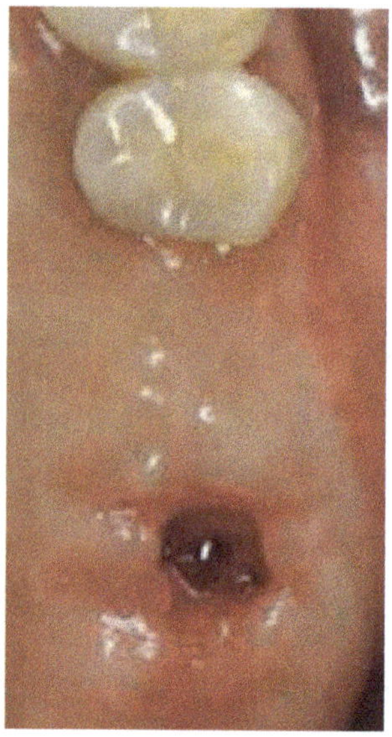

Fig. 3. Oroantral fistula should be corrected before sinus augmentation.

3. Sinus augmentation using crestal approach

Sinus augmentation using the lateral window procedure has been predictable for several decades. However, this procedure has some complications such as postoperative swelling, pain, and a long edentulous healing period. To reduce the complications from the lateral window approach in maxillary sinus augmentation, various crestal approaches such as osteotome mediated sinus floor elevation (OMSFE)[2], piezoelectric internal sinus elevation (PISE)[3-5], hydraulic sinus condensing (HSC) technique[6], internal sinus manipulation (ISM) procedure method[7], and crestal window technique (CWT)[8] and hydrodynamic piezoelectric internal sinus elevation (HPISE)[9-10] have been introduced as alternative to lateral window approach for sinus augmentation.

3.1 Osteotome Mediated Sinus Floor Elevation (OMSFE)

OMSFE technique utilizes osteotome and a surgical mallet to break sinus floor and to compact bone graft into the sinus cavity.

Surgical procedure of OMSFE (Fig. 4-16)

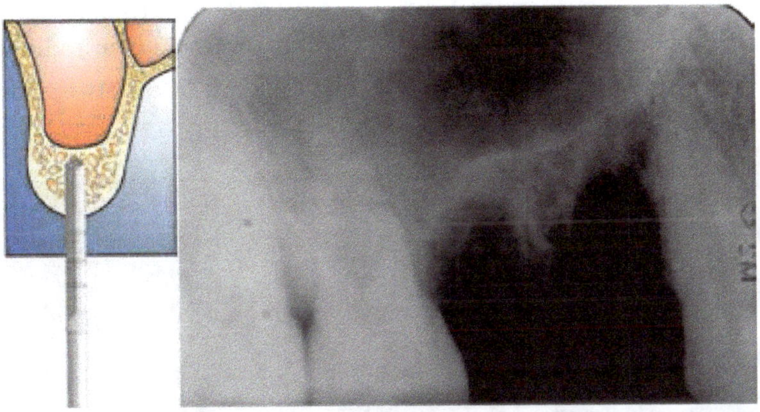

Fig. 4. and 5. A pilot drill is usually used to the depth 1-2mm short to the sinus floor to accommodate osteotome to sinus floor. However as shown on fig 5 , pilot drill is omitted when bone height is less than 2mm from sinus floor at the implant sites

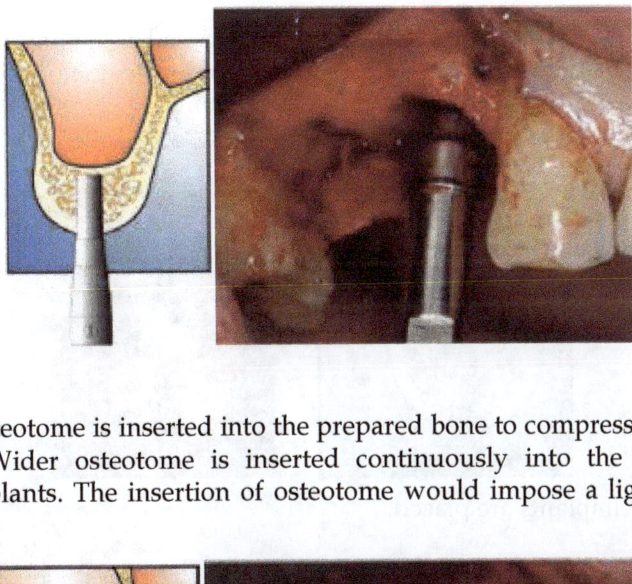

Fig. 6. and 7.

Small diameter osteotome is inserted into the prepared bone to compress sinus floor using a surgical mallet. Wider osteotome is inserted continuously into the prepared bone to accommodate implants. The insertion of osteotome would impose a light pressure on the sinus floor.

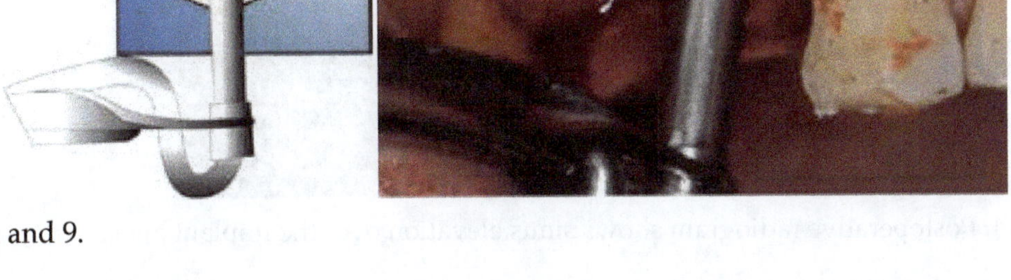

Fig. 8. and 9.

In order to elevate the sinus floor indirectly and provide buffering effect to sinus floor, bone graft material is added using an amalgam carrier. For the graft material, the radiopaque bone grafts, such as mineral allograft or xenograft, are preferred over radiolucent materials such as demineralized allograft.

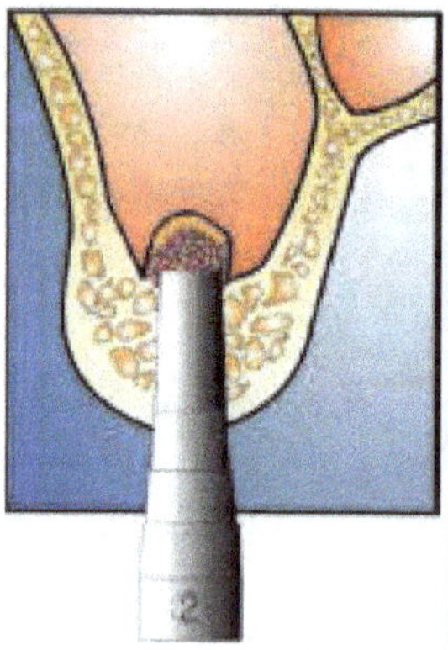
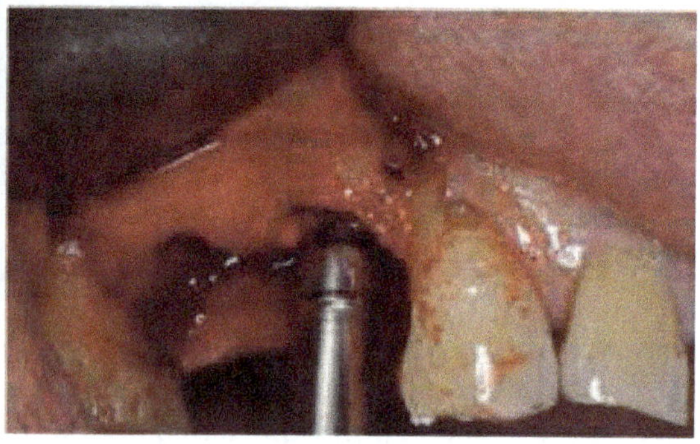

Fig. 10. and 11.

The sinus floor is elevated by repeated bone grafting and osteotome insertion. For sinus floor elevation of 3~4mm, 4~6 times of grafting and osteotome insertion and for the elevation of 5~7mm, 7~10 times of the repetition is required.

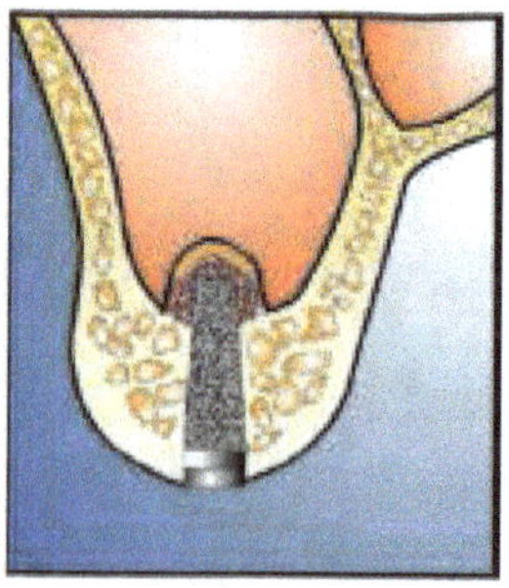
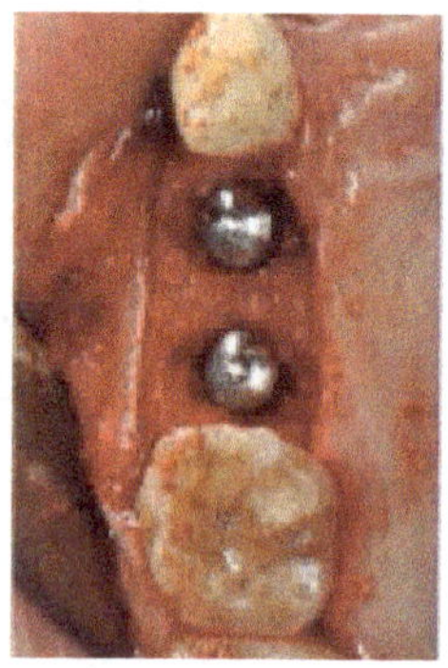

Fig. 12. and 13. The implants are placed.

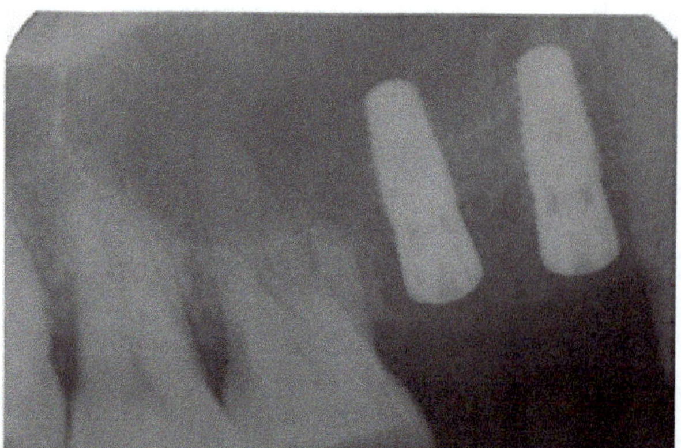

Fig. 14. Postoperative radiogram shows sinus elevation over the implant apex.

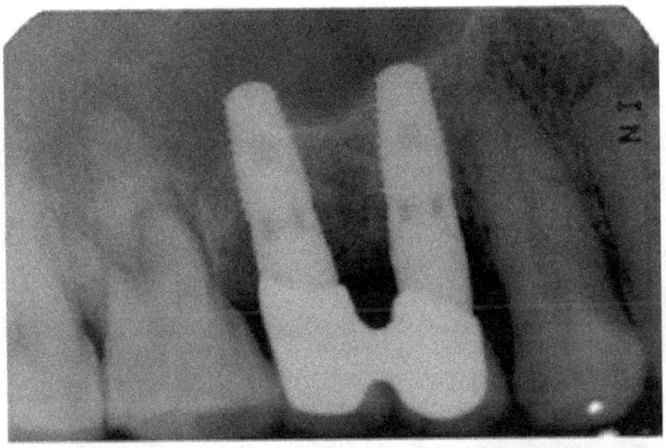

Fig. 15. Final prosthesis was cemented after 6 months healing. New sinus floor is seen in the radiogram.

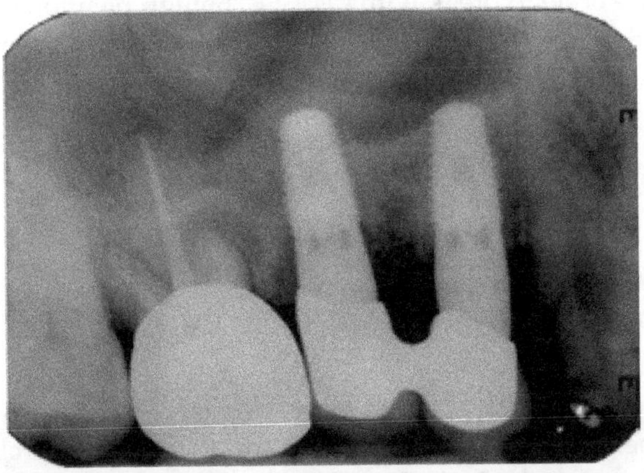

Fig. 16. 2 years after loading. Note newly formed sinus floor.

OMSFE has the advantage of surgical simplicity, resulting in minimal post-operative symptoms. But this technique also has the possibility of complications such as perforation of sinus membrane during bone drilling and bone compaction using osteotome. In addition, benign positional paroxysmal vertigo (BPPV) can be caused by the damage to the internal ear from striking osteotome and surgical mallet when sinus floor is broken.[11-13] It is difficult to break sinus floor in the area of slope of the sinus and in the site of septum with conventional crestal approach, and it could be time consuming and traumatic procedure to the internal ear (Fig 17 and Fig 18). Author experienced one case of BPPV caused from excessive striking of mallet in the anterior slope of sinus cavity in 2000. BPPV is not a common complication but surgeons should avoid excessive force to the surgical mallet when sinus floor is broken. In addition, OMSFE is a blind technique, so sinus augmentation is limited. The OMSFE technique has lower success rates when residual bone height is 4mm or less (when compared to cases with 5mm or more residual bone height).[14]

Sinus membrane integrity should be maintained when performing OMSFE because the membrane perforation causes cessation of sinus floor elevation. It is recommended that drilling should be stopped 1-2mm short to sinus floor in conventional OMSFE but this is not always easy because of magnification of plain radiogram.[6] Accidental sinus membrane perforation can be developed from improper drilling due to magnification of radiogram, improper use of osteotome and excessive compaction of bone graft. Membrane perforation can cause the failure of osseointegration and sinus pathosis. (Fig 19 and Fig 20)

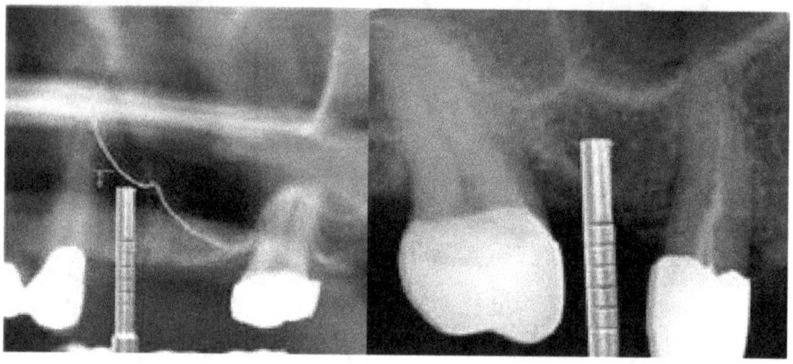

Fig. 17. and 18. Sinus elevation can be difficult at the anterior slope of sinus cavity due to too much remained bone height after initial osteotomy using pilot drill and at the sinus septum because it is very dense bone to break with OMSFE. Benign positional paroxysmal vertigo can be caused by the damage from the internal ear from striking osteotome and surgical mallet to sinus floor at these sites.

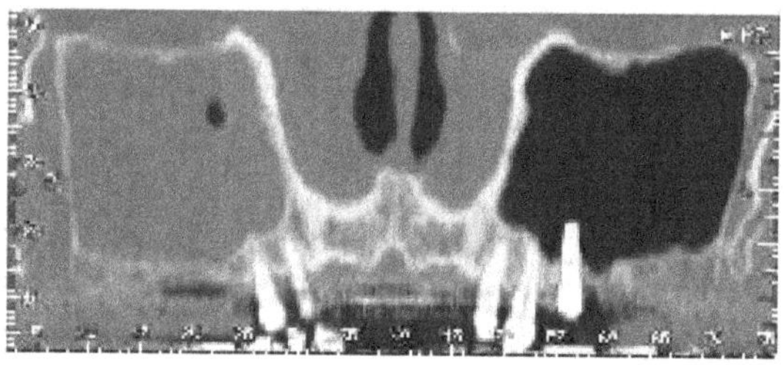

Fig. 19. OMSFE was performed at the site of # 26 and # 27 at private clinic. However membrane was perforated at the both sites. Two implants were placed at the same time. After 6 months healing, # 27 implant was removed because of mobility of implant during uncovering procedure and #26 implant showed the mobility too. The patient was referred to my department for the removal of implant and sinus graft. #26 implant was removed out, followed by sinus graft using lateral window approach. The integrity of sinus membrane should be maintained for successful sinus augmentation when performing OMSFE procedure. Note chronic sinusitis in the right sinus.

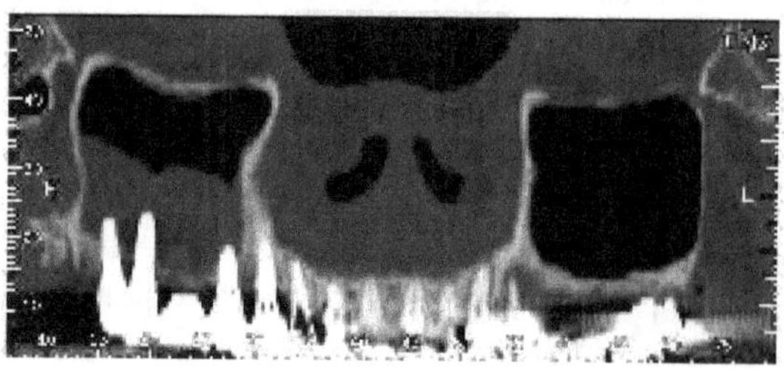

Fig. 20. OMSFE was performed at the both sinus by private clinician. Implants were placed at the same time. All implants placed in the left posterior maxilla were failed due to membrane perforation. She was referred to my department for sinus augmentation in the left sinus. Right sinus shows mucosal thickening due to intrusion of implant in to the sinus cavity. To maintain healthy sinus mucosa, the integrity of sinus membrane should be maintained.

3.2 Piezoelectric internal sinus elevation (PISE)

The PISE and HSC technique are innovative crestal methods which a surgical mallet is not required to break the sinus floor. PISE uses ultrasonic piezoelectric vibration and HSC technique uses high speed diamond bur to break sinus floor directly. These techniques are free from postoperative vertigo, but bone compaction is needed to elevate the sinus membrane. The CWT overcomes the blind nature of conventional OMSFE,[8] but the indication of this technique is limited because this technique is indicated when wide diameter implants (>5mm) are available.

Surgical procedure of PISE (Fig. 21- Fig. 33)

In PISE technique, PISE tip, connected with an ultrasonic piezoelectric device (Surgybone®, Silfradent srl, Sofia, Italy) is used to break the sinus floor. The working head of PISE tip (S028E® tip, Bukbu Dental Co, Daegu, Korea) is 2.8mm wide and 4mm high. A piezoelectric carbide-type tip is more powerful and effective for osteotomy than diamond coated tip. Thanks to selective cut of ultrasonic piezoelectric vibration, the perforation of sinus membrane is very rare when sinus floor is eroded. After braking sinus floor with piezoelectric tip directly, gel or putty conditioned bone graft was prepared to elevate sinus membrane with buffering function. To prepare gel or putty conditioned bone graft, author prefer to mix bovine bone powder (Bio-Cera™, Oscotec Co, Cheonan, Korea) and gel-onditioned allograft (OrthoBlast® II, Isotis Orthobiologics Inc, Irvine, USA). Bovine bone acts as radiopaque material and the gel conditioned allograft acts as buffer during membrane elevation.

The amalgam carrier is used when placing the graft into the narrow socket. A narrow diameter osteotome (usually 2mm in diameter) or PISE tip is inserted to compact the graft in the osteotomy site. After the membrane was elevated properly, the regular diameter implant is placed (3.7-4.0mm wide implant) without additional drilling procedure. To place wide body implant implant site should be widened with drill to accommodate the implant

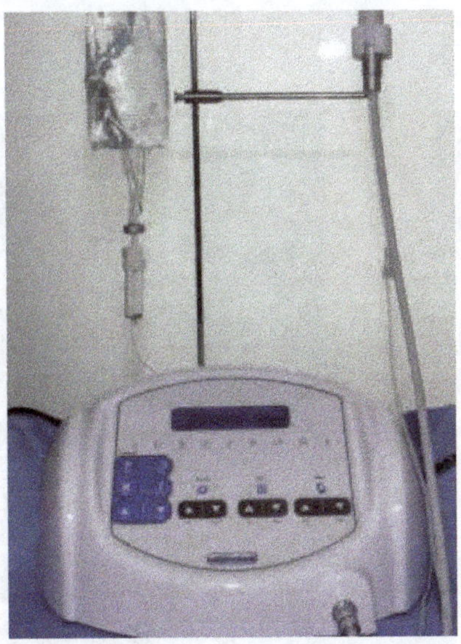

Fig. 21. Ultrasonic piezoelectrci device (Surgybone®, Silfradent srl, Sofia, Italy). This decice works in hard tissue, not in the soft tissue. Therefore membrane perforation is rare when breaking sinus floor.

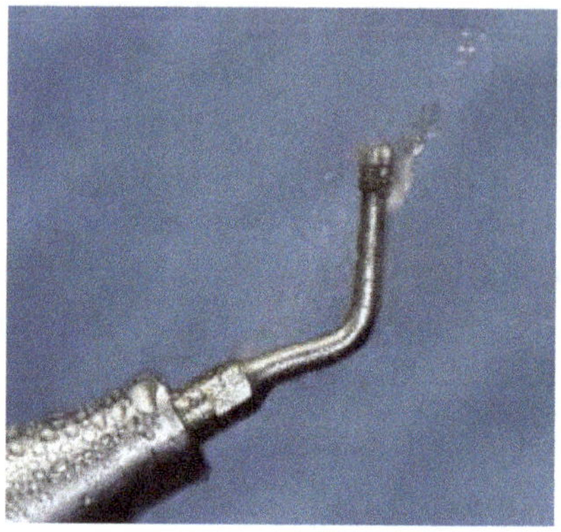

Fig. 22. Carbide type PISE tip (S028E) with external irrigation.

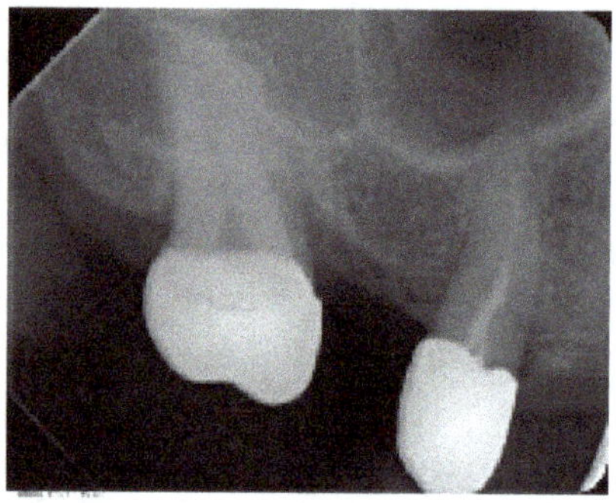

Fig. 23. A periapical radiogram shows high septum in the sinus. The bone around septum is dense, so the breaking of sinus floor using OMSFE technique is time consuming and could be traumatic to internal ear due to heavy striking of mallet. Therefore PISE is applied to break sinus floor directly.

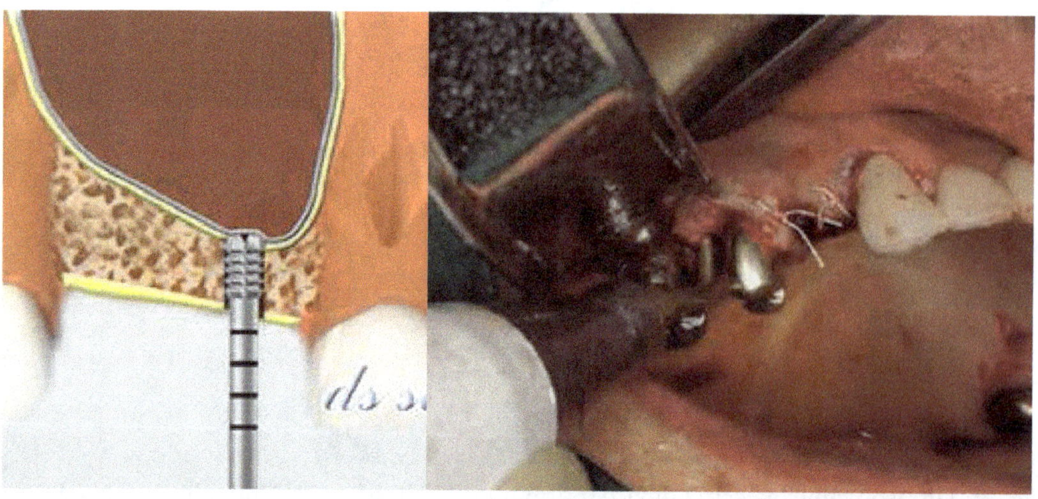

Fig. 24. (left) and Fig. 25. (right). Sinus floor is penetrated with PISE tip directly. A this stage, the exact bone height from alveolar crest to sinu floor is estimated.

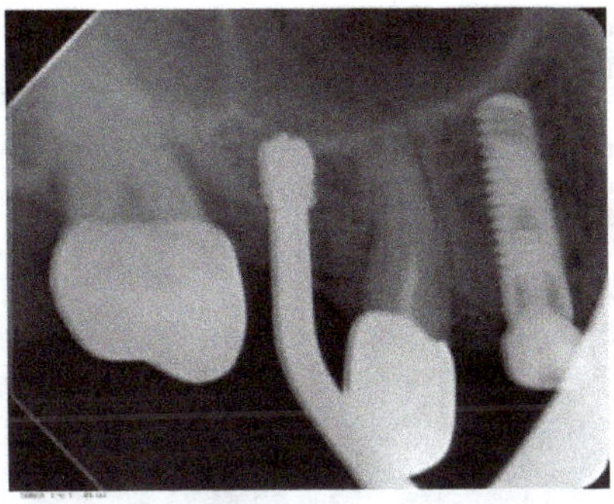

Fig. 26. The sinus floor is completely broken at the implant site by PISE tip. Note the broken sinus floor without membrane perforation.

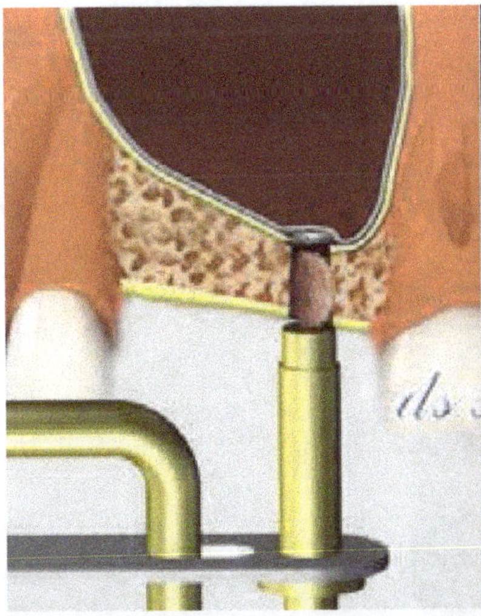

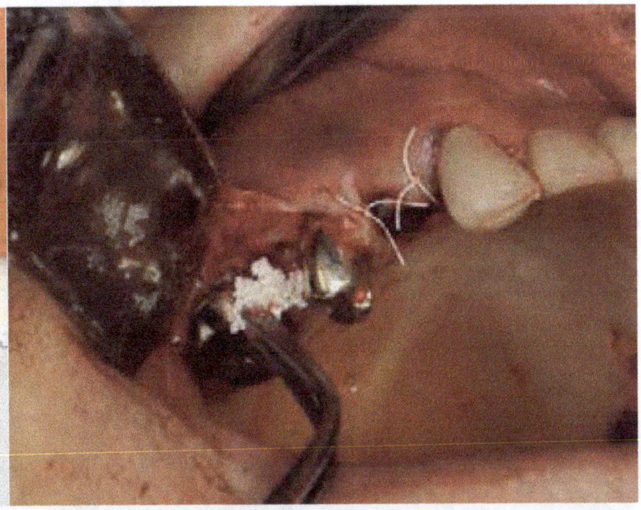

Fig. 27 (left) and Fig. 28. (right). Gel conditioned bone graft materials are carried into the osteotomy site.

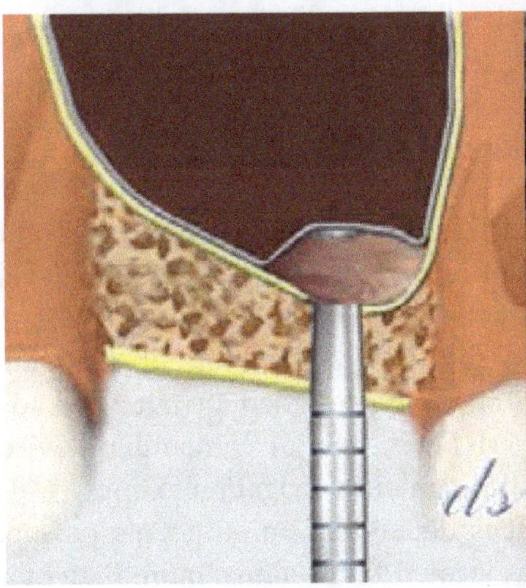

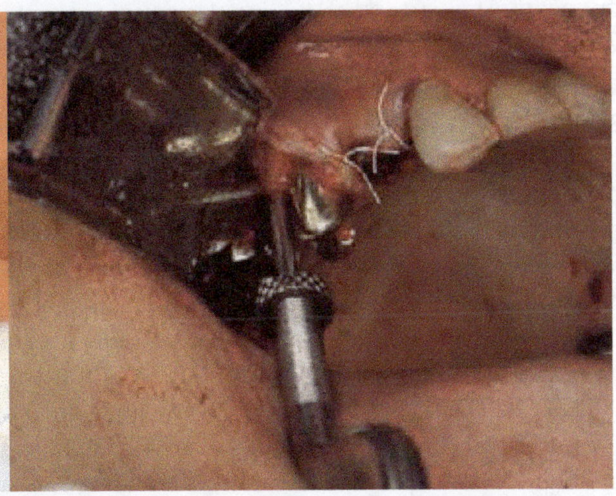

Fig. 26. (left) and Fig. 30. (right). Bone graft is compacted with the narrow osteotome or PISE tip using vibration to elevate sinus membrane.

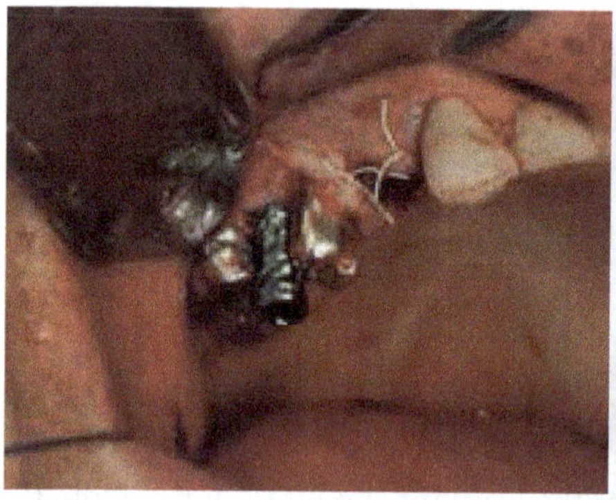

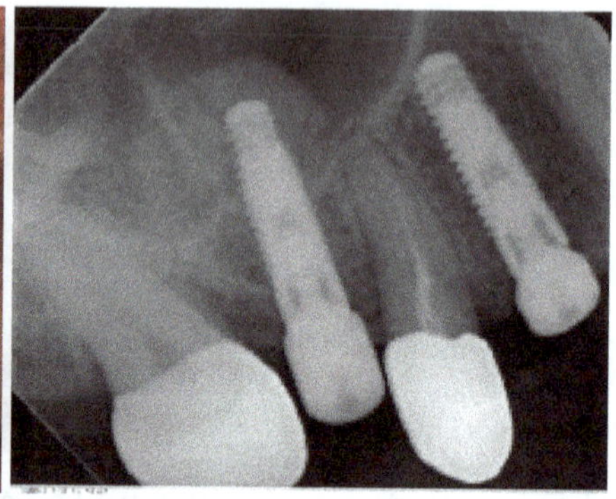

Fig. 31. (left) and Fig. 32. (right). A 3.7mm wide and 13mm high implant is placed without additional drilling procedure. Sinus elevation is seen at the radiogram.

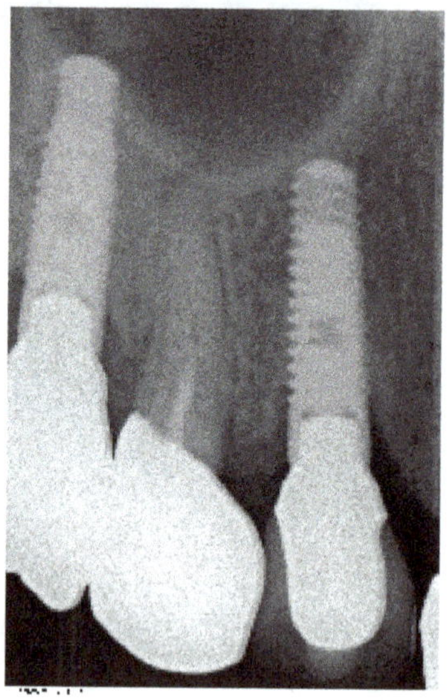

Fig. 33. Final prosthesis is cemented on after 6 months healing. A radiogram indicates sufficient augmentation of the sinus floor.

3.3 Hydrodynamic piezoelectric internal sinus elevation (HPISE)

HPISE is the updated crestal approach from PISE. This technique utilizes ultrasonic piezoelectric vibration to break sinus floor as same as PISE. However, unlike PISE and other conventional crestal approaches, HPISE usually doesn't rely on bone compaction to elevate sinus membrane. HPISE uses water pressure to elevate the sinus membrane. Hydraulic pressure from internal irrigation facilitates gentle and broad elevation of the sinus membrane before bone grafting. The HPISE uses a specially designed tip attached to a piezoelectric ultrasonic unit (Surgybone®, Silfradent srl, Sofia, Italy or compatible device). HPISE tip (S028I®, BukBu Dental Co, Daegu, Korea) allows internal irrigation to apply water pressure to the sinus membrane (Fig 34). Bone graft is dependent on surgeon's personal preference. Bone graft is indicated when heavy cyst is located in the sinus, more than 6mm high sinus elevation is required, implant is not placed simultaneously and postoperative radiopaque image is required to verify sinus elevation.

If the required sinus elevation is minimal (less than 5mm) and implant is placed at the same time, bone graft is not a prerequisite for sinus augmentation. New bone formation is achieved in the new compartment under the elevated sinus membrane thanks to tenting effect. As an alternative to bone graft, collagen sponge or fibrin rich block with concentrated growth factors (CGF®, Medifuge, Silfradent srl, S.Sofia, Italy) can be used. Fibrin rich block with concentrated growth factors can be used to accelerate new bone formation in the sinus

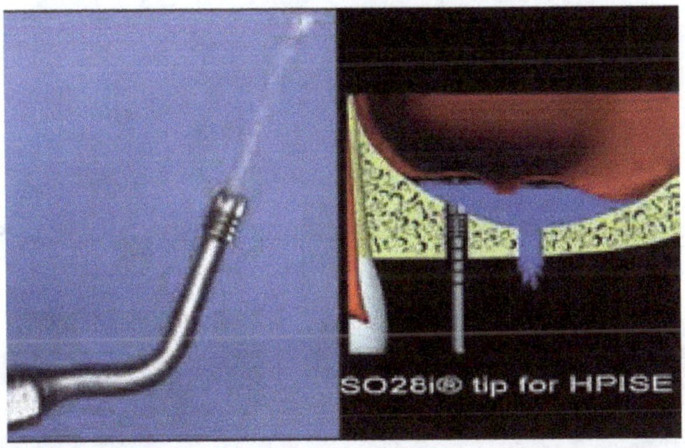

Fig. 34. HPISE (S028I®) tip with internal irrigation. Hydraulic pressure from internally irrigated saline elevates sinus membrane.

Surgical procedure of HPISE without bone graft (Fig. 35- Fig. 47)

As a first step, a 1.6mm wide carbide round insert (S016®, BukBu Dental Co, Daegu, Korea) with external irrigation is used to penetrate sinus floor directly. After breaking the sinus floor with the round tip, a 2.8mm wide HPISE tip is utilized to enlarge the osteotomy site and elevate the sinus membrane using hydraulic pressure. The HPISE tip has 4mm working tip height, and depth indicating lines are marked by 2mm intervals. Hydraulic pressure to the sinus membrane from internally irrigated sterile saline detaches sinus membrane from the sinus floor. Hydraulic pressure is applied for several ten seconds to detach sinus membrane from sinus floor. After the detachment of sinus membrane, surgeons can observe up and down movement of sinus membrane whenever patient takes a breath.
When the diameter of implant is less than 4mm wide, the HPISE insert is the last instrument to make the osteotomy prior to implant placement. Undersizing the osteotomy ensures favorable initial stability of the implant in the posterior edentulous ridge with poor bone quantity and quality. When a wider implant is placed, intermittent drilling is often required to accommodate the wide body implant.

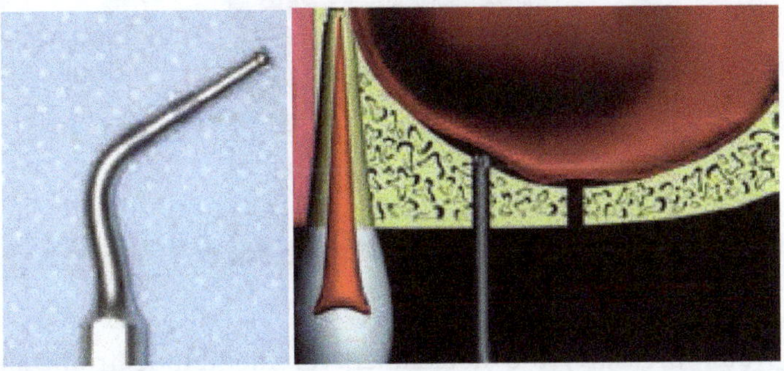

Fig. 35. (left) and Fig. 36. (right). Round carbide tip is used to break sinus floor directly. This tip provides surgeon tactile feeling of sinus membrane.

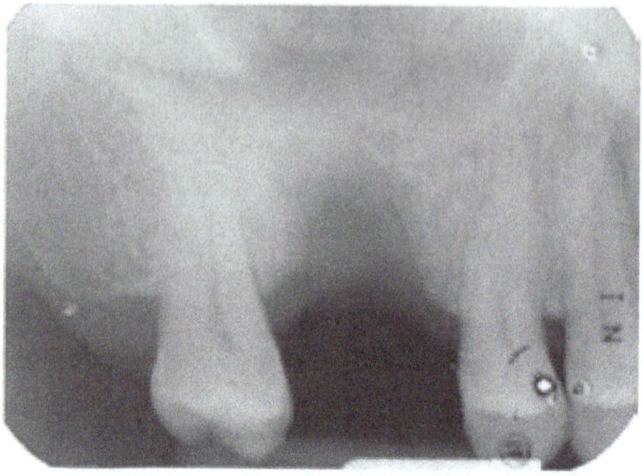

Fig. 37. When remaining bone height at the implant site is very low as shown on this radiogram, round tip can be omitted.

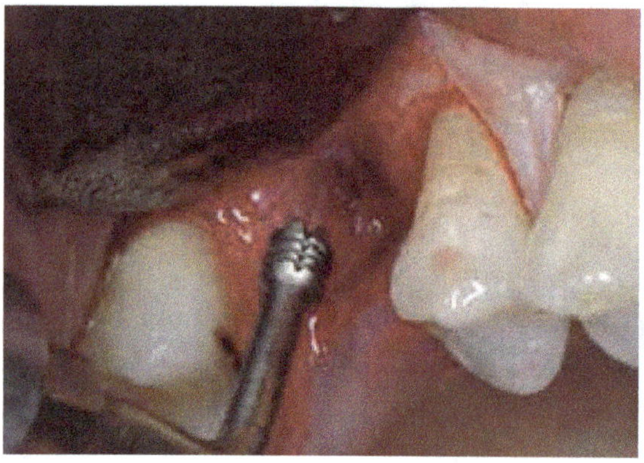

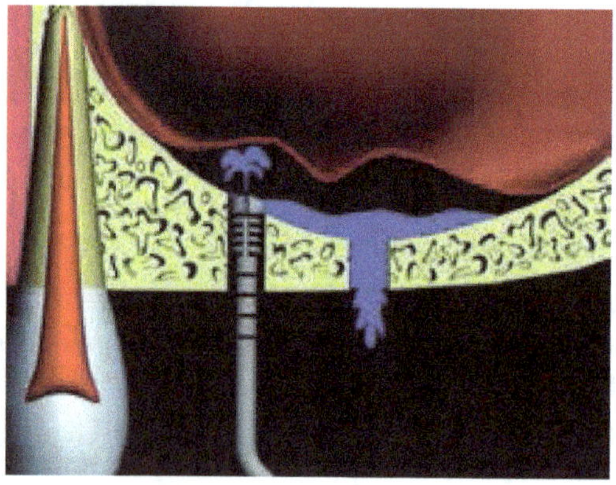

Fig. 38. (left) and Fig. 39. (right). HPISE is inserted to break sinus floor using ultrasonic vibration and elevate sinus membrane using water pressure.

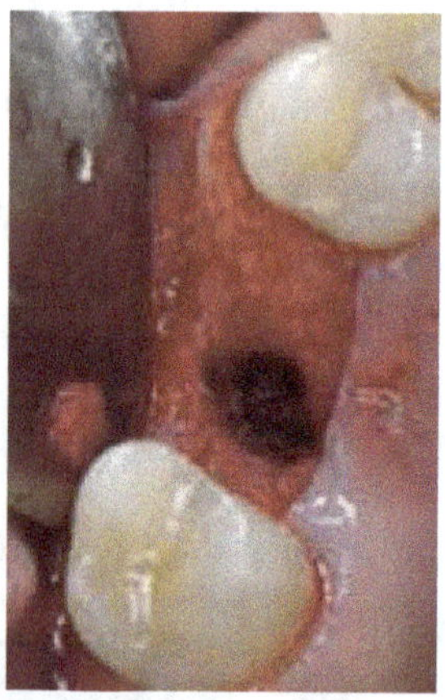

Fig. 40.

After applying water pressure, the detachment of membrane from sinus floor is seen. Surgeon can observe up and down movement of sinus membrane whenever patients take a breath.

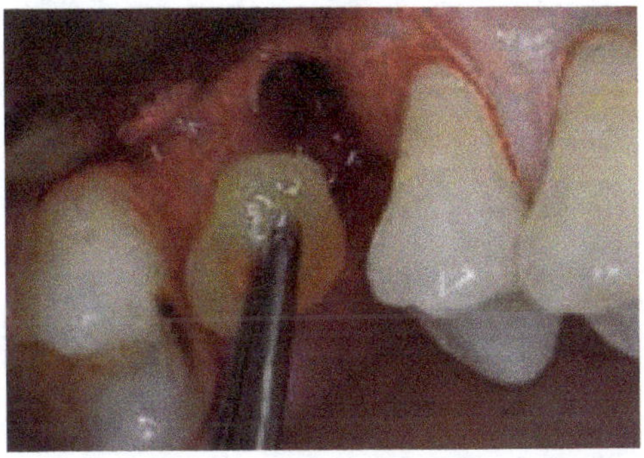

Fig. 41. As alternative to bone graft, CGF alone is inserted in order to accelerate bone reformation in the sinus,

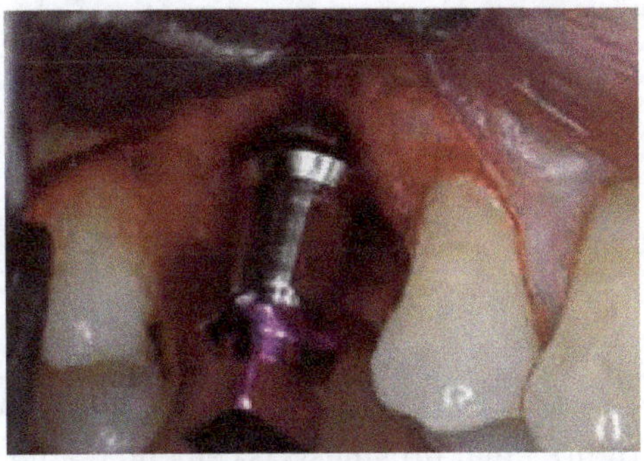

Fig. 42. 4.7mm wide and 11.5mm long HA coated implant is placed at the same time.

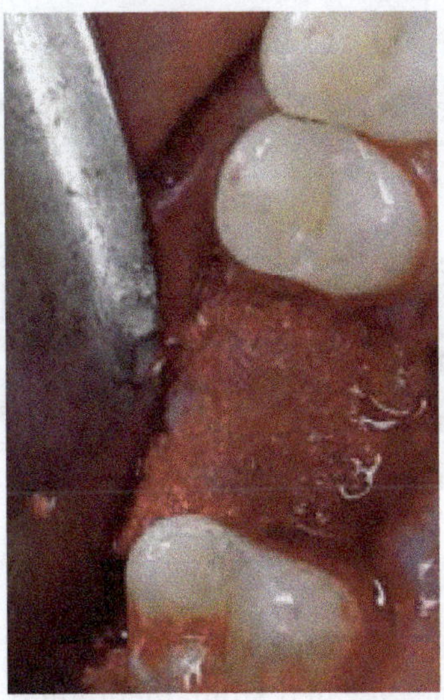

Fig. 43. Bovine bone is grafted in the defect around implant. CGF barrier is covered over the bone graft,

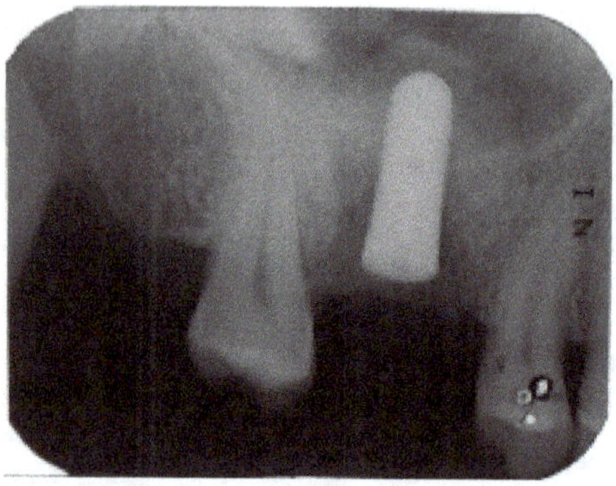

Fig. 44. A radiogram shows membrane elevation without bone graft.

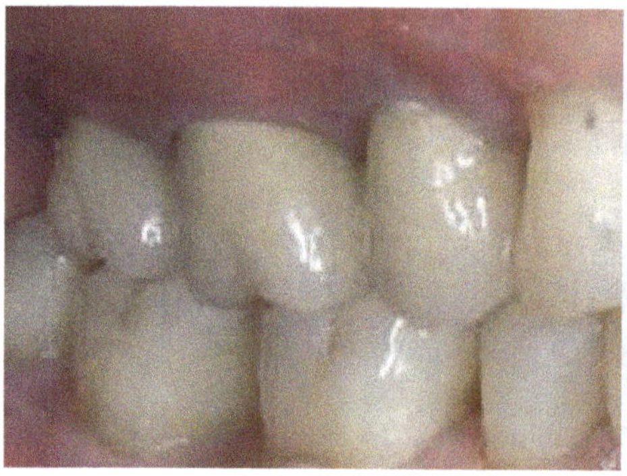

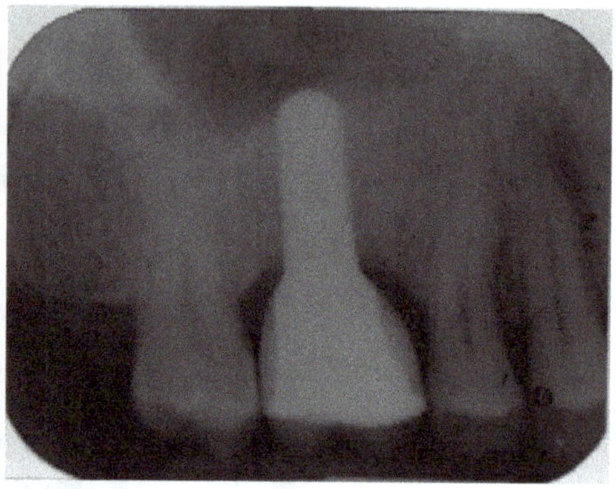

Fig. 45. (left) and Fig. 46. (right). Final prosthesis is cemented after 4 months healing. A radiogram shows sinus augmentation.

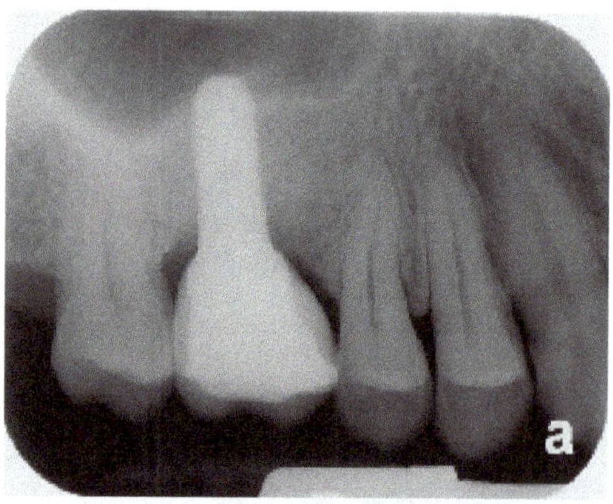

Fig. 47. A radiogram after 18 months loading. New bone formation is evident in the sinus without bone graft.

Surgical procedure of HPISE with bone graft (Fig. 48 – Fig. 60)

After elevating sinus membrane using water pressure, bone graft is optional. Bone graft in the new compartment under the elevated sinus membrane is indicated when heavy cyst is located in the sinus, more than 6mm high sinus elevation is required, implant is not placed simultaneously and postoperative radiopaque image is required to verify sinus elevation.

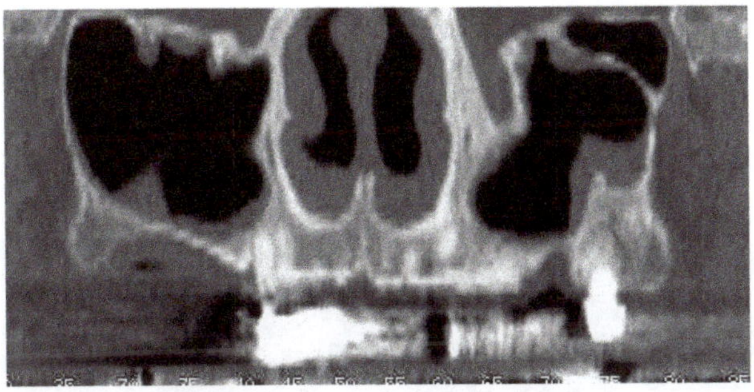

Fig. 48. 69 aged man was referred to my department for sinus and vertical ridge augmentation on the right posterior maxilla. He wants bone augmentation only. A radiogram shows very low bone height on the right posterior maxilla.

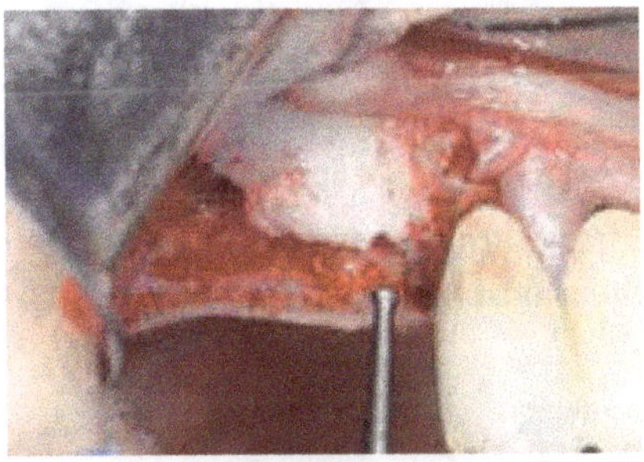

Fig. 49. Round carbide tip is used to break sinus floor at the implant sites.

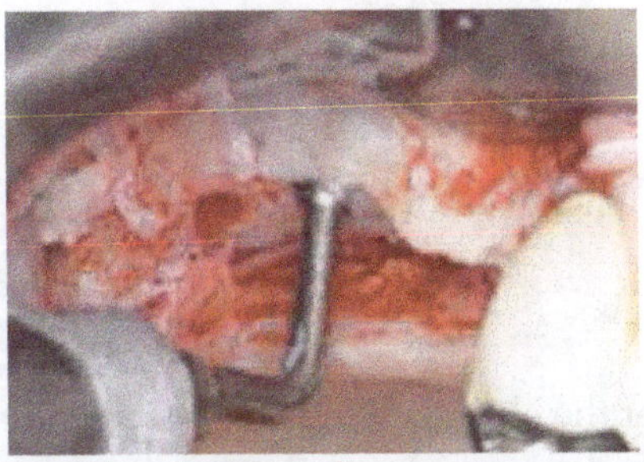

Fig. 50. HPISE tip is inserted into the sinus to elevate sinus membrane with water pressure.

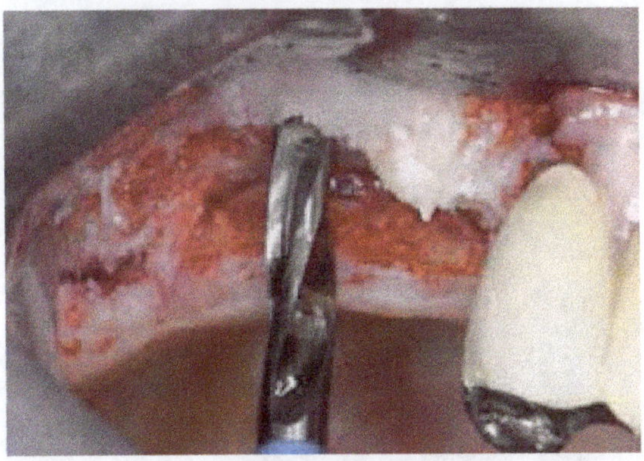

Fig. 51. In order to facilitate bone grafting, 4mm wide implant drill is used to expand the site of bone graft .

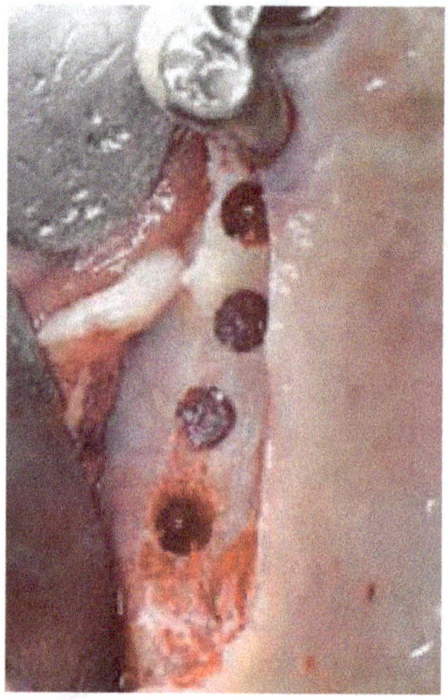

Fig. 52. Note detached sinus membrane from sinus floor. Whenever patient takes a breadth, up and down movement of the membrane is seen.

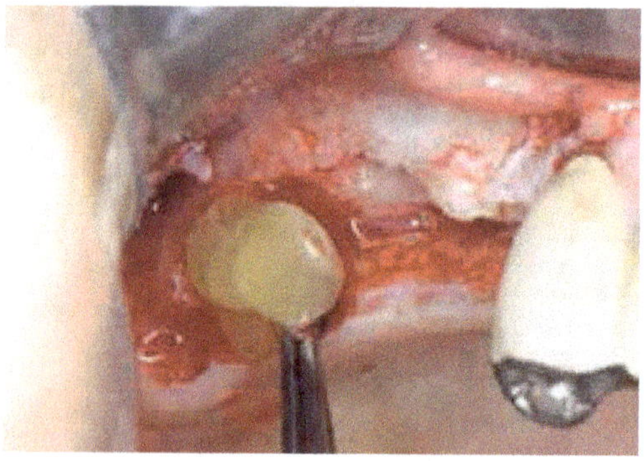

Fig. 53. CGF is inserted under the elevated sinus membrane. The CGF prevents membrane perforation as buffering effect during bone grafting and accelerates bone formation in the sinus.

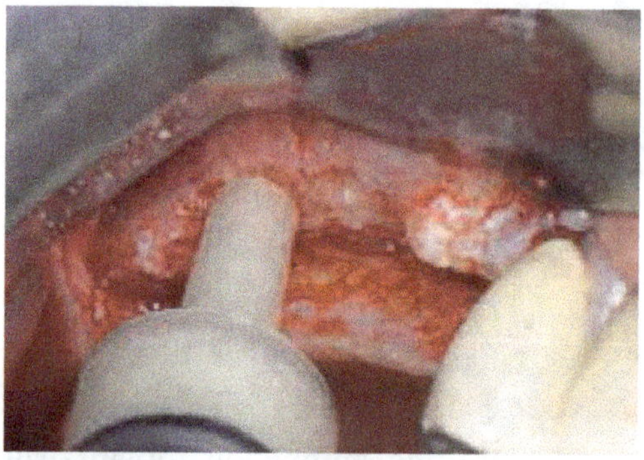

Fig. 54. Gel conditioned allograft is injected into the sinus cavity

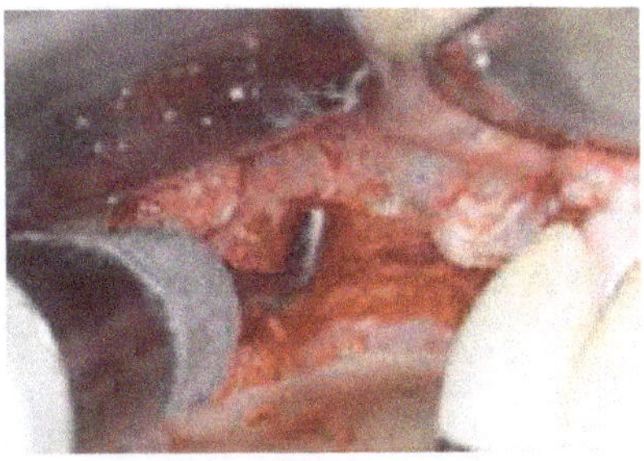

Fig. 55. Bone graft is compacted with HPISE tip

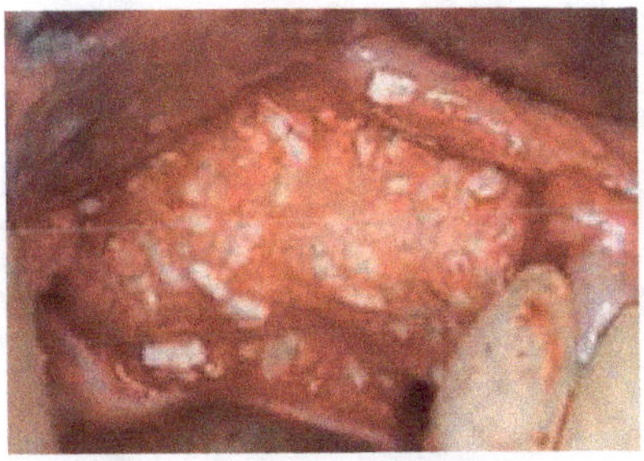

Fig. 56. Vertical bone defect is augmented with the mixture gel conditioned allograft and mineral allograft.

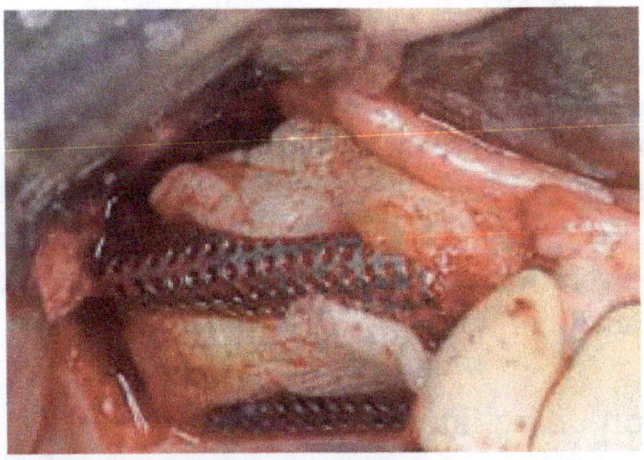

Fig. 57. Ti-mesh is stabilized with bone tack to stabilize bone graft. CGF is covered over the mesh to induce rapid soft tissue healing.

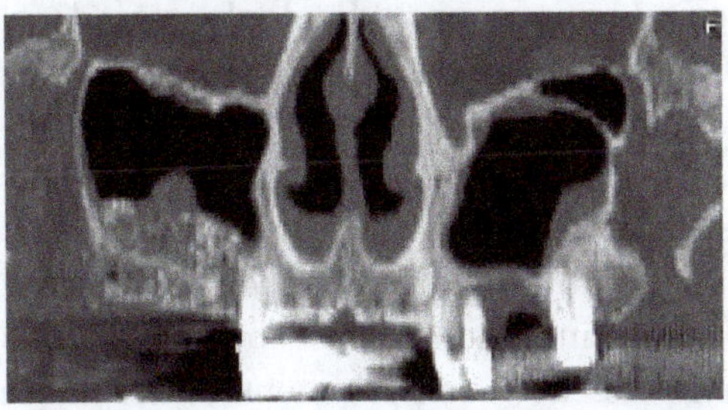

Fig. 58. Postoperative radiogram shows favorable sinus augmentation and ridge augmentation.

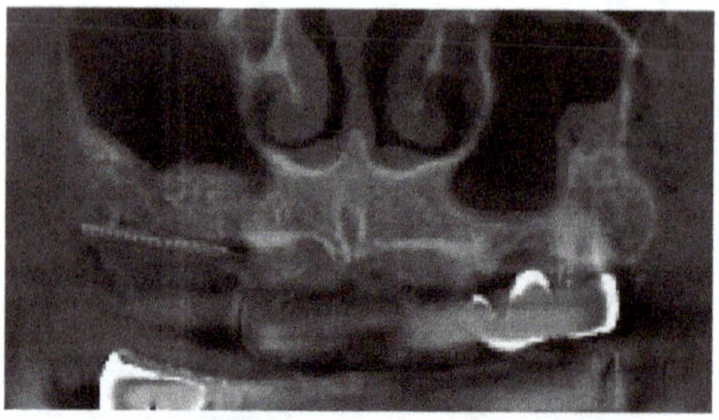

Fig. 59. A radiogram after 6 months healing. Sinus augmentation is evident.

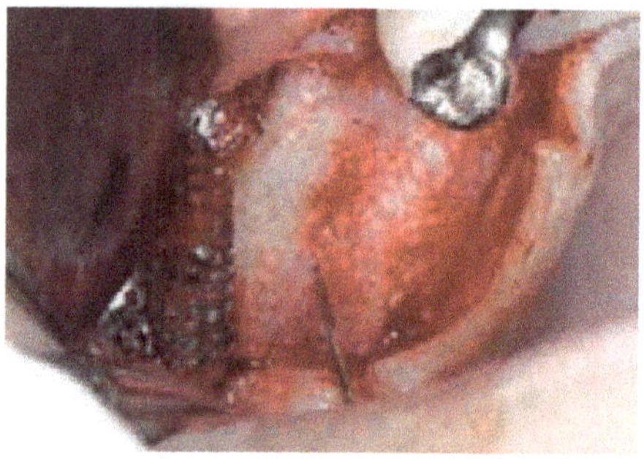

Fig. 60. Ti-mesh is removed after 6 months healing. Favorable idge augmentation is observed. The patient is referred to private clinic for implant placement.

231 implants were placed with HPISE technique at 3 centers from January 2008 to May 2010. 10 implants showed failure. Membrane perforation was developed in 14 implants (6.0% of perforation).CGF alone was inserted in the new compartment under the elevated sinus membrane in 127 implants (54.9%). Bone graft was used in 100 implants (43.2%). Collagen membrane was inserted in 3 implants (1.3%). Hyaloss matrix was used in 1 implant (0.4%). The success rate of implants was 96%. The success rate of HPISE is compatible to lateral window approach. However postoperative patient's discomfort is very minimal than lateral approached sinus augmentation.

4. Sinus augmentation using lateral window approach

Lateral window approach using various bone substitutes have been performed to overcome deficient bone volume on posterior maxillary ridge for decades.[15-17] However some studies reported new bone formation in animal and human's sinus with membrane elevation alone, resorbable gelatin sponge alone, venous blood alone and autologous fibrin gel with concentrated growth factors alone as alternatives to bone materials.[18-25] According to these studies, bone substitutes may not be a prerequisite for sinus augmentation. The function of elevated sinus membrane is controversial, but some studies reported that sinus membrane acted as periosteum and showed osteoinductive potetnial.[26, 27]

Sohn et al reported that significantly higher new bone formation was demonstrated in the sinus without bone graft than inorganic bovine bone grafted sinus.[23] According to this study, bone reformation in the new compartment under the elevated sinus membrane started from elevated sinus membrane and repositioned bony window. Osteoinductive function of sinus membrane seems to be similar to periosteum. Grafted bovine bone acted as only space maker and scaffolding effect in this study. The key for bone reformation in the sinus is not grafting materials but space making under the elevated sinus membrane. Therefore simultaneous implant placement is required to maintain blood clot in the new compartment under the elevated sinus membrane when bone materials are not used.

4.1 New bone formation in the sinus with membrane elevation alone

Lundgren et al first reported radiographic finding of bone reformation in the sinus with membrane elevation alone in human. However the study didn't demonstrate histological evidence to verify new bone formation in the sinus. [18] Palma et al demonstrated histologic evidence to verify new bone formation in the monkey's sinus. According to this study, no differences on new bone formation, implant stability and bone-implant contacts was demonstrated between two groups with and without adjunctive autogenous bone graft.[19]
Sohn et al. first demonstrated histological evidence of new bone formation in human maxillary sinuses with sinus membrane elevation alone and simultaneous implant placement.[22]

Patient selection

Ten sinus surgeries were performed under local anesthesia. The subjects were divided into two groups according to the method of treating the lateral bony window of the sinus. Group A (five cases) used a non-resorbable membrane to seal the lateral window, but a replaceable bony window was used in Group B (five cases) to maintain blood clot in the sinus. The residual bone height of the edentulous site for implant placement varied from 1-9 mm (mean 5 mm). After average six months healing, implants were allowed to connect healing abutment and bone biopsy was performed through the site of previous bony window for histologic evaluation.

Surgical procedure of Group A (with barrier membrane)

A bony window was prepared with round carbide insert (S016®, BukBu Dental, Daegu, Korea) connected with ultrasonic piezoelectric device (Surgybone®, Silfradent srl, Sofia, Italy). After careful elevation of sinus membrane, two 4.2mm wide and 13mm high implants (Seven®, MIS implants Technologies Ltd, Shlomi, Israel) were inserted simultaneously (Fig. 61 - Fig. 62). The bony window was sealed with non-resorbable membrane (Gore-Tex®, W. L. Gore & Associates, INC. Flagstaff, Arizona, USA) and the membrane was stabilized with pin (TiTac™, IMTEC Co., Ardmore, USA) to retain the blood in the sinus (Fig. 63). The bony defect around dental implant was augmented with autogenous bone taken from bony portion of window and gel conditioned allograft (Orthoblast II®, IsoTis OrthoBiologics Inc, California, USA) and covered with a resorbable membrane (Tutoplast Pericardium®) over the bone graft (Fig. 64). Antibiotics (Levofloxacin, 100mg) and analgesics (Zaltoprofen, 80mg), three times a day for seven days, were give to all patients. Postoperative radiographic views were taken to confirm the implant position and to check coagulum formation after surgery (Fig. 65). After average six months healing, the CT scan was taken to evaluate new bone formation in the sinus (Fig. 66 and Fig. 67). Bone biopsy was performed through the site of previous bony window for histologic evaluation (Fig. 68). Follow up radiographic evaluation was continued after the placement of the final prosthetics and at follow-up after loading (Fig. 69 and Fig. 70).

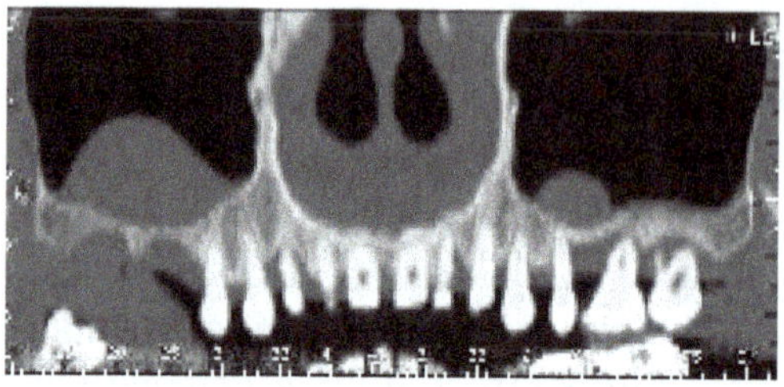

Fig. 61. Preoperative radiogram showing insufficient bone height in the right posterior maxilla.

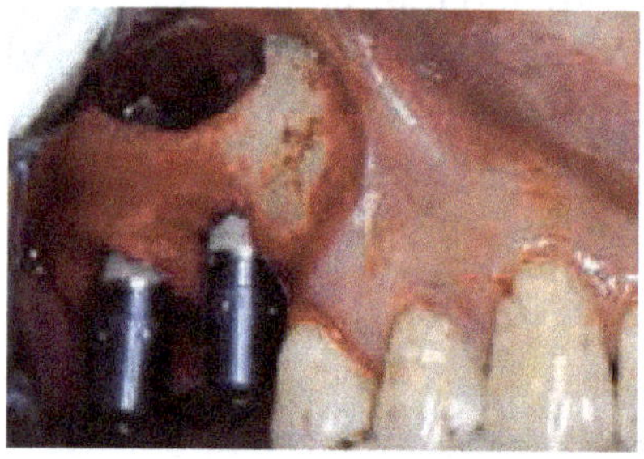

Fig. 62. The preparation of bony window is performed with round carbide tip, connected with ultrasonic piezoelectric device. After careful elevation of sinus membrane, two 13mm high implants is placed simultaneously to maintain space under the elevated sinus membrane.

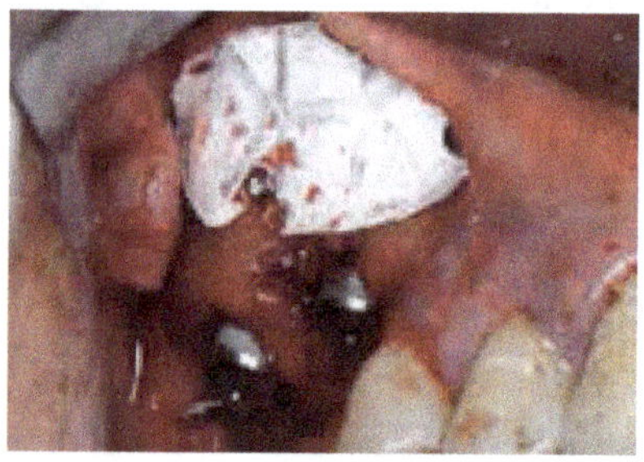

Fig. 63. The bony window is sealed with non-resorbable membrane to retain the blood in the sinus.

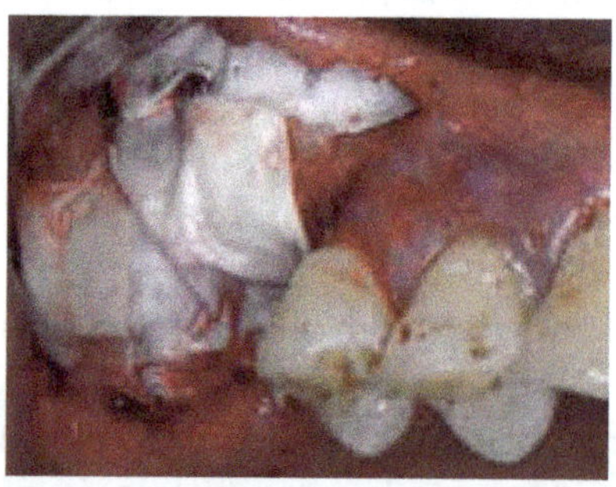

Fig. 64. The bony defect around dental implant is augmented with autogenous bone taken from bony portion of window and gel conditioned allograft, followed by covering with a resorbable membrane.

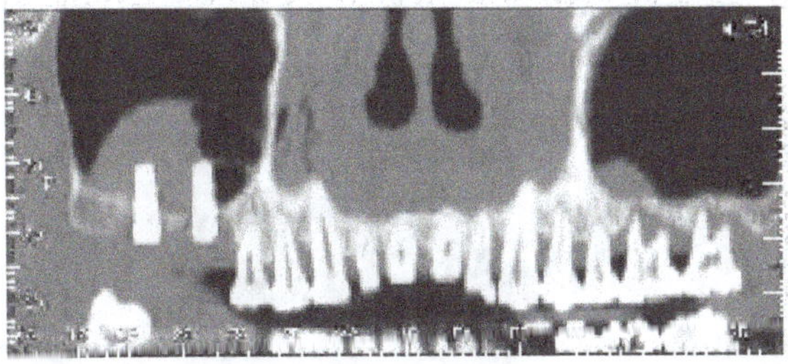

Fig. 65. Postoperative radiogram showing the elevation of sinus membrane.

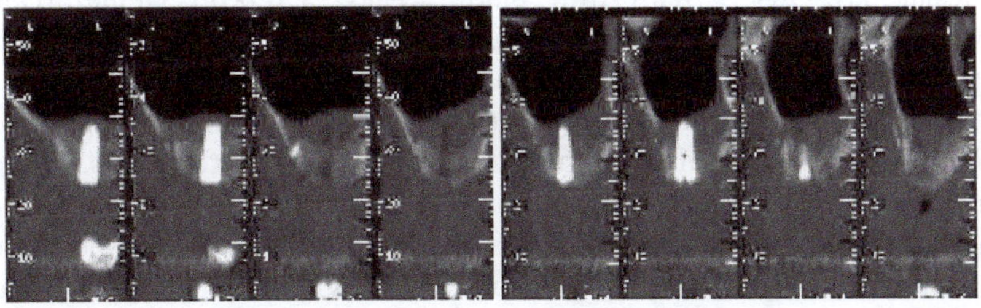

Fig. 66. (left) and 67. (right). CT scan shows bone reformation in the sinus after 6 months healing.

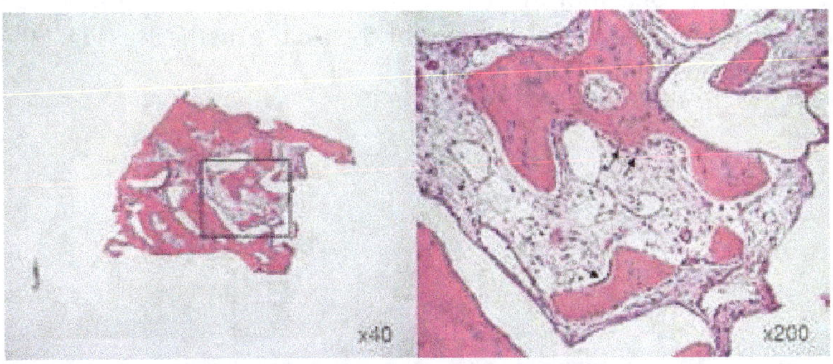

Fig. 68. Bone biopsy showing new bone formation in the sinus. Osteoblats lines along newly formed bone (arrow). (H-E stain).

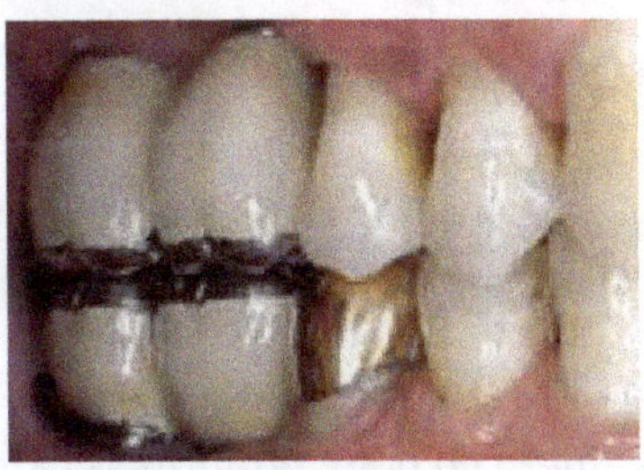

Fig. 69. Final prosthesis

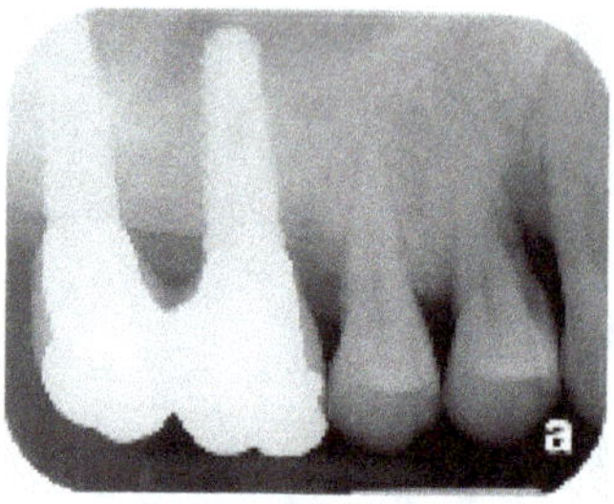

Fig. 70. Two years in function.

Surgical procedure of Group B (with replaceable bony window)

Full thickness mucoperiosteal flap was elevated to expose lateral wall of sinus cavity under local anesthesia. Saw insert with thin blade (S-saw®, BukBu Dental, Daegu, Korea) connected with ultrasonic piezoelectric device (Surgybone®) was tilted to lateral wall of sinus cavity to make replaceable bony window (Fig. 71 and Fig. 72). The bony window was carefully detached from the sinus membrane and the membrane was elevated superiorly very carefully to create new compartment to retain coagulum in the sinus. When membrane perforation was happened, resorbable collagen membrane (Tutoplast Pericardium®, Tutogen Medical GmbH, Neunkirchem am Brand, Germany) was covered over the perforation (Fig. 73 and Fig. 74). Three dental implants (Tapered Screw Vent implant, Zimmer Co) were placed at the same time (Fig. 75). The bony window was repositioned to hold blood in the sinus (Fig. 76). Postoperative care was as same as that of Group A. Postoperative radiograms and CT scans were taken immediately on surgery day and on the day of the uncovering (Fig. 77 - Fig 78). A bone biopsy was taken on the lateral access window area on the uncovering day after a six month healing period (Fig. 79). Follow up radiographic evaluation was continued after the placement of the final prosthetics (Fig. 80 - Fig. 81)

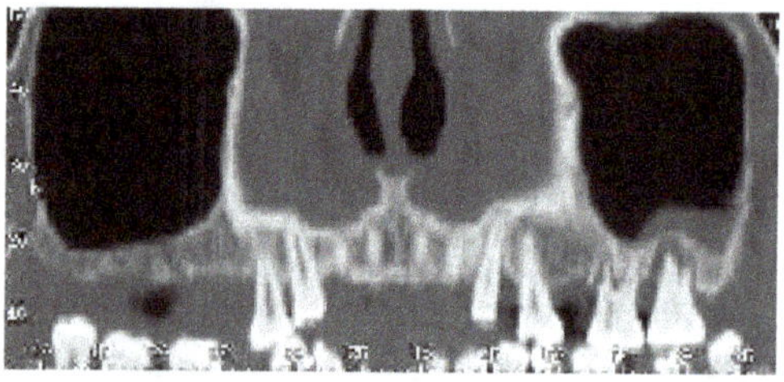

Fig. 71. Preoperative radiogram showing low bone height at right posterior maxilla.

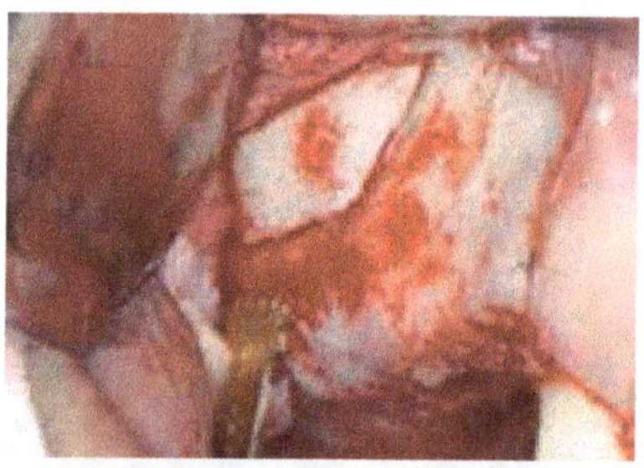

Fig. 72. Replaceable bony window is prepared with saw insert. Tilted osteotomy is made at anterior and inferior osteotomy line. The bony window is carefully detached from the sinus membrane.

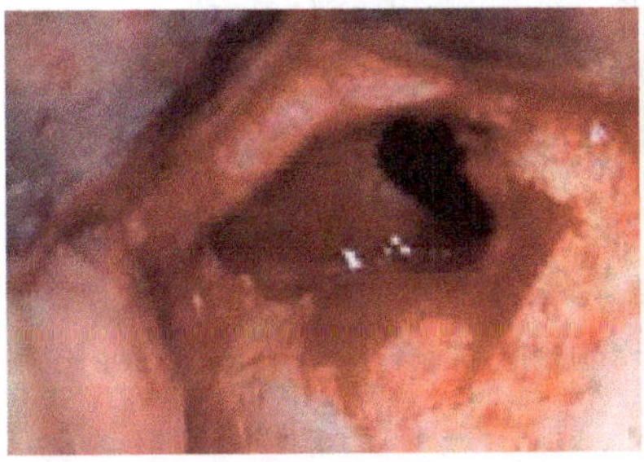
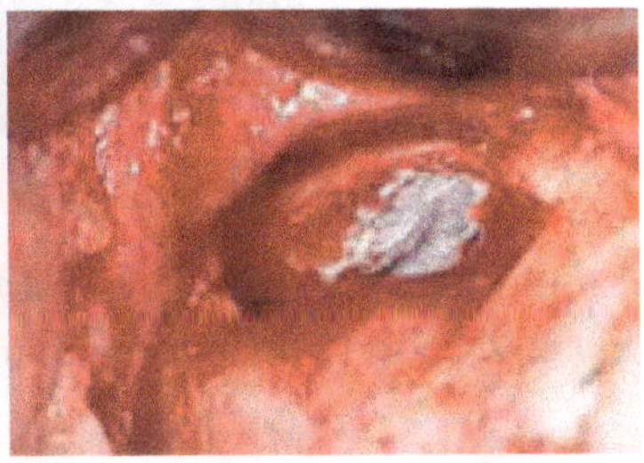

Fig. 73. (left) and Fig. 74. (right). Membrane perforation is happened during the elevation of membrane and resorbable collagen membrane is covered over the perforation.

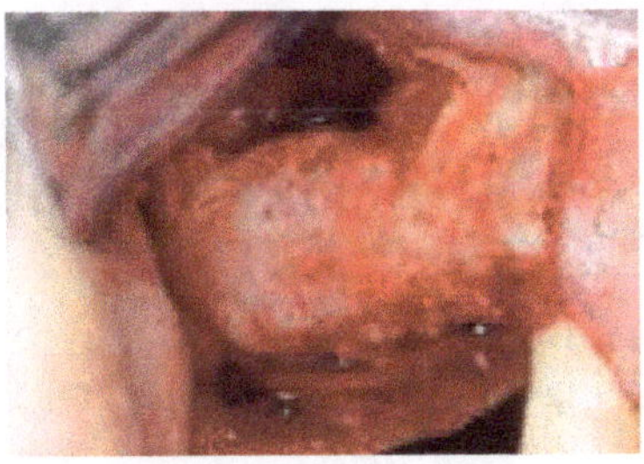

Fig. 75. Three dental implants are placed simultaneously with good stability.

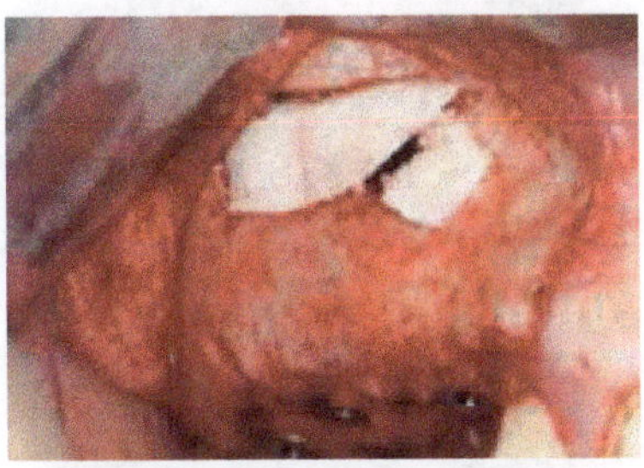

Fig. 76. The bony window is repositioned to seal the window.

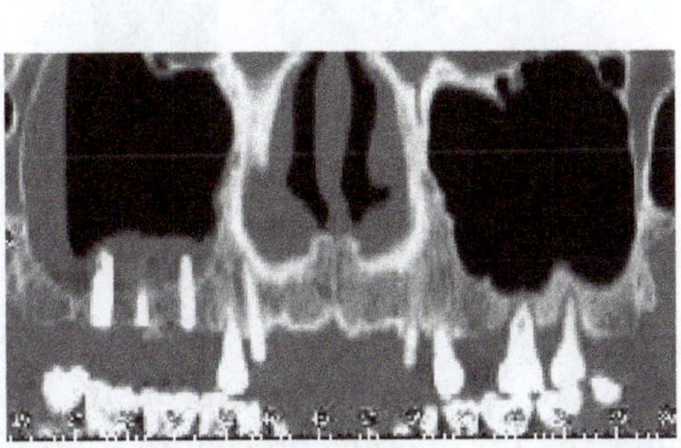

Fig. 77. Postoperative CT scan showing membrane elevation in the sinus.

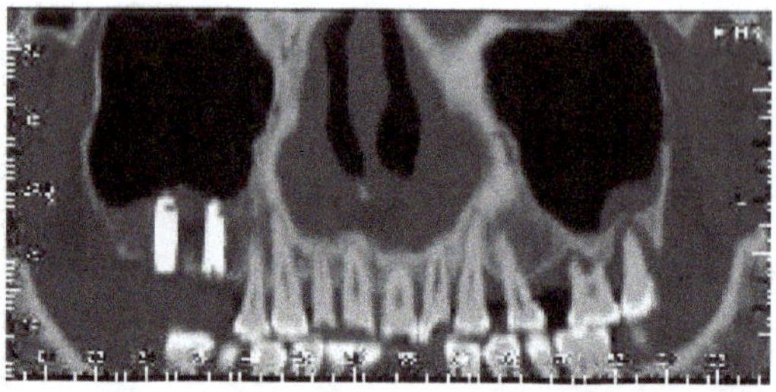

Fig. 78. CT scan shows newly formed bone in the sinus after 6 months healing.

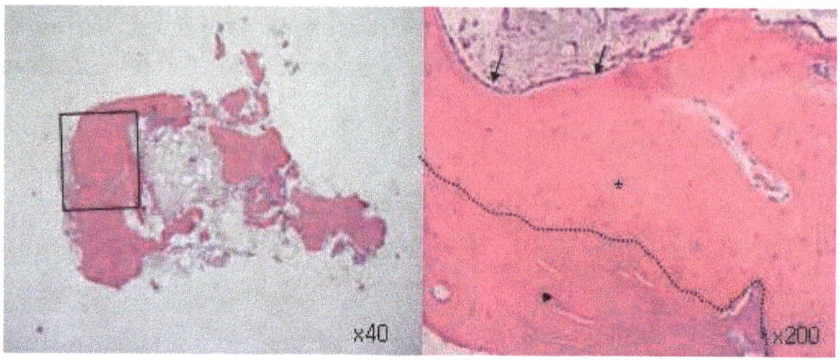

Fig. 79. Bone biopsy taken at the uncovering procedure reveales new bone formation (*) in the sinus. Arrow indicates osteoblasts and triangle indicates the bony portion of window.

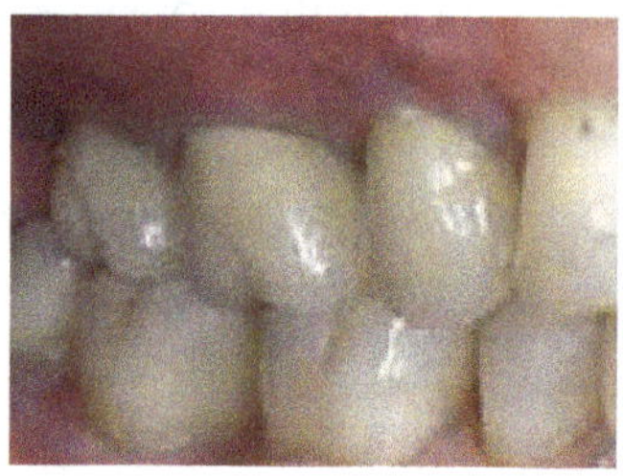

Fig. 80. Final prosthesis.

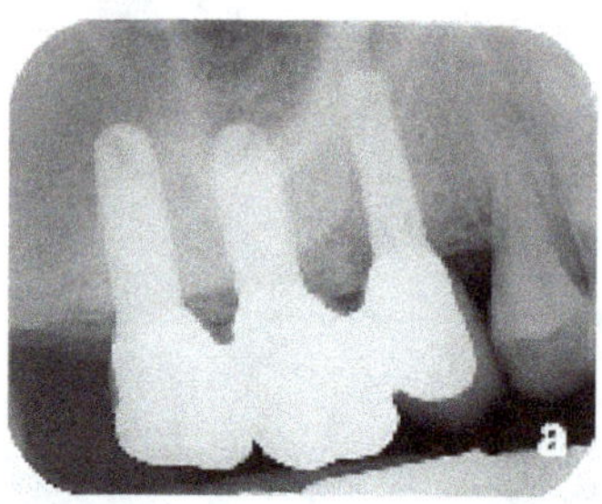

Fig. 81. Radiogram after 3 year and 8 months loading.

Results and discussion

A total of 21 implants were placed simultaneously and no implants showed osseointergration failure after the uncovering procedure. No postoperative infection was developed. All sinuses demonstrated new bone formation through clinical, radiographic and histologic evaluations. All implant supported prosthesis was clinically stable after about 3 year follow-up. There are no differences on new bone formation between two groups. The most important factor is to induce new bone formation in the sinus is to maintain the space of new compartment under the elevated sinus membrane.

To prepare bony window, various cutting devices have been recommended. Rotary bur is a common instrument to make bony window, but high rate of membrane perforation is reported in some studies.[28-30] Some studies reported lower rate of membrane perforation with piezoelectric round tip.[31-33] Current author compared the effect of two types of piezoelectric inserts - round and saw tip - on membrane perforation during creation of lateral bony window.[33] A total rate of membrane perforation using both kinds of piezoelectric insert at 5.51%. The rate of perforation created by the piezoelectric saw (7.14%) was relatively higher than that created by the round diamond insert (2.32%) in this study. But there was no significant difference between the rates for membrane perforation for the two types of piezoelectric inserts. According to this study, the piezoelectric saw insert has some advantages over the round inserts, such as precision, minimal bone loss, and facilitation of precise replacement of the bony window. In addition, replaceable bony window acts as osteoinductive barrier to accelerate new bone formation in the sinus.[23]

4.2 New bone formation in the maxillary sinus using absorbable gelatin sponge alone

Maxillary sinus has a potential to induce new bone formation in the new compartment under the elevated sinus membrane. As demonstrated earlier, bone graft may not be prerequisite for sinus augmentation. So even though resorbable gelatin sponge is inserted in the compartment under the elevated sinus membrane for space making, bone reformation in the sinus is evident.[24,34]

Patient selection

The study consisted of nine patients treated with sinus augmentation with resorbable gelatin sponge membrane and simultaneous implant placement. Seven patients (seven men and two woman), with age ranging from 40 to 75 (a mean age of 55.2 years), were included in this study. Preoperative examinations with panoramic views and dental cone-beam computed topographic scans (Combo®: Pointnix, Seoul, Korea or Implagraphy: Vatec, Kyungi, Korea) were performed. The bone height of remaining alveolar ridge was 1.5~7.2mm (average 4.7 mm). Bilateral sinus surgery was performed in three patients and unilateral sinus surgery was performed in six patients.

Surgical procedures

Prophylactic oral antibiotics, Cefditoren pivoxil (Meiact®; Boryung Parm., Seoul, Korea) 300mg t.i.d. were used routinely, beginning one day prior to the procedure and continuing for seven days. Surgery was performed under local anesthesia through maxillary block anesthesia by using 2% lidocaine that includes 1:100,000 epinephrine. After elevating of full thickness flap, the lateral wall of the maxillary sinus was exposed. Piezoelectric saw with thin blade (S-Saw, Bukbu Dental Co., Diego, Korea), connected to piezoelectric device (Surgybone®, Silfradent srl, Sofia, Italy), was used to create the lateral window of the maxillary sinus. The tilted osteotomy into sinus cavity was performed at anterior and inferior osteotomy line to facilitate the precise replacement of the bony window as a barrier over inserted gelatin sponge in the maxillary sinus (Fig. 82- Fig. 83) . After careful elevation of the sinus membrane, the absorbable gelatin sponge (Cutanplast®, Mascia Brunelli Spa, Viale Monza, Italy) was inserted in the new compartment under the elevated sinus membrane. Twenty two Implants were placed at the same time. The bony portion of lateral window was repositioned to prevent soft tissue ingrowth into the sinus cavity and to promote new bone formation from the lateral wall of maxillary sinus (Fig. 84 - Fig. 87). Preoperative prophylactic antibiotic therapy was continued postoperatively for 7 days and the sutures were removed 14 days postoperatively. After sinus augmentation, postoperative panoramic radiographs and cone-beam CT scans were taken immediately after surgery. An average of 6 months was allowed for the implants to integrate. The implants were then uncovered and panoramic radiographs and dental cone-beam CT scans were obtained to assess the new bone formation around the implants. Follow up radiogram after loading was taken (Fig. 88-92).

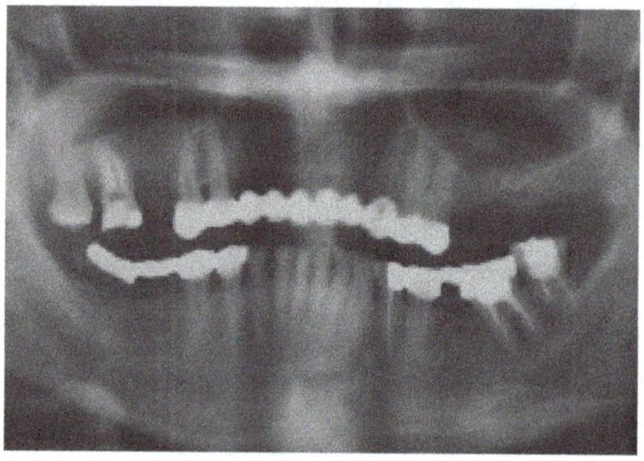

Fig. 82. Preoperative radiogram reveals pneumatization of bilateral maxillary sinus and insufficient bone height in both posterior maxilla.

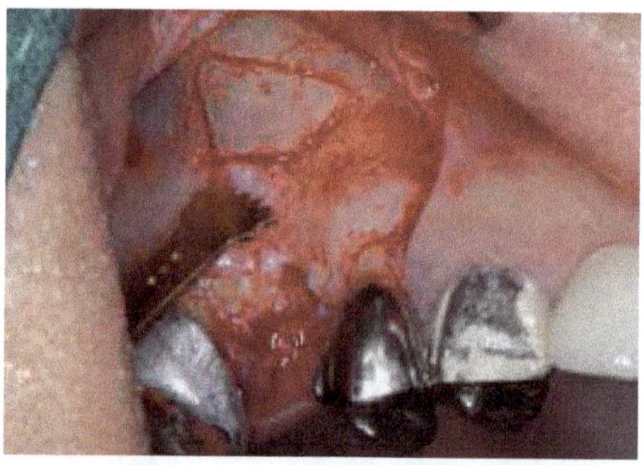

Fig. 83. Replaceable bony window is prepared with piezoelectric saw insert. The tilted osteotomy into the sinus cavity was made to facilitate the precise replacement of the bony window as a barrier over inserted gelatin sponge in the maxillary sinus.

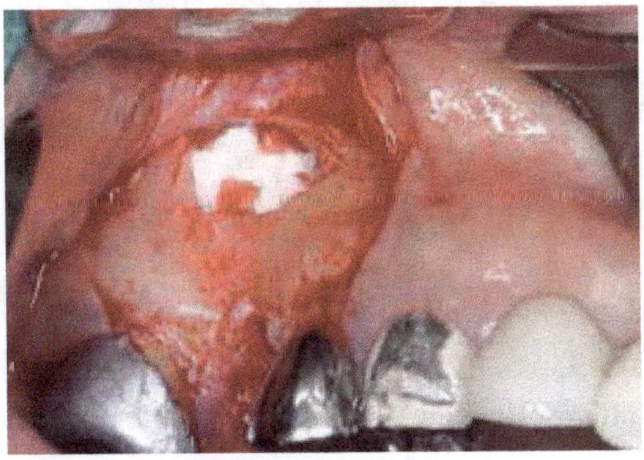

Fig. 84. After careful elevation of sinus membrane, gelatin sponge is inserted in the new compartment under the elevated membrane.

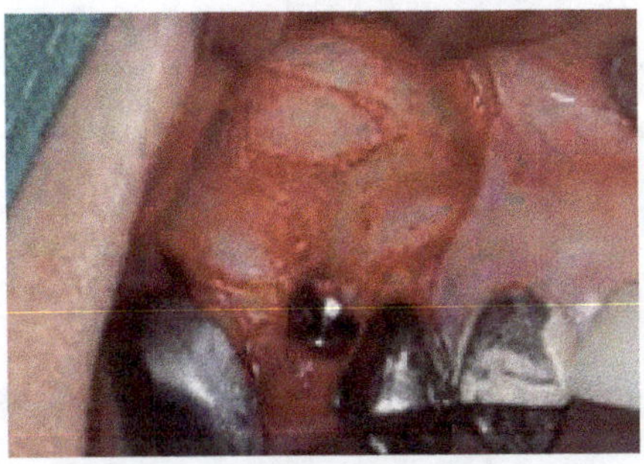

Fig. 85. Implant is placed at the same time and the bony window is repositioned. Ridge augmentation is performed at bony defect around implant.

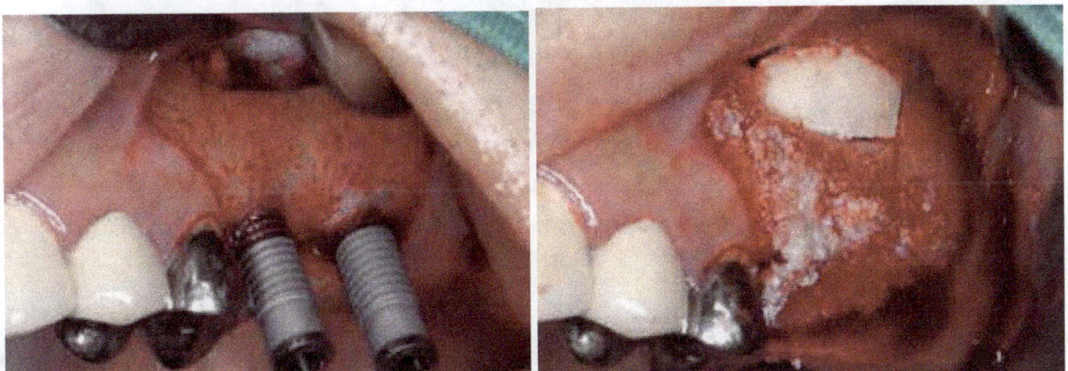

Fig. 86. and Fig. 87. Same procedure is performed in the left sinus.

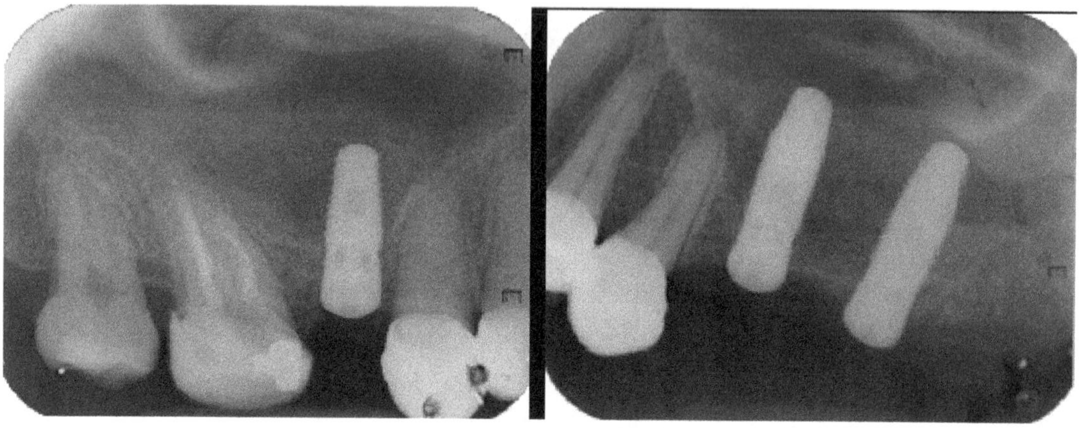

Fig. 88. Postoperative radiograms showing original sinus floor and no radiopaque image in the sinus

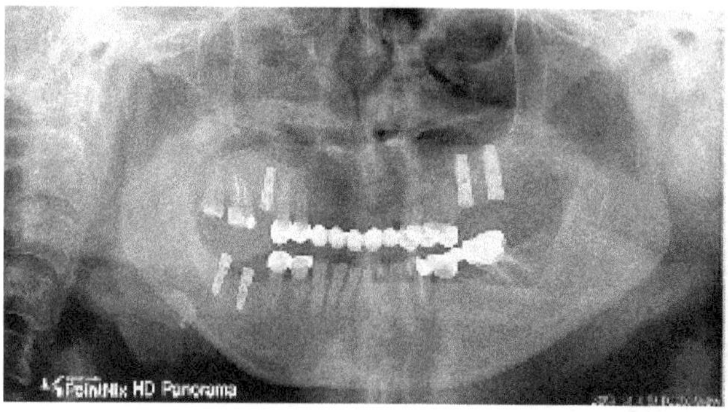

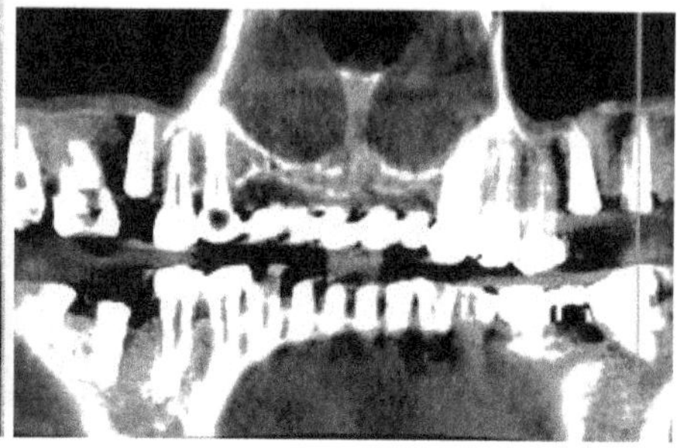

Fig. 89. (left) and Fig. 90. (right). Radiogram taken after 6 months healing reveals bone reformation in the both sinus.

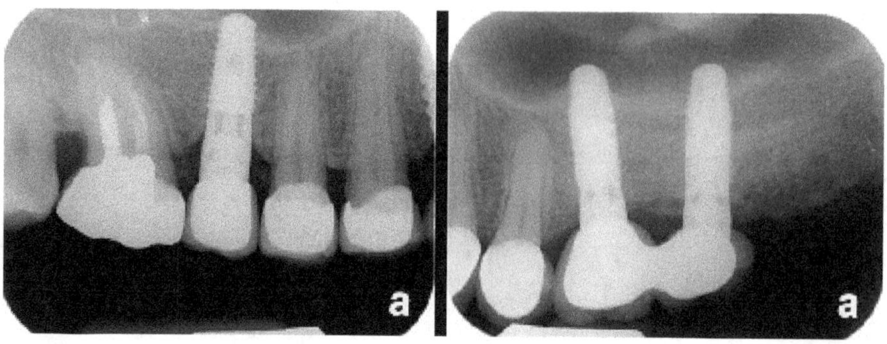

Fig. 91. A radiogram confirming bone reformation in the both sinus after 2 year loading.

Results and discussion

The membrane perforation was developed in two cases. Infection was not developed. New bone formation in the sinus was achieved in all cases using gelatin sponges alone after average six months healing period. Two RBM surfaced implants were failed after the uncovering procedure. The failures came from insufficient initial instability. This study revealed that placement of dental implant with maxillary sinus with gelatin sponge appears to be predictable procedure for sinus augmentation and bone graft is not an essential factor for sinus augmentation.

4.3 Bone reformation in the maxillary sinus using peripheral venous blood alone

As described earlier in this chapter, bone graft is not a prerequisite for sinus augmentation when implant is placed simultaneously. According to Hatano et al and Moon et al's study, [21] The insertion of peripheral venous blood as alternative to graft material can be safely used in maxillary sinus augmentation as demonstrated in this chapter.

Surgical procedure

The surgical procedure is as same as those demonstrated above except for the insertion of venous blood in the new compartment under the elevated sinus membrane (Fig. 92 – Fig. 98)

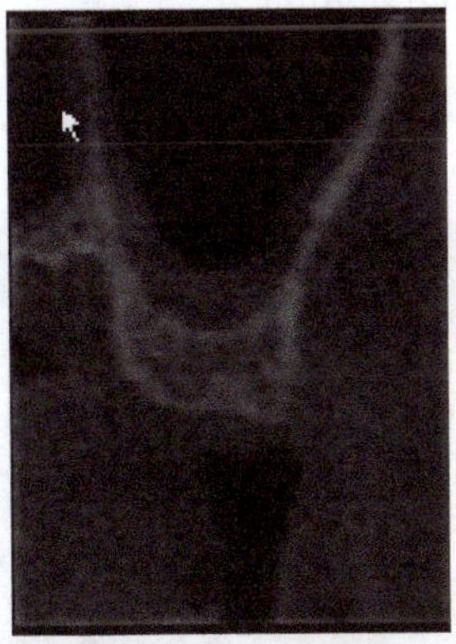

Fig. 92. Preoperative radiogram reveals approximately 6mm bone height at the site of left upper second molar.

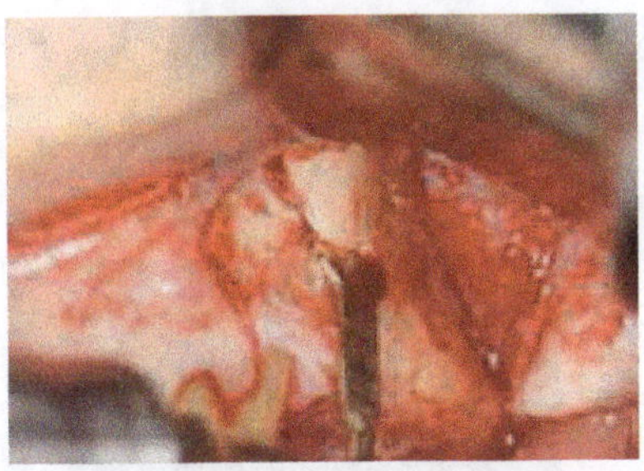

Fig. 93. After the elevation of a mucoperiosteal flap, lateral wall of sinus cavity is exposed. The piezoelectric saw with thin blade (S-Saw, Bukboo Dental Co., Daegu, Korea), connected to piezoelectric device (Surgybone®, Silfradent srl, Sofia, Italy), is used with copious saline irrigation to create the lateral window of the maxillary sinus. The anterior and inferior osteotomy line was created out of perpendicular to the sinus lateral wall, and then superior and posterior osteotomy were made perpendicular to the lateral wall. This design of osteotomy facilitates the precise replacement of the bony window as an osteoinductive barrier over injected venous blood in the maxillary sinus. The bony window was detached carefully to expose the sinus membrane. The sinus membrane is carefully elevated from the sinus floor walls with a manual elevator.

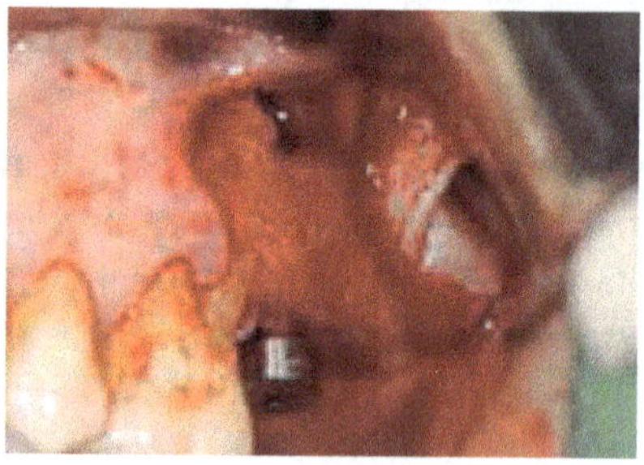

Fig. 94. A 4.1 mm wide and 13 mm high implant (SybronPRO™XRT implants, Sybron implant solution, California, USA) is placed after elevation of the sinus membrane. The collected peripheral venous blood taken from the brachial vein of patient's arm is injected to fill the new compartment of maxillary sinus.

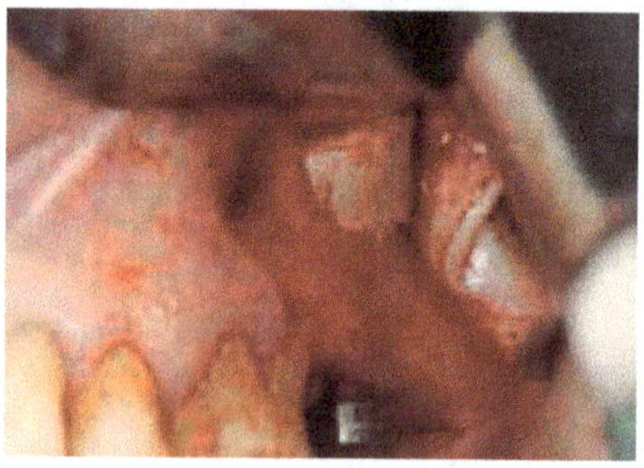

Fig. 95. The detached bony window is repositioned to prevent soft tissue ingrowth into the sinus cavity and to promote new bone formation from the lateral wall of maxillary sinus. This bony widnow acts as osteoinductive barrier.

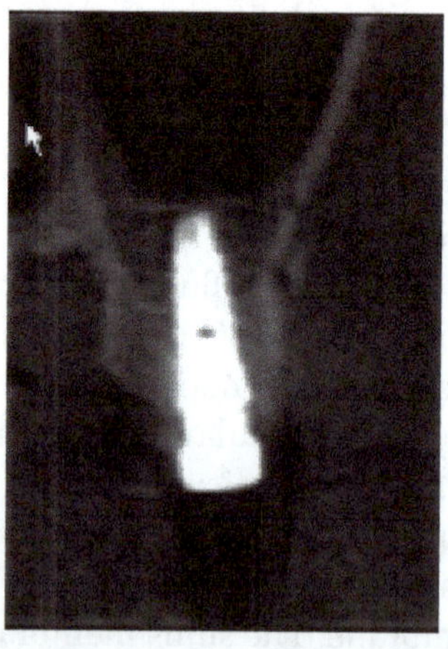

Fig. 96. A postoperative cone-beam CT scans shows venous blood filled sinus.

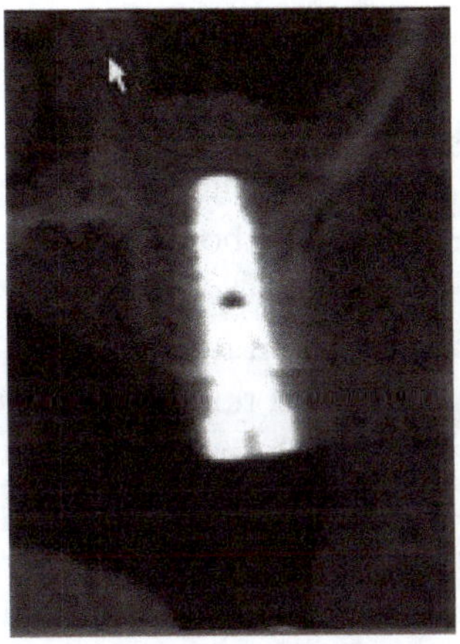

Fig. 97. 6 months healing is allowed for the osseointegration of implant. Cone beam CT shows newly formed bone in the sinus. During uncovering procedure, biopsy specimens is taken with 4 mm wide trephine bur at the site of repositioned bony window.

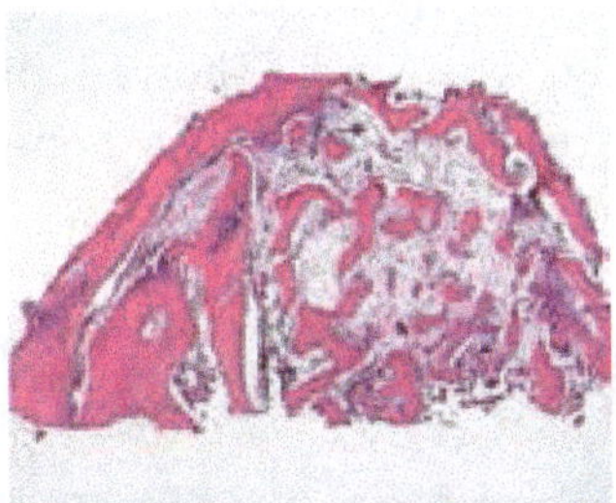

Fig. 98. Bone biopsy reveals active new bone formation. (H-E stain, x 40)

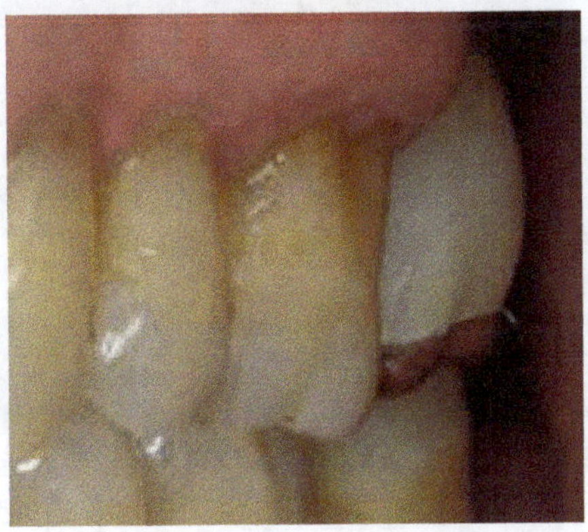

Fig. 99. Final prosthesis.

The peripheral venous blood under the elevated sinus membrane could to induce new bone formation in the maxillary sinus as shown on this case. The presence of a blood clot in healing of circumscribed bone defects was already reported .[36-37] Injection of collected venous blood could be a scaffold for new bone formation in the new compartment under the elevated membrane. The insertion of peripheral venous blood as a graft material can be a viable alternative to bone substitutes and safely used in maxillary sinus augmentation.

4.4 New bone formation in the maxillary sinus using fibrin rich gel with concentrated growth factors alone

Platelet aggregates, such as platelet rich plasma (PRP), platelet rich in growth factors (PRGF), platelet rich fibrin (PRF) and fibrin rich gel with concentrated growth factors alone (CGF) have been used to accelerate new bone formation associated with guided bone regeneration and sinus graft.[38-40] Platelet aggregates are known to contain concentrated growth factors such as transforming growth factor (TGF-β1), Platelet-derived growth factor and vascular endothelial growth factor and release slowly the growth factors. As alternative to bone filler in the sinus, the effect of fibrin rich block with concentrated growth factors (CGF) was already reported.[41] Compared to platelet rich plasma or platelet rich in growth factors, fibrin rich gel with concentrated growth factors is simple to make and doesn't require any synthetic or biomaterials to make gel condition. So it is free from the risk of cross-contamination from bovine thrombin. (Fig 100)

According to current author and colleagues' unpublished study on 61 sinus augmentations using fibrin rich gel with concentrated growth factors alone, fast new bone formation in the sinus was apparent in the all sinus radiographically and histologically.[42] Any significant postoperative complications were not developed. The success rate of implant was 98.2% after average 10 months loading. The study showed that the use of fibrin block with concentrated growth factor acts as alternative to a bone graft and can be a predictable procedure for sinus augmentation.

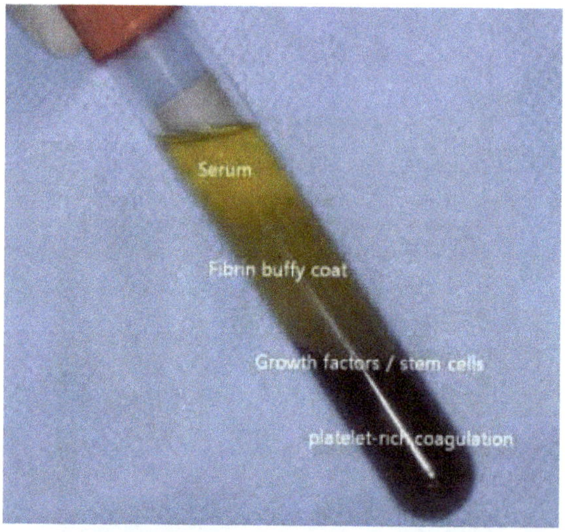

Fig. 100. (left). Fibrin rich block with concentrated growth factors (CGF) made by specific centrifuge (Medifuge®, Silfradent srl, Sofia, Italy). CGF is prepared with 20-60CC of patient's venous blood was taken from patients' vein in patient's forearm before sinus graft is performed. The blood in the test tubes is centrifuged at 2400-2700 rpm using specific centrifuge with a rotor turning at alternated and controlled speed for 12 minutes. The 2nd layer is fibrin buffy coat layer represented by a very large and dense polymerised fibrin block and the 3rd layer is a liquid phase containing the concentrated growth factors, white line cells and stem cells waiting for stimulation and to differentiate into specialized cell types. The second and third layer is known to have high concentration of growth factors. These two layers are inserted into the sinus cavity to accelerate new bone formation.

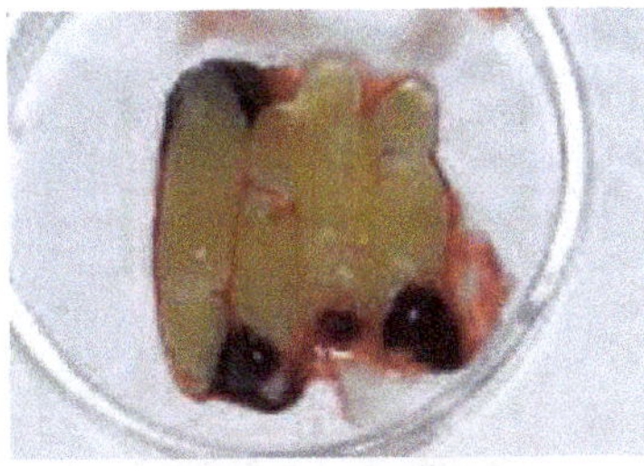

Fig. 101. This Fibrin rich block includes 2nd and 3rd layer of prepared CGF.

Surgical procedure

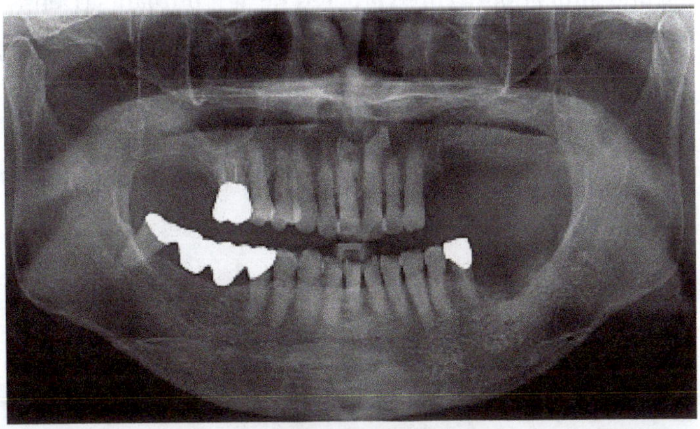

Fig. 102. Preoperative radiogram shows 5-6mm of bone height at left posterior maxilla.

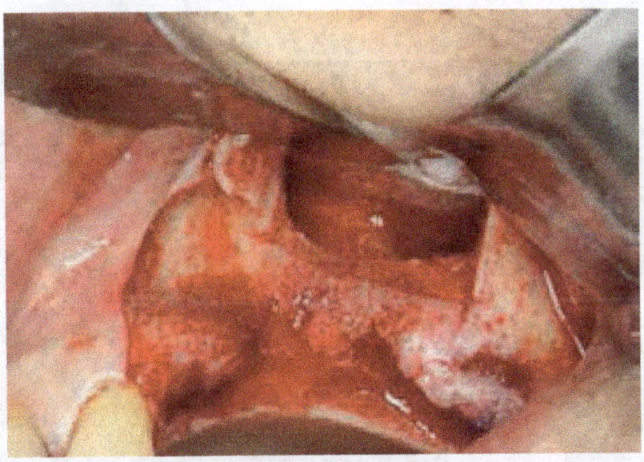

Fig. 103. The piezoelectric saw, connected to ultrasonic piezoelectric device (Surgybone), is used to create the replaceable lateral window of the maxillary sinus. Sinus membrane is carefully elevated to expose medial wall of sinus.

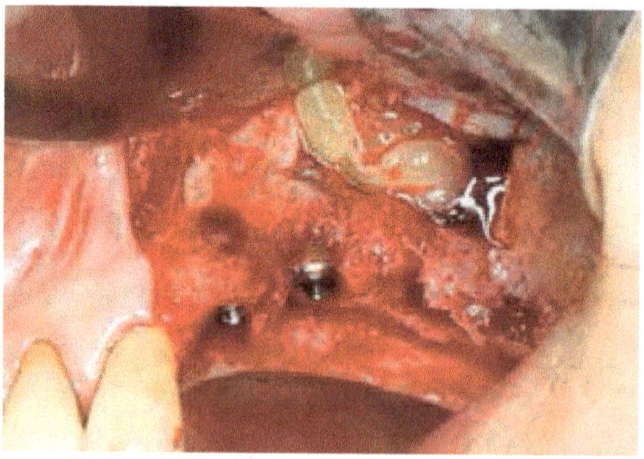

Fig. 104. Four pieces of fibrin rich gel are inserted in the new compartment between the elevated membrane and sinus floor. Three tapered design implants (Dentis implant, Dentis Inc, Daegu, Korea) is placed simultaneously

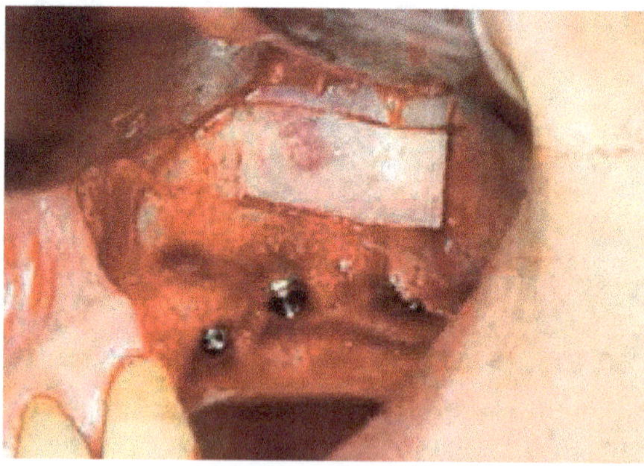

Fig. 105. The bony window was repositioned with stability to seal the window. Guided bone regeneration using mineral allograft and collagen membrane was performed to augment the bony defect around implants.

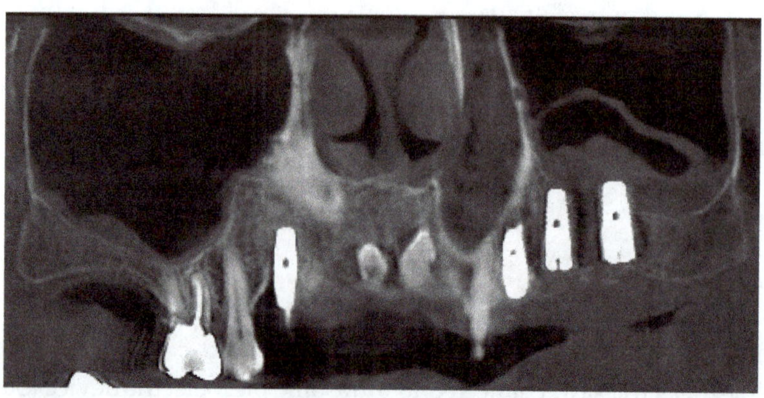

Fig. 106. Postoperative cone beam CT scans showing membrane elevation and implant placement in the left sinus.

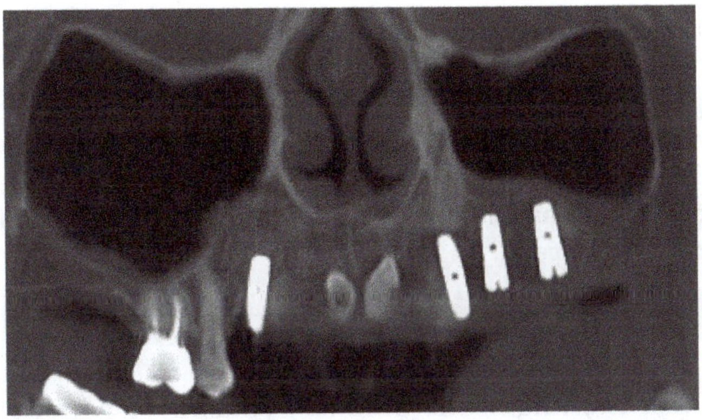

Fig. 107. Radiogram after 5 months healing. Bone reformation is evident in the left sinus

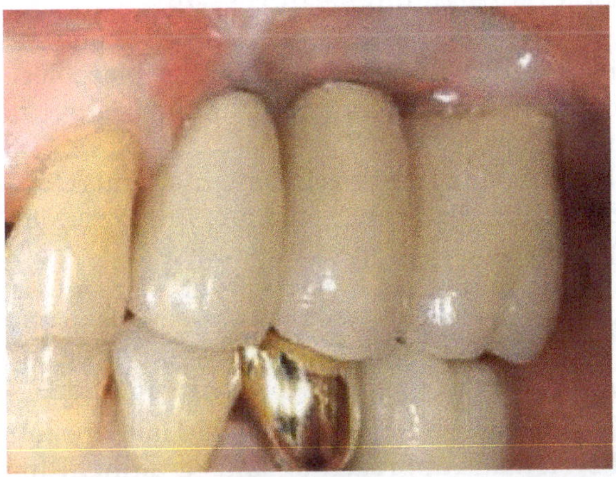

Fig. 108. Final prosthesis after 6 months loading

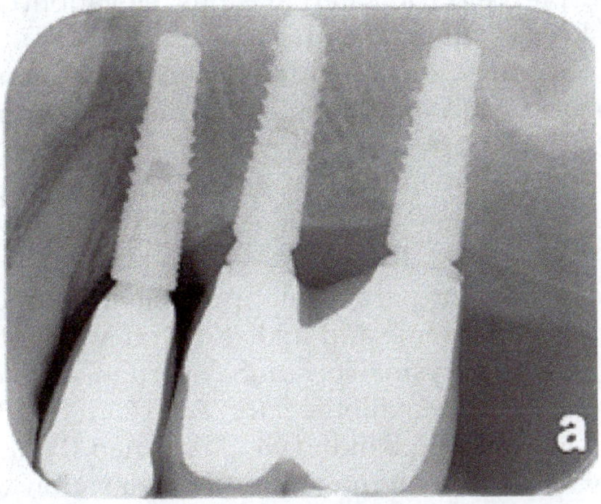

Fig 109. A periapical radiogram after 6 months loading.

As various studies on sinus augmentation without bone graft revealed earlier, bone graft may not be essential factor for sinus augmentation. The key is to maintain new space under the elevated sinus membrane.

No bone added sinus augmentation has many advantages such as

1. Infection is not reported.
2. Significant higher new bone formation is achieved than bone added sinus graft
3. Patient's morbidity is very low because the harvesting of autogenous bone is not required
4. The risk of cross contamination from bovine and human bone is eliminated.
5. Surgical cost can be reduced

5. References

Boyne PJ, James RA. Grafting of the maxillary sinus floor with autogenous marrow and bone. J Oral Surg 1980;38:613-616

Summers RB. The osteotome technique: Part 3-Less invasive methods of elevating the sinus floor. Compendium. 1994;15:698-708.

Sohn DS. Presented at hands on course on piezoelectric bone surgery. 2003;Oct 26.

Sohn DS, Lecture titled with clinical applications of piezoelectric bone surgery. 8th congress of international congress of oral implantologists. Singapore. 2004;Aug.28th.

Sohn DS, Lee JS, An KM, Choi BJ. Piezoelectric internal sinus elevation (PISE) technique: a new method for internal sinus elevation. Implant Dent. 2009;18(6):458-463

Chen L, Cha J. An 8-year retrospective study: 1100 patients receiving 1557 implants using the minimally invasive hydraulic sinus condensing technique. J Periodontol. 2005;76:482-491

Yamada JM, Park HJ. Internal sinus manipulation (ISM) procedure: a technical report. Clin Implant Dent Relat Res. 2007;9(3):128-135

Samuel Lee, Grace Kang, Kwang-Bum park, Thomas Han. Crestal sinus lift: A minimally invasive and systematic approach to sinus grafting. J Implant Adv Clin Dent. 2009;1(1):75-88.

Sohn DS, Moon JW, Ahn KM, et al. Minimally invasive sinus augmentation using hydrodynamic piezoelectric internal sinus elevation(HPISE). Newspaper of Korean Dental Association. 2008;1696:18-19.

Sohn DS, Maupin P, Fayos RP, et al, Minimally Invasive Sinus Augmentation using Ultrasonic Piezoelectric Vibration and Hydraulic Pressure. J Implant Adv Clin Dent. 2010;2.27-40 .

Girolamo MD, Napolitano B, Arullani CA, et al. Paroxysmal positional vertigo as a complication of osteotome sinus floor elevation. Eur Arch Otorhinolarygol. 2005; 262: 631-633.

Peñarrocha M, García A. Benign paroxysmal positional vertigo as a complication of interventions with osteotome and mallet. J Oral Maxillofac Surg. 2006; 64:1324.

Saker M, Oqle O. Benign paroxysmal positional vertigo subsequent to sinus lift via closed technique. J Oral Maxillofac Surg. 2005;63:1385-1387.

Rosen PS, Summers R, Mellado JR, Salkin LM, Shanaman RH, Marks MH, Fugazzotto PA. The bone-added osteotome sinus floor elevation technique: multicenter retrospective report of consecutively treated patients Int J Oral Maxillofac Implants. 1999 ;14(6):853-858

Misch CE. Maxillary sinus augmentation for endosteal implants: organized alternative treatment plans. Int J Oral Implantol. 1987;4:49-58.

Jemt T, Lekholm U. Implant treatment in edentulous maxillae: a 5-year follow-up report on patients with different degrees of jaw resorption. Int J Oral Maxillofac Implants. 1995;10:303-311.

Aghaloo TL, Moy PK. Which hard tissue augmentation techniques are the most successful in furnishing bony support for implant placement? Int J Oral Maxillofac Implants. 2007; 22:49-70.

Lundgren S, Andersson S, Gualini F, et al. Bone reformation with sinus membrane elevation: A new surgical technique for maxillary sinus floor augmentation. Clinical Implant Dentistry and Related Research. 2004; 6(3): 165-173.

Palma VC, Magro-Filho O, de Oliveira JA, et al. Bone reformation and implant integration following maxillary sinus membrane elevation: An experimental study in primates. Clinical Implant Dentistry and Related Research. 2006; 8(1): 11-24.

Nedir R, Bischof M, Vazquez L, et al. Osteotome sinus floor elevation without grafting material: a 1-year prospective pilot study with ITI implants. Clin Oral Implants Res. 2006; 17(6):679-86.

Hatano N, Sennerby L, Lundgren S. Maxillary sinus augmentation using sinus membrane elevation and peripheral venous blood for implant-supported rehabilitation of the atrophic posterior maxilla: case series. Clin Implant Dent Relat Res. 2007;9:150-155.

Sohn DS, Lee JS, Ahn MR, et al. New bone formation in the maxillary sinus without bone grafts. Implant Dent 2008;17:321-331.

Sohn DS, Kim WS, An KM, et al. Comparative histomorphometric analysis of maxillary sinus augmentation with and without bone grafting in rabbit. Implant Dent. 2010;19(3):259-270

Sohn DS, Moon JW, Moon KN, et al. New bone formation in the maxillary sinus using only absorbable gelatin sponge. J Oral Maxillofac Surg. 2010;68(6):1327-1333.

Sohn DS, Moon JW, Moon YS, et al. The use of concentrated growth factor(CGF) for sinus augmentation. The Journal of Oral Implants. 2009;38: 25-38.

Gruber R, Kandler B, Fuerst G, et al. Porcine sinus mucosa holds cells that respond to bone morphogenetic protein (BMP)-6 and BMP-7 with increased osteogenic differentiation in vitro. Clin Oral Implants Res. 2004;15:575-580.

Srouji S, Kizhner T, Ben David D, et al. The Schneiderian membrane contains osteoprogenitor cells: in vivo and in vitro study. Calcif Tissue Int. 2009;84:138-145.

Schwartz-Arad D, Herzberg R, Dolev E. The prevalence of surgical complications of the sinus graft procedure and their impact on implant survival. J Periodontol 2004;75:511–516.

Pikos MA. Maxillary sinus membrane repair: Report of a technique for large perforations. Implant Dent 1999;8:29–34.

Proussaefs P, Lozada J, Kim J, Rohrer MD. Repair of the perforated sinus membrane with a resorbable collagen membrane: A human study. Int J Oral Maxillofac Implants 2004;19:413–420.

Wallace SS, Mazor Z, Froum SJ, Cho SC, Tarnow DP. Schneiderian membrane perforation rate during sinus elevation using piezosurgery: Clinical results of 100 consecutive cases. Int J Periodontics Restorative Dent 2007;27:413–419.

Blus C, Szmukler-Moncler S, Salama M, Salama H, Garber D. Sinus bone grafting procedures using ultrasonic bone surgery: 5-year experience. Int J Periodontics Restorative Dent 2008;28: 221–229.

Sohn DS, Moon JW, Lee HW, et al. Comparison of two piezoelectric cutting inserts for lateral bony window osteotomy: a retrospective study of 127 consecutive sites. Int J Oral Maxillofac Implants. 2010 ;25(3):571-576.

Sohn DS, Moon JW, Moon KN, et al. New bone formation in the maxillary sinus with elevation of sinus membrane and graft of resorbable gelatin sponge : case series report. Implantology 2008; 12-2:26~34.

Moon JW, Son DS, Heo JU, et al. New Bone Formation in the Maxillary Sinus Using Peripheral Venous Blood Alone. Accepted for publication in J Oral Maxillofac Surg.

Melcher AH, Dreyer CJ. Protection of the blood clot in healing of circumscribed bone defects. Journal of Bone Joint Surgery 1962;22:424-429.

Thor A, Rasmusson L, Wennerberg A, Thomsen P, Hirsch JM, Nilsson B, Hong J. The role of whole blood in thrombin generation in contact with various titanium surfaces. Biomaterials. 2007;28:966-974.

Anitua E, Orive G, Pla R, Roman P, Serrano V, Andía I. The effects of PRGF on bone regeneration and on titanium implant osseointegration in goats: a histologic and histomorphometric study. J Biomed Mater Res A. 2009 ;91(1):158-165.

Choukroun J, Diss A, Simonpieri A, Girard MO, Schoeffler C, Dohan SL, Dohan AJ, Mouhyi J, Dohan DM. Platelet-rich fibrin (PRF): a second-generation platelet concentrate. Part V: histologic evaluations of PRF effects on bone allograft maturation in sinus lift. Oral Surg Oral Med Oral Pathol Oral Radiol Endod. 2006;101(3):299-303.

Corigliano M., Sacco L., Baldoni E. CGF- una proposta terapeutica per la medicina rigenerativa. Odontoiatria n°1- anno XXIX- maggio 2010, 69-81. Sohn DS, Moon JW, Moon YS, et al.

The use of concentrated growth factor(CGF) for sinus augmentation. The Journal of Oral Implants. 2009;38: 25-38

Sohn DS, He JU, Kwak DH, et al. Bone regeneration in the maxillary sinus using autologous fibrin rich block with concentrated growth factors alone. Submitted to Implant Dent

Permissions

All chapters in this book were first published by InTech Open; hereby published with permission under the Creative Commons Attribution License or equivalent. Every chapter published in this book has been scrutinized by our experts. Their significance has been extensively debated. The topics covered herein carry significant findings which will fuel the growth of the discipline. They may even be implemented as practical applications or may be referred to as a beginning point for another development.

The contributors of this book come from diverse backgrounds, making this book a truly international effort. This book will bring forth new frontiers with its revolutionizing research information and detailed analysis of the nascent developments around the world.

We would like to thank all the contributing authors for lending their expertise to make the book truly unique. They have played a crucial role in the development of this book. Without their invaluable contributions this book wouldn't have been possible. They have made vital efforts to compile up to date information on the varied aspects of this subject to make this book a valuable addition to the collection of many professionals and students.

This book was conceptualized with the vision of imparting up-to-date information and advanced data in this field. To ensure the same, a matchless editorial board was set up. Every individual on the board went through rigorous rounds of assessment to prove their worth. After which they invested a large part of their time researching and compiling the most relevant data for our readers.

The editorial board has been involved in producing this book since its inception. They have spent rigorous hours researching and exploring the diverse topics which have resulted in the successful publishing of this book. They have passed on their knowledge of decades through this book. To expedite this challenging task, the publisher supported the team at every step. A small team of assistant editors was also appointed to further simplify the editing procedure and attain best results for the readers.

Apart from the editorial board, the designing team has also invested a significant amount of their time in understanding the subject and creating the most relevant covers. They scrutinized every image to scout for the most suitable representation of the subject and create an appropriate cover for the book.

The publishing team has been an ardent support to the editorial, designing and production team. Their endless efforts to recruit the best for this project, has resulted in the accomplishment of this book. They are a veteran in the field of academics and their pool of knowledge is as vast as their experience in printing. Their expertise and guidance has proved useful at every step. Their uncompromising quality standards have made this book an exceptional effort. Their encouragement from time to time has been an inspiration for everyone.

The publisher and the editorial board hope that this book will prove to be a valuable piece of knowledge for researchers, students, practitioners and scholars across the globe.

List of Contributors

Vinicius Nery Viegas, Celso Gustavo Schwalm Lacroix, Rogério Miranda Pagnoncelli and Marília Gerhardt de Oliveira
Pontifícia Universidade Católica do Rio Grande do Sul, Brazil

Shigeto Koyama
Maxillofacial prosthetics Clinic, Tohoku University Hospital Dental Center, Japan

Hiroto Sasaki, Masayoshi Yokoyama, Miou Yamamoto, Naoko Sato and Keiichi Sasaki
Division of Advanced Prosthetic Dentistry, Tohoku University Graduate School of Dentistry, Japan

David Reisberg
The Craniofacial Center, Department of Surgery, The University of Illinois College of Medicine, USA

Feng-ying Yan, Yu-long Shi and Jia-hua Ni
School of Material Science and Engineering, Qingdao University of Science and Technology, China

Fabiano Alvim-Pereira
Federal University of Sergipe (UFS), Lagarto-SE, Brazil

Claudia Cristina Alvim-Pereira
Federal University of Pernambuco (UFPE), Recife-PE, Brazil

Paula Cristina Trevilatto
Pontifical Catholic University of Paraná (PUCPR), Curitiba-PR, Brazil

Mª Angeles Sánchez Garcés, Jaume Escoda-Francolí and Cosme Gay-Escoda
University of Barcelona, Faculty of Dentistry, Spain

Jesus Torres and Juan Carlos Prados-Frutos
Universidad Rey Juan Carlos, Spain

Faleh Tamimi
McGill University, Canada

Mohammad Alkhraisat and Enrique Lopez-Cabarcos
Universidad Complutense, Spain

Argelia Almaguer-Flores and Sandra E. Rodil
Universidad Nacional Autónoma de México, México City

René Olivares-Navarrete
Georgia Institute of Technology, Atlanta, GA, USA

Takayoshi Yamaza and Mizuho A. Kido
Department of Molecular Cell Biology and Oral Anatomy, Graduate School of Dental Science, Kyushu University, Fukuoka, Japan

Smiljana Matić, Novak Stamatović, Zoran Tatić and Aleksandra Petković-Ćurčin
Military Medical Academy, Serbia

José H. Rubo and Vinicius Cappo Bianco
Department of Prosthodontics, Bauru School of Dentistry, University of São Paulo, Bauru, SP, Brazil

Dong-Seok Sohn
Catholic University of Daegu, Daegu, Republic of Korea

Index

www.ingramcontent.com/pod-product-compliance
Lightning Source LLC
LaVergne TN
LVHW062233200926
848484LV00006B/1531